Pass MRCP Part 2

A Problem-based Approach

edited by

Paul Hamilton BSc(Hons) MD FRCP(Edin)
Specialty Registrar, Chemical Pathology (Metabolic Medicine)
Belfast Health and Social Care Trust
Honorary Lecturer, Queens University Belfast
Locum Consultant Physician in General (Internal) Medicine

© 2015 Pastest Ltd
Egerton Court
Parkgate Estate
Knutsford
Cheshire
WA16 8DX

Telephone: 01565 752000

First Published 2015

ISBN: 9781905635948

A catalogue record for this book is available from the British Library. The information contained within this book was obtained by the author from reliable sources. However, while every effort has been made to ensure its accuracy, no responsibility for loss, damage or injury occasioned to any person acting or refraining from action as a result of information contained herein can be accepted by the publishers or author.

At the time of going to press every effort has been made to seek permissions for all images used.

Pastest Online Revision, Books and Courses

Pastest is a well-known, respected provider of medical revision resources. We deliver high levels of customer satisfaction through consistently providing the highest quality online subscriptions, revision books and study courses.

Revision products are available for:

Medical School applicants and undergraduates, MRCP, MRCS, MRCPCH, DCH, GPST, MRCGP, MRCOG, FRCA, Dentistry and Interview Skills.

For further details contact:

Tel: 01565 752000   **Fax: 01565 650264**
www.pastest.co.uk   **enquiries@pastest.co.uk**

Text prepared in the UK by Carnegie Book Production, Lancaster
Printed and bound in the UK by Page Bros., Norwich

Contents

Preface

The recent shift to subspecialisation in medicine has, ironically, come at a time when there is an underlying trend for patients to present to healthcare professionals with complex, multisystem diseases requiring medium- and long-term care. The MRCP examination has been established to identify those physicians who, after a period of training, have acquired sufficient broad-based professional knowledge, skills and attitudes that will enable them to benefit from a period of higher professional training. Therefore physicians in training must demonstrate they have attained a minimum level of knowledge and be able to apply this knowledge to clinical problem solving and clinical practice.

The case studies in this book provide a form of problem-based learning where the physician is presented with a clinical situation that requires resolution. The clinical scenarios are designed to promote active and reflective learning, critical thinking and effective problem solving. Working though the scenarios will provide clinicians with a better understanding of what they know and what they need to practise, and will act as an invaluable revision aid in preparing for part 2 of the MRCP examination.

Professor Gary McVeigh,
Professor of Cardiovascular Medicine,
Queen's University Belfast and Consultant Physician,
Belfast Health and Social Care Trust.

Introduction

Candidates preparing for the MRCP Part 2 examination tend to favour one of two possible revision strategies. Some prefer to systematically digest large quantities of information hoping that, having read widely, they will be in a good position to tackle any problem thrown at them. Others tend to rely on attempting specimen questions. Both approaches have benefits and drawbacks. This book aims to fill a middle-ground, drawing on the strengths of both revision techniques, and in doing so, maximise the efficiency of your preparation for this important examination.

The book is organised into sections based on the topics around which the MRCP Part 2 examination is based. The information is presented in a case-based format, with detailed commentaries outlining the rationale behind the correct answers. The remit of the authors was to cover the major areas of their specialty, either directly in the questions themselves, or by inclusion of the topic in the answers. You will note the highlighting of 'Learning points' throughout the text. These boxes contain information of particular importance. The last chapter of the book comprises a practice examination containing questions from all specialties in random order. You may note that some of the questions are formatted slightly differently from what you might expect in the real examination, for example through the use of occasional 'Which of these options is **not** correct' questions. Although these questions have gone out of favour in college examinations, they are included here to thoroughly test understanding.

No postgraduate study aid can claim to cover every conceivable topic that might come up in an examination. The body of medical knowledge is vast and expanding at a rapid rate. It is my hope however that this book will provide you with an excellent foundation from which to build your knowledge, and perhaps even make you a better doctor in the process.

I would like to express thanks to all the chapter authors who worked hard to produce quality learning material and to Dr Ian Bickle who contributed or sourced many of the radiological images. I am also indebted to the contributors to, and editors of, radiopaedia.org who gave permission for the inclusion of their images in this book. Special thanks go to my wife, Anna, for her patience during the writing process, and to my children Chloe and Jacob to whom I dedicate the book.

P. Hamilton,
February 2015

Contributors

Ian Bickle MB BCh BAO (Hons) FRCR
Consultant Radiologist, Raja Isteri Penigran Anak Saleha Hospital, Bandar seri Begawan, Brunei Darussalam.
Multiple radiological images

Caroline Bleakley MD MRCP (UK)
Specialty Registrar in Cardiology, Belfast City Hospital, Belfast.
Chapter 1 Cardiology

Tomas R Burke MD MRCPI MRCOphth
Specialty Registrar in Ophthalmology, Royal United Hospital, Bath.
Chapter 11 Ophthalmology

Andrea Green MB BCh BAO MRCP (UK)
Specialty Registrar in Respiratory Medicine, Belfast City Hospital, Belfast.
Chapter 13 Respiratory Medicine

Paul Hamilton BSc (Hons) MB BCh BAO (Hons) MD FRCP (Edin)
Specialty Registrar in Chemical Pathology (Metabolic Medicine), Belfast Health and Social Care Trust; Honorary Lecturer, Queen's University Belfast.
Chapter 15 Therapeutics and Toxicology

Stella E Hughes MB BCh BAO MD MRCP (UK) (Neurology)
Consultant Neurologist, Royal Victoria Hospital, Belfast.
Chapter 8 Neurology

Vishal Jayakar MD MRCP (UK) FRCPath
Consultant Haematologist, Kingston Hospital NHS Foundation Trust, Kingston-upon-Thames.
Chapter 6 Haematology

Bee Chan Lee MB BCh BAO (Hons) MRCP (UK)
Consultant Gastroenterologist, Warwick Hospital, Warwick.
Chapter 4 Gastroenterology

Gareth Lewis BSc (Hons) MB MSc Med Ed PhD MRCP (UK)
Specialty Registrar in Renal Medicine, Altnagelvin Area Hospital, Londonderry.
Chapter 9 Nephrology

Emilia Mamwa MB ChB FRCPath DTM&H
Consultant Microbiologist, Doncaster Royal Infirmary, Doncaster.
Chapter 7 Infectious Diseases and Genito-urinary Medicine

Collette McCourt MB BCh BAO MSc Med Ed
Consultant Dermatologist (Locum), Royal Victoria Hospital, Belfast.
Chapter 2 Dermatology

Gavin McDonnell MB BCh BAO (Hons) MD FRCP (Lond)
Consultant Neurologist, Royal Victoria Hospital, Belfast.
Chapter 8 Neurology

Paul H McGurnaghan MB BCh BAO BSc
Specialty Doctor, Infectious Diseases, Royal Victoria Hospital, Belfast.
Chapter 7 Infectious Diseases and Genito-urinary Medicine

Paul McMullan MB BCh BAO MRCP (UK)
Specialty Registrar in Endocrinology / Research Fellow, Royal Victoria Hospital, Belfast.
Chapter 3 Endocrinology and Metabolic Medicine

Katherine A McVeigh MBBS MRCOphth
Specialty Registrar in Ophthalmology, Bristol Eye Hospital, Bristol.
Chapter 11 Ophthalmology

Auleen Miller MB BAO BCh MD FRCP (UK)
Consultant Rheumatologist, Antrim Area Hospital, Antrim.
Chapter 14 Rheumatology

John O'Hare MB BCh BAO (Hons), MRCPsych
Specialty Registrar in Psychiatry, Mater Infirmorum Hospital, Belfast.
Chapter 12 Psychiatry

Anna Ryan MBBS BSc MRCP (UK)
Specialty Registrar in Medical Oncology, Royal Free Hospital, London.
Chapter 10 Oncology and Palliative Medicine

Ciarán Trolan MB BCh MRCP (UK)
Specialty Registrar in Geriatric and General Internal Medicine, Craigavon Area Hospital, Portadown.
Chapter 5 Geriatric Medicine

Normal laboratory values

Haematology

Full blood picture

Haemoglobin (Hb)	
Males	13.5–18 g/dl
Females	11.5–16 g/dl
Mean cell volume (MCV)	76–96 fl
Packed cell volume (PCV)	
Males	0.4–0.54
Females	0.37–0.47
Red cell distribution width (RDW)	12–15%
White cell count (WCC)	$4.0–11.0 \times 10^9/l$
Neutrophils	$2.0–7.5 \times 10^9/l$
Lymphocytes	$1.5–4.0 \times 10^9/l$
Eosinophils	$0.04–0.4 \times 10^9/l$
Monocytes	$0.2–0.8 \times 10^9/l$
Basophils	$0.0–0.1 \times 10^9/l$
Platelets	$150–400 \times 10^9/l$
Reticulocytes	0.5–2.5% of red blood cells
Erythrocyte sedimentation rate (ESR)	
Males	0–15 mm/h
Females	0–22 mm/h
HbA1c (glycated haemoglobin)	3.8–6.4%

Tests of clotting

Activated partial thromboplastin time (APTT)	35–45 s
Prothrombin time (PT)	12–16 s
Fibrinogen	2–4 g/l
Bleeding time	3–9 min
D-dimer	<0.5 mg/l

Haematinics

Iron studies

Iron	11–32 mol/l
Total iron-binding capacity (TIBC)	42–80 mol/l
Ferritin	12–200 µg/l
Folate	>2 µg/l
Vitamin B_{12}	>150 ng/l

Biochemistry

Urea and electrolytes (U&Es)

Sodium (Na^+)	135–145 mmol/l
Potassium (K^+)	3.5–5.0 mmol/l
Urea	2.5–6.7 mmol/l
Creatinine	79–118 µmol/l
	(dependent on muscle mass)
Chloride (Cl^-)	95–105 mmol/l
Bicarbonate (HCO_3^-)	24–30 mmol/l

Liver function tests

Total bilirubin	3–17 µmol/l
Aspartate aminotransferase (AST)	5–35 IU/l
Alanine aminotransferase (ALT)	5–35 IU/l
Alkaline phosphatase (ALP)	30–150 U/l
γ-Glutamyl transpeptidase (GGT)	
Male	11–58 IU/l
Female	7–33 IU/l
Albumin	35–50 g/l

Bone profile

Corrected calcium (Ca^{2+}) (total)	2.10–2.65 mmol/l
Phosphate (PO_4^{3-})	0.8–1.45 mmol/l
Alkaline phosphatase (ALP)	30–150 U/l
Albumin	35–50 g/l

Poisoning

Alcohol	Nil
Carboxyhaemoglobin	<5% of total haemoglobin
Paracetamol	Nil
Salicylates	Nil

NORMAL LABORATORY VALUES

Tumour markers

α-Fetoprotein (AFP)	
<50 years	<10 kU/l
50–70 years	<15 kU/l
70–90 years	<20 kU/l
β Human chorionic gonadotrophin (β-hCG)	<5 U/l
CA125	<35 U/ml
CA19-9	<37 U/ml
Carcinoembryonic antigen (CEA)	<10 ng/ml
Prostate-specific antigen (PSA; males)	
40–49 years	<2.5 ng/ml
50–59 years	<3.5 ng/ml
60–69 years	<4.5 ng/ml
70–79 years	<6.5 ng/ml

Arterial blood gas analysis

pH	7.35–7.45
Arterial partial pressure of oxygen breathing room air (PaO_2)	11–13 kPa
Arterial partial pressure of carbon dioxide breathing room air ($PaCO_2$)	4.7–6.0 kPa
Bicarbonate	24–30 mmol/l
Base excess (BE)	–2 to +2 mmol/l
Anion gap	12–16 mmol/l

Immunoglobulins

IgA	0.8–4.0 g/l
IgG	7.0–14.5 g/l
IgM	0.45–2.0 g/l

Other

Amylase	25–125 U/l
C-reactive protein (CRP)	<10 mg/l
Creatine kinase (CK)	
Male	25–195 IU/l
Female	25–170 IU/l
CK-MB	<25 IU/l
Globulin	18–36 g/l
Lactate	0.5–2.0 mmol/l
Lactate dehydrogenase (LDH)	70–250 IU/l
N-terminal pro-brain natriuretic protein (NT-proBNP)	<125 pmol/l
Osmolality (plasma)	280–300 mosmol/kg

pH   7.35–7.45
Total protein   60–80 g/l
Troponin I   <0.1 μg/l
Troponin T   <0.03 μg/l
Urate   0.15–0.50 mmol/l

Endocrinology

Cortisol
    9am   200–700 nmol/l
    10pm   50–250 nmol/l
Free thyroxine (T_4)   7.6–19.7 pmol/l
Thyroid-stimulating hormone (TSH)   0.4–4.5 mU/l
Total thyroxine (T_4)   70–140 nmol/l

Therapeutic drug levels

Digoxin (6 hours post-dose)   0.8–2.0 nmol/l
Lithium   0.5–1.5 mmol/l

Cerebrospinal fluid

Glucose   2.5–4.4 mmol/l
                                    (two-thirds of plasma value)
Red cell count (RCC)   0/mm^3
Total protein   <0.45 g/l
White cell count (WCC)   <5/mm^3

Urine

Creatinine clearance
    Male   85–125 ml/min
    Female   75–115 ml/min
Metanephrines   <5.5 μmol/day
Osmolality   250–1250 mosmol/kg
Protein   <0.2 g/day

Sweat

Chloride   <60 mmol/l

Image credits

Figure 5.4: Dr Ahmed Abdrabou, Ain-Shams University, Egypt

Figure 8.1: Dr Frank Gaillard, Royal Melbourne Hospital, Melbourne, Australia

Figure 8.3: Image provided courtesy of epilepsy.com

Figure 9.8: Dr Kris Holte, Specialty Registrar in Dermatology, Belfast Health and Social Care Trust.

Figure 11.1: Reproduced with kind permission of *Retinal Physician*, PentaVision LLC

Figure 11.2: Visuals Unlimited, Inc./Chris Barry/Getty Images

Figure 13.2: Dr Jeremy Jones, Royal Hospital for Sick Children, Edinburgh, UK

Figure 13.3: Dr David Cuete, Santiago, Chile

Figure 13.4: Dr Yi-Jin Kuok, Perth, Australia

Figure 13.6: Dr Frank Gaillard, Royal Melbourne Hospital, Melbourne, Australia

Figure 14.1: Dr Jeremy Jones, Royal Hospital for Sick Children, Edinburgh, UK

Figure 16.4: Dr Frank Gaillard, Royal Melbourne Hospital, Melbourne, Australia

Figure 16.5: Dr Yen-Chung Liu, Kwangchow, China

CHAPTER 1

Cardiology

Caroline Bleakley

CASE 1

A 38-year-old lady is admitted complaining of a week-long history of chest
tightness. She has no risk factors for coronary artery disease and has no past
medical history of note other than a bout of an influenza-like illness around four
weeks ago. Her ECG is shown in Figure 1.1.

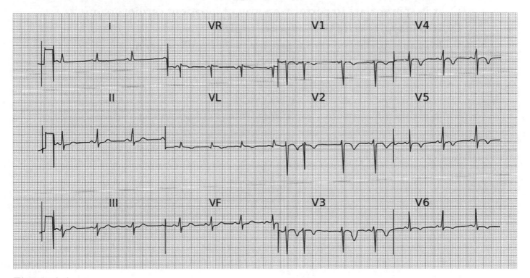

Figure 1.1

Blood testing reveals: High sensitivity troponin T 456 ng/litre, C-reactive protein
31 mg/litre, Full blood picture normal.

There is no evidence of pulmonary oedema on a chest X-ray, but she is noted to
have a few beats of non-sustained ventricular tachycardia on monitoring. What is
the most likely diagnosis?

- A. **Unstable angina**
- B. **Acute myocardial infarction**
- C. **Myocarditis**
- D. **Pericarditis**
- E. **Cardiomyopathy**

CASE 2

A 73-year-old man is seen in the emergency department having been referred by his GP for assessment of an irregular heartbeat. He has a history of hypertension and type 2 diabetes, but is otherwise in good health. He had attended his GP with symptoms of a chest infection but had not experienced any palpitations. The irregular pulse was detected as part of a routine physical examination.

On examination his heart rate is 100 bpm and a 12-lead ECG shows atrial fibrillation (AF). Blood testing reveals: C-reactive protein 54 mg/litre, white cells 11×10^9/litre.

A chest X-ray does not show any consolidation or pulmonary oedema. Which of the following is not true?

A. It is appropriate to start anticoagulation
B. It is appropriate to arrange an outpatient cardioversion
C. It is appropriate to perform an urgent inpatient cardioversion
D. It is inappropriate to commence aspirin
E. It is appropriate to commence a rate-controlling agent

CASE 3

A 40-year-old man with no history of cardiac disease has been brought to the emergency department complaining of palpitations which awoke him from his sleep. He is assessed by the triage nurse who records his heart rate as 184 bpm and blood pressure of 126/82 mmHg. A 12-lead ECG is shown in Figure 1.2. Which of these drugs is most likely to result in an adverse outcome for the patient?

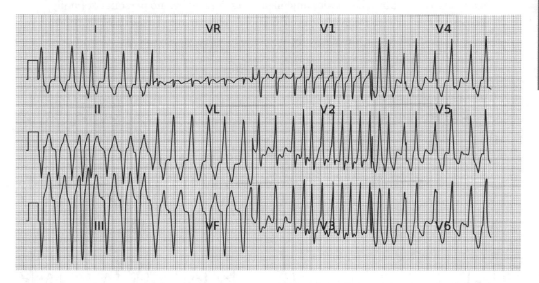

Figure 1.2

   A. **Beta blocker**
   B. **Digoxin**
   C. **Calcium channel blocker**
   D. **Adenosine**
   E. **Amiodarone**

CASE 4

A 31-year-old man develops chest pain while playing football and is brought by ambulance to the emergency department. On arrival he complains of a 3-day history of intermittent chest pain which peaked during the game today and was associated with some shortness of breath. In the department he is still in pain but finds relief in sitting forward and breathing shallowly. He is normotensive with a heart rate of 108 bpm. He denies any illicit drug use and has no personal or family history of cardiac disease. A 12-lead ECG shows widespread ST elevation, as shown in Figure 1.3. Which of the following would be most suggestive of an ischaemic origin to his symptoms?

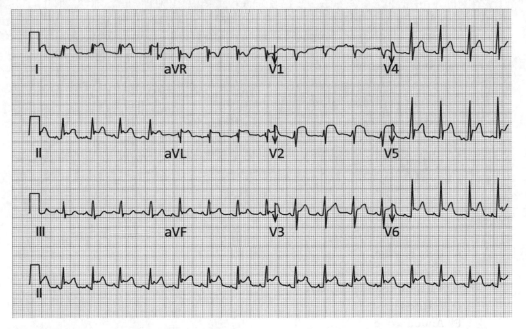

Figure 1.3

    A. Concave ST elevation globally
    B. PR depression
    C. PR elevation in AVR
    D. Reciprocal ST depression in the inferior leads
    E. Concave ST elevation in a specific territory

CASE 5

A 73-year-old lady attends a cardiology outpatient clinic for follow-up of aortic stenosis. She is usually in good health but has recently begun to complain of shortness of breath on walking to the shops and has had two episodes of feeling faint. She does not describe any chest pain or palpitations and her GP started her on a diuretic without any real improvement in symptoms. You review her most recent echocardiogram, which had been performed three weeks before this appointment. This shows that the mean gradient across her aortic valve is 30 mmHg while the valve orifice is 0.7 cm^2. Her last study had shown a mean gradient of 29 mmHg with a valve orifice of 1.3 cm^2. You also notice that her left ventricular function has deteriorated from an ejection fraction of 60% to 37%. What is the most appropriate course of action for this lady?

    A. **Refer for aortic valve replacement**
    B. **Increase the dose of her diuretic**
    C. **Repeat her echocardiogram in six months**
    D. **Arrange an exercise stress test (EST)**
    E. **Start spironolactone**

CASE 6

A 42-year-old lady is referred by her GP for investigation of shortness of breath on exertion. She gives a 6-month history of increasing dyspnoea without chest pain. There are no risk factors for cardiac disease and she is a lifelong non-smoker with no past medical history. A chest X-ray shows some prominence of the pulmonary arteries but no oedema and a 12-lead ECG is normal. A surface echocardiogram later shows moderate tricuspid regurgitation with an estimated pulmonary artery pressure of 54 mmHg with normal biventricular function. Pulmonary function testing is normal apart from a reduction in DLCO to 55% predicted. Right heart catheterisation demonstrates a normal pulmonary capillary wedge pressure and left ventricular end-diastolic pressure with a pulmonary artery pressure of 60 mmHg. What is the most complete diagnosis?

    A. **Pulmonary venous hypertension**
    B. **Pulmonary arterial hypertension**
    C. **Right ventricular cardiomyopathy**
    D. **COPD**
    E. **Tricuspid regurgitation**

CASE 7

A 76-year-old man is seen at the outpatient clinic with progressive dyspnoea. Six months ago he had been able to walk a mile each day, but he has taken to driving this distance recently. He is known to have heart failure on the basis of a myocardial infarction ten years ago. He has never had angina and is a non-smoker. Currently he is short of breath on walking around 30 yards. He sleeps on three pillows and notices that his ankles have become swollen recently. His GP had increased his diuretic without any effect and he is already on maximal doses of an ACE inhibitor, β blocker and spironolactone. His 12-lead ECG is shown in Figure 1.4 and a chest X-ray reveals mild pulmonary congestion. Echocardiography reveals a drop in ejection fraction from 45 to 25% in the last 12 months. Which of the following statements is false?

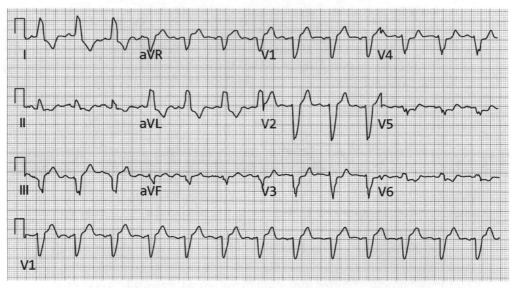

Figure 1.4

A. He has New York Heart Association class III heart failure
B. His BNP will be elevated
C. He may be considered for cardiac resynchronisation therapy (CRT)
D. His LV function is too low to be considered for CRT
E. He may be considered for an ICD

CASE 8

A 27-year-old man collapses suddenly while playing basketball and dies despite prolonged resuscitation. He had no family history of cardiac disease; however, his grandfather had died while swimming. A post-mortem examination identifies the cause of death as a thoracic aortic dissection and notes his tall habitus with evidence of lens dislocation. The family are keen to know whether there may be an inherited trait and whether his sister should be screened. Which statement is true?

A. There is no need for the sister to be screened
B. The cause of death is most likely sporadic
C. This condition is a result of a fibrillin gene mutation
D. There may be downward dislocation of the lens
E. No other family members will be affected

CASE 9

A 70-year-old man with a history of mitral valve prolapse is admitted with rigors and fever. No source of infection is identified after clinical assessment, but two sets of blood cultures are positive for viridans streptococci. A transthoracic echocardiogram shows mild mitral regurgitation and a trans-oesophageal echo identifies a small mobile mass on the anterior leaflet tip. He is started on intravenous antibiotic therapy and his fever settles within seven days. What is the most appropriate course of treatment?

A. He may require follow-up colonoscopy for possible bowel cancer
B. IV antibiotics are recommended for at least four weeks
C. He should be referred immediately for mitral valve replacement
D. He does not require a prolonged course of antibiotics
E. He can go home with oral antibiotics

CASE 10

A 36-year-old man attends his GP for a routine medical examination for his work insurance. He reports no symptoms and is a keen sportsman; however, his blood pressure is recorded as 152/92 mmHg. Which of the following would be an appropriate next step?

A. Start an ACE inhibitor
B. Start a thiazide diuretic
C. Arrange a 24-hour ambulatory BP monitor
D. Repeat his blood pressure in six months
E. Start a calcium channel blocker

CASE 11

A 60-year-old man experiences severe central chest pain while mowing his lawn. He delays contacting his GP until his wife arrives home 30 minutes later. An ambulance is sent immediately by the GP and on arrival the paramedics record the ECG shown in Figure 1.5 and administer anti-platelet therapy.

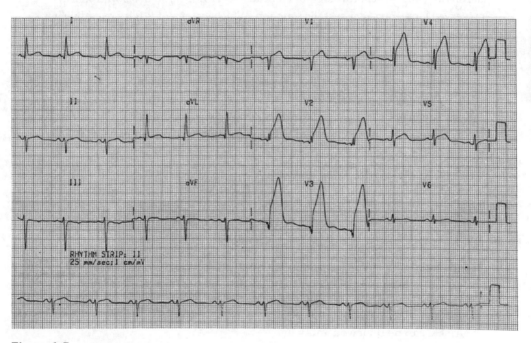

Figure 1.5

Which of the following has the most prognostic benefit for this man at this stage?

A. **Immediate thrombolysis**

B. **Half-dose thrombolysis and immediate transfer to a primary percutaneous coronary intervention centre**

C. **Full-dose thrombolysis and immediate transfer to a primary percutaneous coronary intervention centre**

D. **A glycoprotein IIb/IIIa inhibitor**

E. **Immediate transfer to a primary percutaneous coronary intervention centre**

CASE 12

An 80-year-old lady experiences progressive dyspnoea while gardening. Six months ago she could have easily gardened for a few hours every day; however, she is now short of breath after only 20 minutes. She does not complain of any chest discomfort but does now also experience palpitations. Her ECG confirms atrial fibrillation, and an echocardiogram identifies severe mitral stenosis with well-preserved left ventricular systolic function. Which statement is false regarding her management?

A. **Warfarin should be considered**
B. **She may require a trans-oesophageal echocardiogram**
C. **She may be considered for mitral valve replacement**
D. **She may be considered for mitral balloon valvuloplasty**
E. **Stress testing is indicated before consideration of surgery**

CASE 13

A 64-year-old man is known to have moderate mitral regurgitation (MR) and attends for routine follow-up. His most recent echocardiogram now shows severe regurgitation with a left ventricular ejection fraction of 55%. He remains asymptomatic. Which statement is true?

A. **He can be reviewed annually**
B. **Repair of the valve will not be possible**
C. **He should wait until symptoms develop to consider surgery**
D. **He should be considered for valve repair or replacement**
E. **Medication is of no benefit**

CASE 14

A 52-year-old man seeks advice regarding anticoagulation for atrial fibrillation (AF). He has a history of hypertension and has type 2 diabetes. He is keen to explore the option of newer anticoagulants rather than warfarin, which he has heard requires intensive monitoring. Which of the following is not true?

A. Dabigitran is contraindicated in diabetes
B. Apixaban and rivaroxaban are factor Xa inhibitors
C. Dabigatran is a thrombin IIa inhibitor
D. Rivaroxaban is licensed for deep venous thrombosis/pulmonary embolism (DVT/PE) prophylaxis and treatment
E. None of these agents is licensed for stroke prevention in AF in the setting of a prosthetic heart valve

CASE 15

A young man who has just returned from Thailand presents with acute dyspnoea and pleuritic chest pain. On examination his heart rate is 121 bpm, blood pressure 90/60 mmHg and oxygen saturation 94% on room air. He has been well recently with no cough or flu prodrome and his chest X-ray is unremarkable. Routine bloods are sent urgently and a 12-lead ECG is performed (see Figure 1.6).

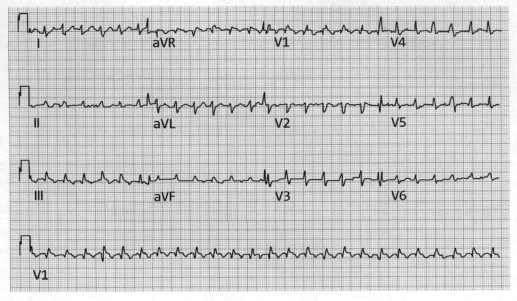

Figure 1.6

Which of the following is not appropriate in his initial management?

  A. Calculate his Wells score
  B. Perform a CT pulmonary angiogram
  C. Perform an echocardiogram
  D. Systemic hypotension should be corrected
  E. He should receive thrombolysis before any further investigation

CASE 16

You see a 54-year-old lorry driver at the outpatient clinic three weeks following his presentation with an acute coronary syndrome and percutaneous coronary intervention to his left anterior descending coronary artery with a drug-eluting stent. He has no significant residual disease and his LV function was only mildly impaired on a pre-discharge echo. What advice would you give him regarding his anti-platelet therapy?

A. He can safely stop clopidogrel after four weeks but remain on aspirin lifelong

B. Aspirin can be discontinued after four weeks but clopidogrel must continue lifelong

C. Aspirin and clopidogrel can be discontinued after six months

D. Aspirin should continue lifelong but clopidogrel can be discontinued after 12 months

E. Both aspirin and clopidogrel can be discontinued after 12 months

CASE 17

You are contacted by the relative of an inpatient to discuss the need for an implantable cardiac defibrillator (ICD). The patient himself is a 43-year-old man who presented with a large anterior ST elevation myocardial infarction (MI) and underwent primary percutaneous coronary intervention to his left anterior descending coronary artery. He has been stable with no arrhythmias since his presentation five days ago, but his echo has shown severe left ventricular systolic dysfunction with an ejection fraction of 25%. He is currently New York Heart Association (NYHA) class II and his ECG shows normal sinus rhythm with narrow QRS complexes. What is correct regarding his need for an ICD?

A. He should receive an ICD before discharge

B. He should receive an ICD only if his ejection fraction falls below 20%

C. His need for an ICD should be reassessed after four weeks

D. He should receive a cardiac resynchronisation therapy (CRT) defibrillator on account of his poor left ventricular (LV) function

E. He does not require an electrophysiological (EP) study before considering an ICD

CASE 18

A young female driver has had an implantable cardiac defibrillator (ICD) implanted for arrythmogenic right ventricular cardiomyopathy, she had documented non-sustained ventricular tachycardia on a Holter monitor and a family history of sudden cardiac death. What advice would you give her regarding driving?

A. She should not drive for one month
B. She should not drive for six months
C. She is now not allowed to drive again
D. She can drive in 12 months if the ICD has not delivered any therapy
E. She can drive in one week

CASE 19

You are asked to review a 40-year-old man with trisomy 21 who has been admitted with a suspected chest infection. His family are able to tell you that he attended cardiology as a child but has not been reviewed since. He is dyspnoeic at rest and profoundly hypoxic even with full oxygen therapy. You note that there is no evidence of consolidation on his chest X-ray and his inflammatory markers are normal as is his d-dimer. There is evidence of congestion on his chest X-ray but very few crepitations on auscultation, although he is markedly oedematous and desaturates quickly off oxygen. You arrange an urgent echocardiogram which shows right heart dilatation with an estimated pulmonary artery pressure of 130 mmHg with good left ventricular function. What is the likely mechanism of right heart failure?

A. Myocardial infarction
B. Pulmonary embolism
C. Chest sepsis
D. Eisenmenger syndrome
E. Asthma

CASE 20

You review a 70-year-old lady who has been admitted with dyspnoea. She describes progressive shortness of breath on exertion to the extent that she is now short of breath after 30 m. She has also been propping herself up in bed with three pillows and has noticed swelling of her ankles. Her NT-proBNP concentration is > 1000 ng/litre, but her echo shows normal left ventricular systolic function. Which additional information is likely to be most useful?

A. **Echo assessment of left ventricular diastolic function**
B. **Pulmonary function testing**
C. **Chest X-ray**
D. **CT pulmonary angiogram**
E. **High-resolution CT chest**

CASE 21

You review a 24-hour Holter recording from a gentleman you had seen at the outpatient clinic who you suspected had a recent transient ischaemic attack (TIA). He has a history of hypertension but was otherwise well. The recording shows a single 60-second episode of atrial fibrillation. What is the most appropriate next step?

A. **Calculate his CHA_2DS_2VASc and HASBLED scores**
B. **Commence him on warfarin**
C. **Commence him on a novel anticoagulant**
D. **Advise him that 60 seconds of atrial fibrillation is below the threshold for treatment in the current treatment guidelines**
E. **Arrange a further 24-hour Holter recording**

CASE 1

C: Myocarditis

The diagnosis of myocarditis (inflammation of the myocardium) is often confused with an acute coronary syndrome (ACS) as both can present with chest discomfort together with ECG changes and a rise in troponin levels.

> ### Learning point
>
> The clue to the diagnosis of myocarditis rather than an infarct will be in the history. A patient who is younger with no risk factors for coronary artery disease and perhaps a history of a recent coryzal or flu-like illness should raise suspicions of this diagnosis. Myocarditis most commonly is of infectious aetiology, with viral causes being particularly likely. More rarely, cases may be due to autoimmune activity such as in connective tissue diseases and sarcoidosis.

Diagnosis may involve the following:

- ✦ echocardiography: to assess ventricular function
- ✦ cardiac MRI: typical patterns of enhancement are seen with myocarditis and this modality can be used to guide endomyocardial biopsy
- ✦ coronary angiography: to exclude coronary artery disease
- ✦ endomyocardial biopsy: provides a tissue diagnosis.

Complications can arise from myocarditis and are largely due to the development of an acute cardiomyopathy. Some patients develop severe left ventricular systolic dysfunction, ventricular arrhythmias and high degrees of atrioventricular block. In some cases the cardiomyopathy does not recover.

Treatment of myocarditis is dependent on the presence or absence of left ventricular (LV) dysfunction. Those who escape without LV impairment can be managed with simple pain relief while the acute phase settles. Those with LV impairment require standard heart failure therapy, similar to any patient presenting with heart failure. This would typically include a diuretic, β blocker, angiotensin-converting enzyme (ACE) inhibitor and aldosterone antagonist.

CASE 2

C: It is appropriate to perform an urgent inpatient cardioversion

Atrial fibrillation is one of the most common problems encountered in cardiology. It affects 1.5–2% of adults and those over the age of 40 have a 25% lifetime risk of developing the condition. Causes of AF are multiple: alcohol, ischaemic heart disease, hypertension, valvular heart disease (especially mitral valve disease, which frequently causes the left atrium to dilate, so predisposing to AF) and hyperthyroidism.

The mechanism of stroke risk in AF is sometimes not well appreciated. Fibrillation of the atria (in contrast to their coordinated contraction) increases blood stasis within these chambers, most specifically within the left atrial appendage (LAA). It is this structure which is the main source of clot formation in AF. Hence a trans-oesophageal echo may be carried out to identify the LAA and any evidence of clot within it before cardioversion is performed in patients who have not been adequately anticoagulated.

Learning point

Cardioversion should be considered for all patients with newly diagnosed AF. Novel oral anticoagulant drugs are now being used routinely in this setting as an alternative to warfarin. While warfarin compliance can be checked using the International Normalised Ration (INR), there is no such comparable test for NOACs and patients must be informed of the increased risk of stroke during cardioversion if compliance has been lacking in the weeks leading up to the procedure. Current guidelines recommend three weeks of anticoagulation before conversion in order to reduce the risk of embolisation from a pre-existing clot in the heart. Four weeks of therapy is needed post-cardioversion even if the procedure has been successful.

Much confusion surrounds rate-controlling agents in AF. In a person with paroxysmal or persistent AF, an anti-arrythmic agent may be used to prevent episodes of AF. Such agents include amiodarone, sotalol, flecainide and propafenone. Flecainide and propafenone are not used in patients with left ventricular impairment, a history of coronary artery disease or for those over the age of 65 years as they may be detrimental and ironically pro-arrythmic in such circumstances. For those already in permanent AF there is no point in prescribing an anti-arrythmic agent as the patient is already permanently in the arrhythmia. In these patients a simple rate-controlling agent is appropriate; β blockers are the most commonly used drug class for this purpose.

continued

Catheter ablation of AF is currently only recommended for those who remain symptomatic of their AF despite medical therapy. Although highly publicised, the success rates are around 80% after two procedures. There is no role for this procedure at present in asymptomatic patients.

CASE 3

D: Adenosine

This man has presented with a broad complex tachycardia which may cause confusion as to whether the diagnosis is that of ventricular tachycardia (VT) or supraventricular VT (SVT) with aberrant conduction. In this case the diagnosis is atrial fibrillation (AF) with Wolff–Parkinson–White (WPW) pattern, or in other terms, AF conducted via an accessory pathway.

Learning point

There are certain features on the ECG that distinguish this from VT. First, the rhythm is irregular with no consistency between complexes. Second, the bundle branch pattern in lead V1 (in this case right bundle branch) is not seen in VT. The patient's history is also important in determining the cause of the tachycardia. A young man with no history of ischaemic heart disease (IHD) is more likely to present with SVT with aberrant conduction. In those with a history of IHD, 95% of broad complex tachycardias will be ventricular in origin due to previous scar formation from an old myocardial infarction (MI) or an impaired and dilated ventricle.

Administering adenosine in this case in an attempt to distinguish SVT from VT will result in blocking of the atrioventricular (AV) node and subsequent 1 : 1 conduction of the AF from the atria to the ventricles via the accessory pathway. As the actual atrial rate of AF is commonly 200–300 bpm, this 1 : 1 conduction caused by blocking of the AV node quickly results in a ventricular rate of 200–300 bpm, which may result in ventricular fibrillation.

CASE 4

D: Reciprocal ST depression in the inferior leads

The diagnosis is pericarditis rather than ST elevation MI (STEMI). This is a young man with no antecedent cardiac disease who describes the typical features of pericardial rather than ischaemic chest pain, ie positional pain that is often pleuritic in nature. The ECG is classic of pericarditis with two very specific features relating to the PR interval.

Learning point

PR segment elevation in AVR is very specific for pericarditis, while PR depression in the other leads is considered pathognomonic of pericarditis. In this instance you should not see reciprocal ST depression as you may see in a STEMI, a feature which suggests ischaemia in a specific coronary artery territory. The changes associated with pericarditis tend not to be confined to such territorial parts of the pericardium, meaning ST elevation is frequently present in all leads.

The importance for management is that the incorrect diagnosis of a STEMI in this situation may lead to the administration of thrombolysis, which would almost certainly result in a pericardial effusion. Given the classic presentation, and features of this man's presentation he should have an echocardiogram, which may show an echo bright pericardium in keeping with pericarditis. Colchicine has been shown to reduce the risk of recurrent episodes and patients should generally receive up to six weeks of therapy. Less than 1% of patients with acute pericarditis go on to develop constrictive pericarditis. Echo features in keeping with constrictive pericarditis rather than a restrictive cardiomyopathy include a septal bounce indicative of ventricular interdependence, higher mitral annular tissue Doppler velocity and diastolic flow reversal in the hepatic veins.

CHAPTER 1 ANSWERS

CASE 5

A: Refer for aortic valve replacement

Aortic stenosis (AS) is increasing in prevalence as the population ages. It is a degenerative disease of the aortic valve resulting in calcium deposition on the valve leaflets which then restricts leaflet mobility. It is graded as mild, moderate and severe depending on the area of the valve orifice and the mean gradient across the valve. Severe stenosis is classified as a valve area of < 1 cm^2 and a mean gradient of > 40 mmHg.

Learning point

In this case, the valve area of 0.7 cm^2 is in keeping with severe stenosis; however, the mean gradient is lower than would be expected for a severe stenosis. This is a case of low-flow aortic stenosis where the new impairment of left ventricular (LV) function means that the now failing ventricle cannot generate sufficient force to expel blood up the outflow tract and through the aortic valve with as much vigour as when the ventricular function was preserved. This is a common cause of confusion and often leads to erroneous labelling of aortic stenosis as moderate. One should always check LV function when assessing aortic stenosis and, if the ventricle is impaired, then the valve area is a more reliable indicator of the severity of stenosis. In these circumstances, a stress test such as a dobutamine stress echo can reveal the true gradient by increasing LV work.

The natural course of AS is for the valve to progressively tighten. Nearly all patients with severe AS develop symptoms within five years. The annual rate of sudden cardiac death in this asymptomatic group is around 1%.

Class 1 indications for valve replacement are:

✦ severe AS with symptoms

✦ severe AS in those undergoing coronary artery bypass grafting (CABG). (There is little point in opening the patient's chest for CABG to then have to re-open the same wound when the valve needs to be replaced.)

✦ severe AS in those undergoing surgery on the aorta or other heart valves

✦ severe AS and evidence of LV systolic dysfunction (EF < 50%).

Other indications are as outlined in Table 1.1.

Indication	Class of evidence
AVR is indicated in patients with severe AS and any symptoms related to AS.	I
AVR is indicated in patients with severe AS undergoing CABG surgery of the ascending aorta or another valve.	I
AVR is indicated in asymptomatic patients with severe AS and systolic LV dysfunction (LVEF < 50%) not due to another cause.	I
AVR is indicated in asymptomatic patients with severe AS and an abnormal exercise test showing symptoms on exercise clearly related to AS.	I
AVR should be considered in high-risk patients with severe symptomatic AS who are suitable for TAVI, but in whom surgery is favoured by a 'heart team' based on the individual risk profile and anatomic suitability.	IIa
AVR should be considered in asymptomatic patients with severe AS and an abnormal exercise test showing fall in blood pressure below baseline.	IIa
AVR should be considered in patients with moderate AS undergoing CABG surgery of the ascending aorta of another valve.	IIa
AVR should be considered in symptomatic patients with low-flow, low-gradient (< 40 mmHg) AS with normal EF only after careful confirmation of severe AS.	IIa
AVR should be considered in symptomatic patients with severe AS, low flow, low gradient with reduced EF and evidence of flow reserve.	IIa
AVR should be considered in asymptomatic patients with normal EF and none of the above-mentioned exercise test abnormalities, if the surgical risk is low, and one or more of the following findings is present: ✦ very severe AS defined by a peak transvalvular velocity > 5.5 m/s, or ✦ severe valve calcification and a rate of peak transvalvular velocity progression ≥ 0.3 m/s per year.	IIa
AVR may be considered in symptomatic patients with severe AS low-flow, low-gradient and LV dysfunction without flow reserve.	IIb
AVR may be considered in asymptomatic patients with severe AS, normal EF and none of the above-mentioned exercise test abnormalities, if surgical risk is low, and one or more of the following findings is present ✦ markedly elevated natriuretic peptide levels confirmed by repeated measurements and without other explanations ✦ increase of mean pressure gradient with exercise by > 20 mmHg ✦ excessive LV hypertrophy in the absence of hypertension.	IIb

Table 1.1: Indications for aortic valve replacement in aortic stenosis[1]

continued

Note the use of 'classes of recommendations' in this table and throughout this chapter. Class I recommendations relate to situations where there is evidence and/or general agreement that a given treatment or procedure is beneficial, useful or effective. Class II recommendations are when there is conflicting evidence and/or a divergence of opinion about the usefulness/efficacy of a given treatment or procedure (class IIa – the weight of evidence/opinion is in favour of usefulness/efficacy; class IIb – less well established). Class III recommendations relate to when there is evidence or general agreement that a measure is not useful/effective and which, in some cases, may be harmful.

In clinical practice the decision is heavily influenced by patient co-morbidity and patient choice. Transcatheter aortic valve implantation (TAVI) is now considered a viable alternative in patients who are deemed at high operative risk. The procedure involves placing a valve via a catheter into position across the existing valve, and then inflating a balloon to crush the native valve and expand the new percutaneous valve into its position. Thirty-day mortality is in the region of 5–7%[2] and many patients require insertion of a permanent pacemaker after the procedure due to trauma to the conduction system caused during positioning of the new valve. These figures are felt to be favourable considering the inevitable mortality in those who do not receive a replacement.

CASE 6

B: Pulmonary arterial hypertension

This is a classic presentation of pulmonary arterial hypertension (PAH), which affects women more than men. Chest X-ray findings are non-specific but may show enlargement of the pulmonary arteries. The ECG tends not to reveal anything abnormal, other than perhaps right bundle branch block if the right ventricle has started to fail or dilate.

Learning point

An easily performed test that can point to the diagnosis is pulmonary function testing, which classically shows a reduction in transfer factor without significant restriction or obstruction. A normal DLCO makes pulmonary hypertension unlikely while a DLCO of < 50% predicted is a very high mortality indicator. Right heart catheterisation can be very informative in determining if left-sided heart disease is a likely cause of the pulmonary hypertension. The pulmonary capillary wedge pressure is used as a surrogate of left atrial pressure (the left atrium is not accessible from the venous circulation) and if normal, indicates absence of significant mitral valve disease or LV dysfunction, which are a cause of pulmonary venous hypertension.

The Dana-Point classification of pulmonary hypertension divides causes into groups (see Table 1.2).

> **Group 1:** Pulmonary arterial hypertension (PAH)
>
> Causes: Idiopathic, inherited, drug-induced, connective tissue disease, HIV, portal hypertension, congenital heart disease, persistent pulmonary hypertension of the newborn, pulmonary veno-occlusive disease
>
> **Group 2:** Pulmonary hypertension due to left heart disease
>
> Causes: Systolic dysfunction, diastolic dysfunction, valve disease
>
> **Group 3:** Pulmonary hypertension due to lung disease
>
> Causes: COPD, interstitial lung disease, sleep-disordered breathing
>
> **Group 4:** Chronic thromboembolic pulmonary hypertension
>
> **Group 5:** Pulmonary hypertension with unclear multi-factorial mechanisms

Table 1.2: Dana-Point classification of pulmonary hypertension[3]

CHAPTER 1 ANSWERS

Learning point

The importance of identifying the cause is in order to guide treatment. Familial pulmonary hypertension has an autosomal dominant inheritance pattern and a grave mortality in the young with an untreated median survival of under three years. Group 1 patients are most likely to respond to vasodilator therapy while group 2 patients (those with left-sided heart disease) will be made worse by this therapy. Therefore, vasodilators are offered to group 1 patients only. Therapy may include an endothelin receptor blocker and a phosphodiesterase inhibitor.

Response to therapy can be followed by a functional assessment such as a 6-minute walk test and a pulmonary arterial pressure assessment such as an echocardiogram. The PA pressure should fall as therapy takes effect. Beware the patient whose PA pressure is falling but who feels no better. The onset of right ventricular dysfunction can lower the pressure owing to inability of the failing right ventricle to generate significant pressure into the pulmonary artery.

For those with chronic thromboembolic pulmonary hypertension, pulmonary thrombectomy is associated with a good outcome if they survive surgery (operative mortality is 3–5%).

CASE 7

D: His LV function is too low to be considered for CRT

Heart failure symptoms are classified according to the New York Heart Association (NYHA) scoring system (see Table 1.3).

> Class I: no limitation of ordinary activity
>
> Class II: symptoms during ordinary activity
>
> Class III: symptoms during less than ordinary/minimal activity
>
> Class IV: symptoms at rest

Table 1.3: New York Heart Association (NYHA) scoring system for heart failure symptoms

This man has NYHA class III symptoms. Brain natriuretic peptide (BNP) is a marker of LV dysfunction and will be elevated in this case. Caveats in its use include the fact that it may be elevated in those with renal impairment, obesity, sepsis, cirrhosis and pulmonary hypertension. Large randomised trials have consistently demonstrated the mortality benefit of ACE inhibitors, angiotension receptor blockers, diuretics, β blockers and aldosterone anatagonists in heart failure and these should be combined in maximal doses in all patients, as tolerated by blood pressure.

Learning point

In CRT, the aim is to place pacemaker leads in the right ventricle and epicardially, via the coronary sinus, to the lateral wall of the left ventricle and thereby resynchronise the dysynchronous ventricular contractions which characterise wide left bundle branch block (LBBB) morphology heart failure. A third lead is placed in the right atrium as with any dual chamber pacemaker. CRT has been shown to improve symptoms and survival in carefully selected patients who meet the criteria described in Table 1.4.

Indication for cardiac resynchronisation therapy	Level of evidence
CRT is indicated in patients with heart failure whose EF is < 35%, with LBBB and a QRS duration > 150 ms, who exhibit NYHA class II–IV symptoms and who are on adequate medical therapy	Ia
CRT should be considered in patients with heart failure whose EF is < 35%, with LBBB and a QRS duration > 120 ms, who exhibit NYHA class II–IV symptoms and who are on adequate medical therapy	Ib
CRT should be considered in patients with heart failure whose EF is < 35%, with non-LBBB and a QRS duration > 150 ms, who exhibit NYHA class II–IV symptoms and who are on adequate medical therapy	IIa
CRT should be considered in patients with heart failure whose EF is < 35%, with non-LBBB and a QRS duration > 120 ms, who exhibit NYHA class II–IV symptoms and who are on adequate medical therapy	IIb
CRT is not recommended in heart failure patients with a QRS duration of < 120 ms	III

Table 1.4: Indications for cardiac resynchronisation therapy[4]

CASE 8

C: This condition is a result of a fibrillin gene mutation

This man died as a result of an undiagnosed aortic aneurysm which subsequently ruptured.

Learning point

The diagnosis is likely to be Marfan syndrome, which results from a defect in the fibrillin-1 (*FBN-1*) gene. Marfan syndrome is an autosomal dominant condition affecting connective tissue. It occurs in approximately 1 in 4000 individuals in Western populations. Prognosis is largely dependent on the development of cardiovascular complications such as aortic pathology and valvular heart disease. An ascending aortic diameter of ≥ 45 mm is an indication for surgical treatment of the aorta in Marfan syndrome.

The 2010 Revised Ghent Nosology for Marfan syndrome suggests seven rules in the diagnosis of Marfan syndrome[5] (see Table 1.5).

In the absence of family history:	In the presence of family history:
Aortic root dilatation Z score ≥ 2 AND ectopia lentis	Ectopia lentis AND family history of Marfan syndrome
Aortic root dilatation Z score ≥ 2 AND *FBN-1*	A systemic score ≥ 7 points AND family history of Marfan syndrome
Aortic root dilatation Z score ≥ 2 AND systemic score ≥ 7 points	Aortic root dilatation Z score ≥ 2 AND family history of Marfan syndrome
Ectopia lentis AND *FBN-1* mutation with known aortic pathology	

Table 1.5: The 2010 Revised Ghent Nosology for Marfan syndrome

In each of the scenarios shown in Table 1.5, features suggestive of Shprintzen–Goldberg syndrome, Loeys–Dietz syndrome, or Ehlers–Danlos syndrome must be excluded and genetic testing (eg *TGFBR1/2*, collagen biochemistry, COL3A1) should be performed.

Systemic features to look for are listed below.[5]

Wrist sign

Thumb sign

Pectus carinatum

Pectus excavatum

Chest asymmetry

Hind-foot deformity

Flat foot

Spontaneous pneumothorax

Dural ectasia

Protucio acetabulae

Scoliosis or thoracolumbar kyphosis

Reduced elbow extension

Facial features

Skin striae

Severe myopia

Mitral valve prolapse

Reduced upper segment/lower segment

Increased arm span/height

CHAPTER 1 ANSWERS

CASE 9

B: IV antibiotics are recommended for at least four weeks

This is a case of infective endocarditis (IE) of a native mitral valve and current guidelines recommend four weeks of IV antibiotics in such cases. In prosthetic valves six weeks of IV antibiotics is recommended. The Duke criteria are the most widely used in the diagnosis of infective endocarditis:

Definite endocarditis:	Possible endocarditis:	Not endocarditis:
2 major criteria	1 major + 1 minor criteria	Alternative source of sepsis
OR	OR	Resolution of symptoms and signs with < 4 days of antibiotics
1 major + 3 minor criteria	3 minor criteria	No evidence of endocarditis at surgery
OR		Does not meet criteria for possible IE
5 minor criteria		

Major criteria:

+ Blood culture positive for IE

+ Typical micro-organism consistent with IE from two separate blood cultures: viridans streptococci, *Streptococcus bovis*, HACEK group, *Staphylococcus aureus*, or community-acquired enterococci in the absence of a primary focus

+ Micro-organisms consistent with IE from persistently positive blood cultures defined as follows: at least two positive cultures of blood samples drawn > 12 h apart; or all of three or a majority of > 4 separate cultures of blood (with first and last sample drawn at least 1 h apart)

+ Single positive blood culture for *Coxiella burnetii* or anti-phase 1 IgG antibody titre > 1 : 800

+ Evidence of endocardial involvement

+ Echocardiogram positive for IE (TOE recommended for patients with prosthetic valves, with 'possible IE' by clinical criteria or complicated IE [paravalvular abscess]; TTE as first test in other patients)

Minor criteria:

+ Predisposition, predisposing heart condition, or IV recreational drug use

+ Fever

+ Vascular phenomena: major arterial emboli, septic pulmonary infarcts, mycotic aneurysm, intracranial hemorrhage, conjunctival hemorrhages, and Janeway lesions

+ Immunologic phenomena: glomerulonephritis, Osler's nodes, Roth's spots, and rheumatoid factor

+ Microbiological evidence: positive blood culture but does not meet a major criterion or evidence of active infection with organism consistent with IE

Table 1.6: Duke criteria for diagnosing infective endocarditis[6]

Staphylococcus aureus followed by viridans streptococci and coagulase negative staphylococci are the three most common causal organisms in IE. *S. aureus* has a particularly poor prognosis. Some organisms are notoriously difficult to grow from culture samples including *Aspergillus, Brucella, Coxiella burnetii, Chlamydia* and HACEK (*Haemophilus, Aggregatibacter, Cardiobacterium, Eikenella* and *Kingella*) bacteria. *Streptococcus bovis* infection can be associated with underlying bowel malignancy. Surgery for IE is usually only indicated in the presence of consequent heart failure, valve destruction, overwhelming sepsis or to prevent recurrent systemic embolisation.

A recent update to the National Institute for Health and Clinical Excellence (NICE) guidance for endocarditis prophylaxis has removed the recommendation to administer antibiotics before routine dental work in those with predisposing conditions to infective endocarditis (see Table 1.7). The caveat to this is that antibiotics should be administered if active infection is seen in the mouth or gums.

CHAPTER 1
ANSWERS

> Do not offer antibiotic prophylaxis against infective endocarditis:
> - ✦ to people undergoing dental procedures
> - ✦ to people undergoing non-dental procedures at the following sites: upper and lower gastrointestinal tract
> - ✦ genito-urinary tract; this includes urological, gynaecological and obstetric procedures, and childbirth
> - ✦ upper and lower respiratory tract; this includes ear, nose and throat procedures and bronchoscopy.

Table 1.7: Antibiotic prophylaxis for those at risk of endocarditis[7]

CASE 10

C: Arrange a 24-hour ambulatory blood pressure monitor

Hypertension is an abnormal elevation of the BP within the arterial system, the vast majority (90–95%) of which is related to no identifiable cause and is therefore termed essential hypertension. In the UK, one quarter of the adult population has hypertension, rising to half of those over the age of 60 years. Globally, almost one third of the population in developed countries is known to have hypertension. A direct correlation exists between the magnitude of hypertension and cardiovascular risk, and for patients aged 40–70 years, each increase of 20 mmHg in systolic BP or 10 mmHg in diastolic BP results in a doubling of risk. Conversely, a 2 mmHg reduction in systolic pressure would translate into a 10% lower stroke mortality and 7% reduction in ischaemic heart disease or other vascular mortality. Current grades of hypertension as defined by the European Society of Cardiology (ESC) are listed in Table 1.8.

Grade of hypertension	Clinic systolic pressure (mmHg)	Clinic diastolic pressure (mmHg)	Ambulatory pressure average daytime reading (mmHg)
High–normal	130–139	85–89	–
1	140	90	135/85
2	160	100	150/95
3	180	110	–

Table 1.8: ESC definitions of hypertension. The diagnosis of grade 1 or 2 hypertension requires both a clinic measurement and ambulatory monitoring

Learning point

The 2011 NICE guidelines for the management of hypertension advise therapy for BP reduction if clinic readings are ≥ 140/90 mmHg together with ambulatory readings of greater than 135/85 mmHg. This represents a lowering of the threshold for therapeutic intervention from the 2006 guidelines, which had advocated treatment in those with readings ≥ 140/90 mmHg together with a calculated ten-year CVD risk of ≥ 10%, existing CVD or evidence of target organ damage.

In a change to NICE's previous guidance from 2006, the 2011 guideline includes a recommendation that hypertension should be confirmed by 24-hour ambulatory blood pressure monitoring (ABPM) rather than relying on measurements taken exclusively in a clinic setting.

According to the 2013 ESC guidelines, the recommended first agent can be any of an ACE inhibitor (or an angiotensin receptor blocker if the former is poorly tolerated or contraindicated), a calcium channel blocking agent, a thiazide type diuretic or a β blocker. The 2011 NICE guidelines still advocate ACE inhibitor or angiotensin receptor blocker in Caucasians < 55 years and a calcium channel blocker or diuretic in Black patients and those > 55 years.

CASE 11

E: Immediate transfer to a primary percutaneous coronary intervention centre

Primary percutaneous coronary intervention (PPCI) is a class 1 indication in acute ST elevation MI (STEMI) with superiority over thrombolysis if delivered promptly and by an expert. The 2012 ESC guidelines on the management of STEMI advise the following targets:[8]

- ✦ First medical contact to first ECG ≤ 10 min.
- ✦ First medical contact to reperfusion therapy:
    - ✧ for fibrinolysis ≤ 30 min
    - ✧ for primary PCI ≤ 90 min (≤ 60 min if the patient presents within 120 min of symptom onset or directly to a PCI-capable hospital).

The guidelines advocate the following with respect to reperfusion therapy (including primary PCI):

- ✦ Reperfusion therapy is indicated in all patients with symptoms of < 12 h duration and persistent ST-segment elevation or (presumed) new left bundle branch block.
- ✦ Reperfusion therapy (preferably primary PCI) is indicated if there is evidence of ongoing ischaemia, even if symptoms may have started > 12 h beforehand or if pain and ECG changes have been stuttering.
- ✦ There is currently no role for facilitated PCI, ie full- or half-dose lysis followed by immediate PPCI.

The role of dual anti-platelet therapy (DAPT) has been overcomplicated in recent years with the arrival of newer agents. The ESC has attempted to simplify this as follows:

- ✦ If the patient has no contraindications to prolonged DAPT.
- ✦ Drug-eluting stents (DES) should be preferred over bare metal stents (BMS).
- ✦ DAPT is recommended with aspirin together with one of the following ADP-receptor blockers:
    - ✧ prasugrel in clopidogrel-naive patients, if no history of prior stroke/TIA and age < 75 years
    - ✧ ticagrelor
    - ✧ clopidogrel, if prasugrel or ticagrelor are not available or contraindicated.
- ✦ An injectable anticoagulant must be used:
    - ✧ bivalirudin is preferred over heparin and a GPIIb/IIIa blocker
    - ✧ enoxaparin may be preferred over unfractionated heparin
    - ✧ unfractionated heparin must be used in patients not receiving either bivalirudin or enoxaparin.

CASE 12

E: Stress testing is indicated before consideration of surgery

Mitral stenosis (MS) is still most commonly a result of rheumatic fever. Patients may be asymptomatic for many years before developing symptoms. A valve area of < 1 cm² with a mean gradient of > 10 mmHg is considered severe (see Table 1.9).

	Aortic stenosis	Mitral stenosis	Tricuspid stenosis
Valve area (cm²)	< 1.0	< 1.0	–
Indexed valve area (cm²/m² BSA)	< 0.6	–	–
Mean gradient (mmHg)	> 40[a]	> 10[b]	≥ 5
Maximum jet velocity (m/s)	> 4.0[a]	–	–
Velocity ratio	< 0.25	–	–

Table 1.9: Indications for surgery in cardiac valvular stenosis[1]

Stress testing is indicated in patients who are asymptomatic or whose symptoms are equivocal or out of keeping with the severity of MS. Dobutamine or exercise echocardiography may provide additional information by assessing changes in mitral gradient and pulmonary pressures during stress.[1]

In asymptomatic patients survival is good up to ten years. Symptom progression can be highly variable with sudden deterioration usually precipitated by pregnancy or complications such as AF. Symptomatic patients have a poor prognosis without intervention.[1]

Interventions include:
+ Percutaneous mitral commissurotomy (PMC): Good initial results, defined as valve area > 1.5 cm² with no mitral regurgitation (MR) > 2/4, are achieved in over 80% of cases. Clinical follow-up data confirm the late efficacy of PMC: event-free survival ranges from 30 to 70% after 10–20 years.

+ Mitral valve replacement: The most common surgery for MS (~95%). Operative mortality ranges from 3 to 10% and correlates with age, functional class, pulmonary hypertension and presence of CAD. Long-term survival is related to age, functional class, AF, pulmonary hypertension, preoperative LV/RV function and prosthetic valve complications.[1]

continued

Learning point

Intervention should only be performed in patients with clinically significant MS (valve area ≤ 1.5 cm^2). Intervention should be performed in symptomatic patients. Most patients with favourable valve anatomy currently undergo PMC. PMC should be considered as an initial treatment for selected patients with mild to moderate calcification or unfavourable subvalvular apparatus, who have otherwise favourable clinical characteristics, especially in young patients in whom postponing valve replacement is particularly attractive.

The ESC guidance on intervention in MS is outlined in Figure 1.7.

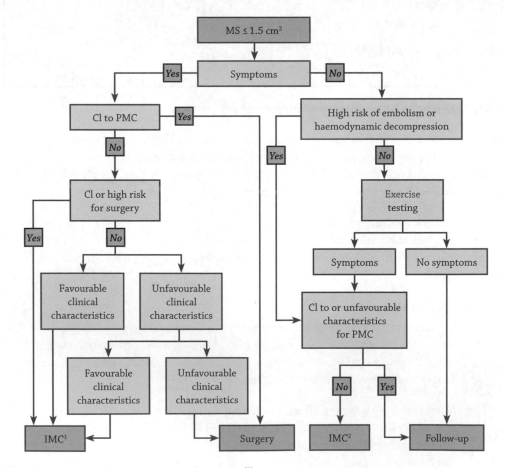

Figure 1.7: Interventions in mitral stenosis[1]

CASE 13

D: He should be considered for valve repair or replacement

This man is asymptomatic with severe MR and a falling left ventricular ejection fraction.

Learning point

MR will usually flatter left ventricular function, making it look better than it is due to the ventricle being able to expel blood both forwards through the aortic valve and backwards through the regurgitant mitral valve. Therefore, any fall in EF in MR should raise an alarm.

Echocardiographic criteria for the definition of severe valve regurgitation – see below.

	Aortic regurgitation	Mitral regurgitation	Tricuspid regurgitation
Qualitative			
Valve morphology	Abnormal flail large coaptation defect	Flail leaflet/ruptured papillary muscle/ large coaptation defect	Abnormal flail large coaptation defect
Colour flow regurgitant jet	Large in central jets, variable in eccentric jets	Very large central jet or eccentric jet adhering, swirling and reaching the posterior wall of the left atrium	Very large central jet or eccentric wall impinging jet
CW signal or regurgitant jet	Dense	Dense/triangular	Dense/triangular with early peaking (peak < 2 m/s in massive TR)
Other	Holodiastolic flow reversal in descending aorta (EDV > 20 cm/s)	Large flow convergence zone	–

continued

	Aortic regurgitation	Mitral regurgitation		Tricuspid regurgitation
Semiquantitative				
Vena contracta width (mm)	> 6	≥ 7 (> 8 for biplane)		≥ 7
Upstream vein flow	–	Systolic pulmonary vein flow reversal		Systolic hepatic vein flow reversal
Inflow	–	E-wave dominant ≥ 1.5 m/s		E-wave dominant ≥ 1 m/s
Other	Pressure half-time < 200 ms	TVI mitral/TVI aortic > 1.4		PISA radius > 9 mm
Quantitative		Primary	Secondary	
EROA (mm²)	≥ 30	≥ 40	≥ 20	≥ 40
R Vol (ml/beat)	≥ 60	≥ 60	≥ 30	≥ 45
+ enlargement of cardiac chambers/ vessels	LV	LV, LA		RV, RA, inferior vena cava

CW, continuous wave; EDV, end-diastolic velocity; EROA, effective regurgitant orifice area; LA, left atrium; LV, left ventricle; PISA, proximal isovelocity surface area; RA, right atrium; RV, right ventricle; R Vol, regurgitant volume; TR, tricuspid regurgitation; TVI, time–velocity integral.

Table 1.10: Echocardiographic criteria for the definition of severe valve regurgitation[1]

CASE 14

A: Dabigitran is contraindicated in diabetes

The introduction of the novel oral anticoagulant agents (NOACs) has caused some confusion. Designed to offer an alternative to warfarin, these agents have been promoted as likely to appeal to younger patients on the basis that no blood testing is needed to monitor their efficacy.

	Dabigatran	Rivaroxaban	Apixaban
Mode of action	Direct thrombin (factor IIa) inhibitor	Factor Xa inhibitor	Factor Xa inhibitor
Time to peak action	2–3 h	2–4 h	3–4 h
Half-life	12–14 h	5–9 h (up to 13 h in elderly)	12 h
Dosage	150 mg BD (75 mg BD if renal impairment)	20 mg OD (15 mg OD in renal impairment) (Acute DVT/PE 15 mg BD for 21 days then 20 mg OD)	5 mg BD (2.5 mg BD if age > 80 years/body weight 60 kg/renal impairment)
Reduced eGFR	Contraindicated if < 30 ml/min	Contraindicated if < 15 ml/min Caution if 15–29 ml/min	Contraindicated if < 15 ml/min Caution if 15–29 ml/min

Table 1.11: Characteristics of novel oral anticoagulant agents

The advantage is greater lifestyle flexibility; however, the significant disadvantage is the lack of reversibility of these agents should the patient experience a significant bleed. As yet only rivaroxaban has been licensed for prophylaxis and treatment of DVT/PE, while apixaban and dabigatran are licensed for the prophylaxis of DVT in patients who have undergone elective knee or hip replacement surgery.

There are no prospective data on the safety of cardioversion in patients receiving NOACs. Observational data from the three large trials (RE-LY, ROCKET-AF and ARISTOTLE) did not show any difference in the number of strokes or systemic embolisms, and the stroke rate was comparable with that in earlier trials with other forms of anticoagulation, with or without trans-oesophageal echocardiography guidance.[9, 10, 11] Management of major bleeding in those taking the new agents is hindered by lack of an antidote but should

continued

involve stopping the drug together with general haemostatic measures, such as mechanical compression, fluid replacement and blood products such as packed red cells, fresh frozen plasma or platelets. A haematologist should be contacted. (See Figure 1.8.)

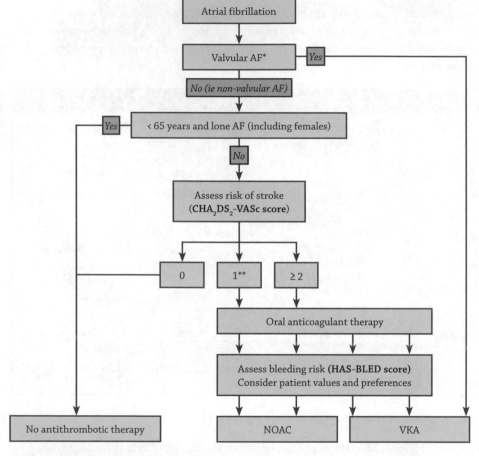

* Includes rheumatic valvular AF, hypertrophic cardiomyopathy, etc

** Antiplatelet therapy with asprin plus clopidogrel, or – less effectively – asprin only, may be considered in patients who refuse any OAC

Figure 1.8: ESC guidance on anticoagulation for atrial fibrillation[12]

CASE 15

E: He should receive thrombolysis before any further investigation

The Wells score is a useful indicator of the likelihood of pulmonary embolism (PE) (see Table 1.12).

Variable	Points
Predisposing factors	
Previous DVT/PE	+1.5
Recent surgery/immobilisation	+1.5
Cancer	+1
Symptoms	
Haemoptysis	+1
Clinical signs	
Heart rate > 100 bpm	+1.5
Clinical signs of DVT	+3
Clinical judgement	
Alternative diagnosis less likely than PE	+3
Clinical probability	**Total**
Low	0–1
Intermediate	2–6
High	≥ 7

Table 1.12: Wells score

If the likelihood is that the diagnosis is PE, patients must be classified as either high risk or not high risk depending on the presence of shock and hypotension.

Learning point

Patients presenting with shock or hypotension who are suspected to have high-risk PE (early mortality > 15%) require immediate diagnostic testing to decide on the appropriateness of thrombolysis or embolectomy (if thrombolysis is contraindicated or fails). Thrombolysis is not usually indicated for non-high-risk patients. CT scanning and echocardiography are the most useful diagnostic tools. Echocardiography will identify right ventricular overload and strain. Troponin elevation in acute PE is secondary to right ventricular overload and injury, and is a further sign that thrombolysis may be necessary.

CASE 16

D: Aspirin should continue lifelong but clopidogrel can be discontinued after 12 months

Current guidelines advocate 12 months of dual anti-platelet therapy following a presentation with acute coronary syndrome whether the patient is revascularised or not. In the case of stenting, the type of stent used is not discriminated between as the guidelines advise 12 months of dual anti-platelet therapy with both drug-eluting and bare metal stents. After 12 months, clopidogrel may be safely discontinued but aspirin should continue lifelong.

In the case of elective percutaneous coronary intervention, it may be possible to discontinue clopidogrel after one month following the use of a bare metal stent. If, however, a drug-eluting stent is used then 12 months of dual anti-platelet therapy is required.

CASE 17

C: His need for an ICD should be reassessed after four weeks

In patients who have had a myocardial infarction (MI), current guidance advises waiting for four weeks after the event before making a decision about the need for an ICD. ICDs may be used for either primary or secondary prevention of sudden cardiac death in those who have had an infarct. Indications are listed below.[13]

Primary prevention:

✦ At least four weeks after the MI, all of the following must be satisfied to proceed with an ICD:

　✧ left ventricular ejection fraction (LVEF) < 35%

　✧ NYHA class < IV

　✧ non-sustained ventricular tachycardia (NSVT) on Holter recording

　✧ positive EP study for inducible VT.

✦ At least four weeks after the MI, both of the following must be satisfied to proceed with an ICD:

　✧ LVEF < 30%.

　✧ Widened QRS ie > 120 ms

Secondary prevention:

✦ ICD is indicated in:

　✧ survivors of out-of-hospital (OOH) cardiac arrest due to ventricular tachycardia/ventricular fibrillation (VT/VF)

　✧ prolonged VT with haemodynamic compromise

　✧ prolonged VT without haemodynamic compromise but with an LVEF< 35% and NYHA class < IV.

CASE 18

A: She should not drive for one month

Strict rules regarding driving must be followed for patients with ICDs. The Driving and Vehicle Licensing Agency has clear guidance for class 1 and class 2 (HGV) drivers[14] (see Table 1.13).

Class of license	Duration of driving ban
Class 1	
ICD for primary prevention	1 month
ICD for secondary prevention	6 months
Appropriate therapy from the device	Can drive after 6 months if changes to medication were made that are likely to prevent recurrent events
Inappropriate therapy from the device	Can drive after 1 month if no further events
Lead revision	1 month
Box change	1 week
Class 2 (HGV)	
ICD	Loss of class 2 license

Table 1.13: DVLA guidance for class 1 and class 2 (HGV) drivers

CASE 19

D: Eisenmenger syndrome

This man with Down syndrome has Eisenmenger syndrome secondary to untreated congenital heart disease. His normal blood results rule out the other distracting answers and there is no clinical evidence of asthma.

Down syndrome is most commonly associated with atrioventricular and ventricular septal defects (VSDs), both of which result initially in left to right shunts. VSDs may be muscular or membranous depending on whereabouts they lie in the ventricle (muscular VSDs lie more distal, membranous VSDs lie just beneath the atrioventricular valves).

CHAPTER 1 ANSWERS

Learning point

A common pitfall is to assume that the right heart is the victim in VSD left to right shunting, when in fact the volume overload is on the left heart and therefore it is the left ventricle that dilates (the right ventricle is in systole during left to right shunting and therefore cannot be overloaded). The consistent increased flow through the lungs eventually causes irreversible damage to the pulmonary vasculature bed, which raises pulmonary artery pressures and causes the shunt to reverse. The development of a right to left shunt is termed Eisenmenger syndrome and results in cyanosis.

General consensus is that once Eisenmenger has been established, defect closure is pointless. Defect closure before shunt reversal is key.

CASE 20

A: Echo assessment of left ventricular diastolic function

This lady describes the classic features of heart failure and her NT-proBNP is raised in keeping with the diagnosis being that of heart failure. Her echocardiogram, however, shows normal left ventricular function. Do not let this put you off the most likely diagnosis.

CHAPTER 1
ANSWERS

Learning point

Just because she does not have systolic dysfunction does not rule out diastolic dysfunction (a failure of the heart to relax properly rather than to contract properly).

Diastolic heart failure is referred to as heart failure with preserved ejection fraction (HFPEF). The history is not in keeping with any of the other distractors and a chest X-ray is likely only to confirm pulmonary oedema rather than offer a diagnosis. Echo assessment of left ventricular diastolic function is therefore likely to yield the diagnosis in this case. Mitral annular tissue velocities and mitral inflow patterns can identify diastolic dysfunction. HFPEF presents similarly to systolic dysfunction clinically, but currently there is no evidence for benefit of any of the usual heart failure medications. Patients ordinarily are treated with diuretics, ACE inhibitors, β blockers and an aldosterone antagonist, as these have been shown to be of benefit in systolic heart failure and physicians feel obliged to commence anti-failure therapy.

CASE 21

A: Calculate his CHA$_2$DS$_2$VASc and HASBLED scores

The European Society of Cardiology has defined atrial fibrillation (AF) as shown in Table 1.14.[15]

Paroxysmal AF	Recurrent self-terminating lasting > 30 s and < 7 days
Persistent AF	Lasting > 7 days or terminated by electrical or chemical conversion
Permanent AF	Longstanding AF resistant to electrical or chemical conversion
Silent AF	Asymptomtic AF discovered incidentally

Table 1.14: European Society of Cardiology definitions for atrial fibrillation (AF)

Stroke prevention in AF is key to the management. In the case described here, it is important to calculate the CHA$_2$DS$_2$VASc and HASBLED scores to balance the risk of bleeding from anticoagulation against the risk of stroke. A CHA$_2$DS$_2$VASc score of ≥ 2 should prompt the prescription of anticoagulation if the HASBLED score is not raised. A CHA$_2$DS$_2$VASc of 1 should prompt consideration of anticoagulation with patient preference taken into account. Anticoagulation is not usually recommended for a score of 0 (see Table 1.15).

Risk factor	Score
Congestive heart failure	1
Hypertension	1
Age ≥ 75 years	2
Diabetes	1
Stroke/TIA/thromboembolism	2
Vascular disease	1
Age 64–75 years	1
Sex (females)	1

Table 1.15: CHA$_2$DS$_2$VASc scoring system

References

1. The Joint Task Force on the Management of Valvular Heart Disease of the European Society of Cardiology (ESC) and the European Association for Cardio-Thoracic Surgery (EACTS). 2012. Guidelines on the management of valvular heart disease (version 2012). European Heart Journal, 33, 2451–2496

2. Moat N E. 2011. Long-Term Outcomes After Transcatheter Aortic Valve Implantation in High-Risk Patients With Severe Aortic Stenosis: The U.K. TAVI (United Kingdom Transcatheter Aortic Valve Implantation) Registry. Journal of the American College of Cardiology, 58, 2130–2138

3. Simonneau G et al. 2009. Updated clinical classification of pulmonary hypertension. Journal of the American College of Cardiology, 54, S43–S54

4. The Task Force on cardiac pacing and resynchronization therapy of the European Society of Cardiology (ESC). 2013. 2013 ESC Guidelines on cardiac pacing and cardiac resynchronization therapy. European Heart Journal, 34, 2281–2329

5. Loeys B et al. 2010. The revised Ghent nosology for the Marfan syndrome. Journal of Medical Genetics, 47, 476–485

6. Baddour L et al. 2005. Infective Endocarditis. Circulation, 111, e394–433

7. NICE. 2008. Prophylaxis against infective endocarditis. Antimicrobial prophylaxis against infective endocarditis in adults and children undergoing interventional procedures. NICE clinical guideline 64. www.nice.org.uk/guidance/cg64

8. The Task Force on the management of ST-segment elevation acute myocardial infarction of the European Society of Cardiology. 2012. ESC Guidelines for the management of acute myocardial infarction in patients presenting with ST-segment elevation. European Heart Journal, 33, 2569–2619

9. Nagarakanti R et al. 2011. Dabigatran vs warfarin in patients with atrial fibrillation: an analysis of patients undergoing cardioversion. Circulation, 123, 131–136

10. Flaker G et al. 2012. Apixaban and warfarin are associated with a low risk of stroke following cardioversion for AF: results from the ARISTOTLE Trial. European Heart Journal, 33 (Abstract Supplement), 686

11. Piccini J P and Stevens S. 2012. Outcomes following cardioversion and atrial fibrillation ablation in patients treated with rivaroxaban and warfarin in the ROCKET-AF trial. Circulation, 126, A19281

12. Camm A et al. 2012. Focused update of the ESC Guidelines for the management of atrial fibrillation. European Heart Journal, 33, 2719–2747

13. ESC Guidelines on cardiac pacing and cardiac resynchronization therapy. 2013. European heart journal, 34, 2281–2329

14. DVLA. 2014. Medical guidelines for professionals. www.gov.uk/current-medical-guidelines-dvla-guidance-for-professionals

15. Brignole M et al. 2013. ESC guidelines on cardiac pacing and cardiac resynchronization therapy. European Heart Journal, 34, 2281–2329

CHAPTER 2

Dermatology

Collette McCourt

CASE 1

A ten-year-old girl presents with a painful rash on the lower legs and buttocks one week following a sore throat. On examination, there are non-blanching violaceous papules as shown in Figure 2.1.

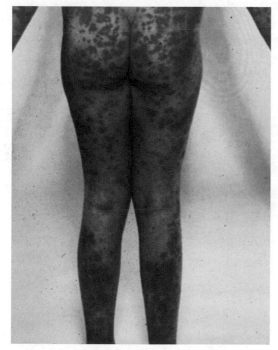

Figure 2.1

What is the most likely diagnosis?

    A. Measles

    B. Chickenpox

    C. Henoch–Schönlein purpura (IgA vasculitis)

    D. Scarlet fever

    E. Rubella

CASE 2

A 66-year-old lady with a 6-year history of dialysis-dependent kidney failure presents with a painful rash on the right thigh and lower leg. She has been on warfarin for four years and her anticoagulation has been stable. On examination of the thigh and lower leg, tender plaques with surrounding retiform purpura and central necrosis are noted.

Blood tests reveal: Haemoglobin 122 g/litre, White cells 5.4×10^9/litre, Eosinophils 0.3×10^9/litre, Platelets 478×10^9/litre, INR 2.3, Corrected calcium 2.84 mmol/litre, Phosphate 1.9 mmol/litre, Parathyroid hormone 18.5 pmol/litre, Anticardiolipin antibodies: IgG 28 U/ml, IgM 10 U/ml.

What is the most likely diagnosis?

    A. **Antiphospholipid antibody syndrome**
    B. **Calciphylaxis**
    C. **Cholesterol embolisation**
    D. **Coumarin skin necrosis**
    E. **Thromboembolism from arteriovenous fistula**

CASE 3

A 26-year-old man with a 4-year history of Crohn's disease presents with a rapidly enlarging painful ulcer on the right lower leg. He describes a small pustule, which had enlarged rapidly over one week (see Figure 2.2).

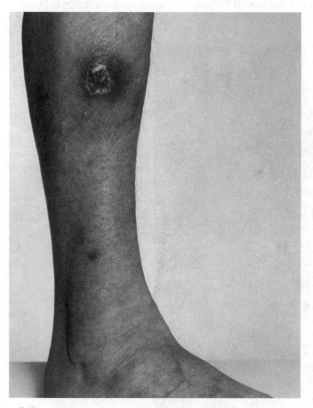

Figure 2.2

What is the most appropriate initial management?

A. **Oral flucloxacillin**
B. **Topical fusidic acid**
C. **Topical terbinafine**
D. **Oral steroids**
E. **Surgical debridement**

CASE 4

A 55-year-old man presents with a 6-week history of an itchy rash, which began on the inner aspect of his wrists and ankles and gradually progressed to involve his lower back. He is not on regular medication. On examination there is a bilaterally symmetrical rash consisting of polygonal violaceous papules with overlying lacy white streaks (see Figure 2.3).

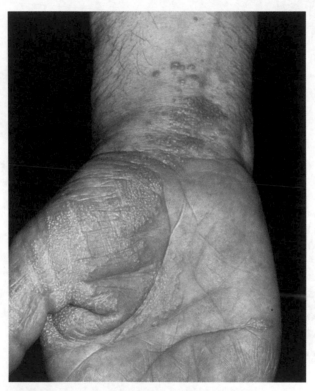

Figure 2.3

What is the most likely diagnosis?

    A. **Pityriasis rosea**
    B. **Guttate psoriasis**
    C. **Tinea corporis**
    D. **Tinea versicolor**
    E. **Lichen planus**

CASE 5

A 25-year-old man with a history of newly diagnosed coeliac disease presents with an extremely itchy rash on his buttocks, elbows and knees. On examination he has a rash consisting of excoriations and vesicles on the extensor surfaces (see Figure 2.4).

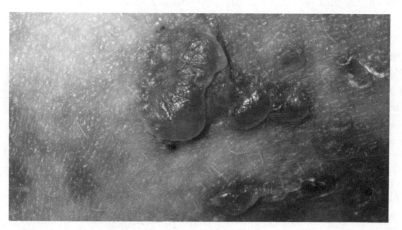

Figure 2.4

What is the treatment of choice for the skin disease?

    A. **Oral steroids**
    B. **Topical terbinafine**
    C. **Topical steroids**
    D. **Dapsone**
    E. **Oral flucloxacillin**

CASE 6

A 25-year-old woman presents with a 10-year history of a facial rash. Previous treatments have included 3-month courses of both doxycycline and erythromycin, in combination with topical retinoids and benzoyl peroxide. She has been on Dianette® (cyproterone acetate and oestrogen) for three months with no benefit. Examination of her skin reveals moderate acne with scarring.

What is the next appropriate step in management?

A. **Topical steroids**
B. **Work-up for isotretinoin**
C. **A 3-month course of trimethoprim**
D. **Topical benzoyl peroxide/clindamycin**
E. **Metformin**

CASE 7

A 79-year-old retired gardener presents with a 3-month history of a rapidly enlarging lesion on his right ear pinna. On examination, a tender nodule is noted on the superior aspect of the pinna (see Figure 2.5).

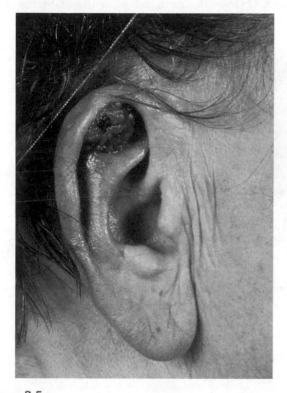

Figure 2.5

What is the most likely diagnosis?

    A. **Basal cell carcinoma**

    B. **Squamous cell carcinoma**

    C. **Epidermal cyst**

    D. **Bowen's disease**

    E. **Actinic keratosis**

CASE 8

An 18-year-old woman presents with a 5-day history of fever, shortness of breath and a non-productive cough. This was associated with a rash, which started on her hands and feet and spread along her limbs towards the chest and back. She has also developed lesions in her mouth. On examination, a rash consisting of discrete 'targetoid' erythematous macules and papules is noted on her arms, legs and face (see Figure 2.6).

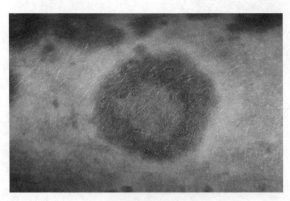

Figure 2.6

Investigations reveal: Haemoglobin 96 g/litre, White cells 5.0 × 109/litre, Platelets 150 × 109/litre, Blood film: red cell agglutination, Sodium 136 mmol/litre, Potassium 4.4 mmol/litre, Urea 3.0 mmol/litre, Creatinine 56 µmol/litre, Bilirubin 24 µmol/litre, AST 70 U/litre, ALT 76 U/litre, ALP 114 U/litre, Albumin 37 g/litre.

Chest X-ray: left middle lobe consolidation.

What is the most likely diagnosis?
- A. **Mycoplasma pneumonia**
- B. **Lyme disease**
- C. **Legionnaires' disease**
- D. **Streptococcal pneumonia**
- E. **Influenza**

CASE 9

A 42-year-old lady with hepatitis C (on triple therapy: telaprevir, ribavirin and pegylated interferon) was referred to dermatology with the new onset of a blistering rash on her dorsal hands. Before the onset of the rash she had been on holiday in Spain. On examination she had multiple crusted erosions, scars, milia and tense blisters on her dorsal hands and forearms (see Figure 2.7).

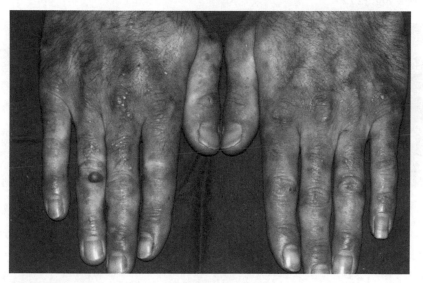

Figure 2.7

What is the most appropriate investigation?

- A. **Genetic testing for HFE gene**
- B. **Skin swab for herpes simplex virus PCR**
- C. **Skin scrapings for mycology**
- D. **Urinary porphyrins**
- E. **Skin swab for bacterial culture**

CASE 10

A 57-year-old lady is referred to dermatology with an itchy rash on her face, scalp, chest and hands. She has no history of skin disease. She describes 5 kg of weight loss and difficulty getting out of a chair. On examination, a violaceous oedematous rash is noted over the periorbital area and cheeks (including the nasolabial folds) with scaly violaceous papules overlying the interphalengeal joints of the dorsal hands (see Figure 2.8).

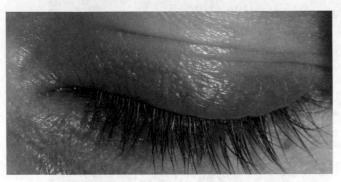

Figure 2.8

What is the most appropriate initial investigation from the options given?

A. **Creatine kinase**
B. **Urinalysis**
C. **Anti-double-stranded DNA**
D. **Direct microscopy of skin scrapings**
E. **Patch testing to contact allergens**

CASE 11

A 13-year-old girl attends the outpatient clinic as an emergency. One week following a coryzal illness and sore throat, she describes the sudden onset of a rash affecting her trunk and limbs. On examination she has a widespread rash consisting of multiple small 4–5 mm pink to red scaly papules and plaques on her torso, arms and legs (see Figure 2.9).

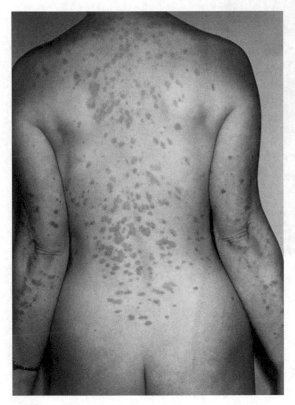

Figure 2.9

What is the diagnosis?

    A. **Atopic dermatitis**
    B. **Henoch–Schönlein purpura**
    C. **Guttate psoriasis**
    D. **Lichen planus**
    E. **Pityriasis versicolor**

CASE 12

A six-year-old girl presents with the sudden onset of an oval-shaped area of alopecia on her scalp noted by her parents overnight. No hair loss has been noted elsewhere. She is otherwise healthy and well, and there is no family history of note (see Figure 2.10).

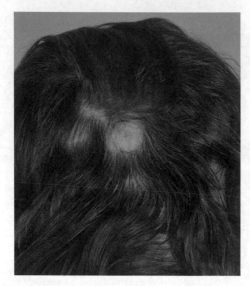

Figure 2.10

What is the most likely diagnosis?

- A. **Telogen effluvium**
- B. **Tinea capitis**
- C. **Alopecia totalis**
- D. **Alopecia areata**
- E. **Trichotillomania**

CASE 13

A 25-year-old lady presents with whitening of the skin around her hands, eyes and mouth. She has a past history of type 1 diabetes. On examination, symmetrical depigmented patches with well-demarcated borders are noted on the hands, perioral and periocular areas. On Wood's light examination no fluorescence is noted.

What is the most appropriate management for this condition?

A. Topical terbinafine
B. High-factor (SPF 50 with high UVA) sunscreen
C. Oral itraconazole
D. Monitoring only
E. Topical selenium sulfide shampoo

CASE 14

A 17-year-old girl presents to your clinic with numerous brown marks on her trunk and limbs, which have been enlarging with growth. On examination, 15 macules are noted as shown in Figure 2.11.

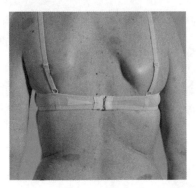

Figure 2.11

In which of the following disorders are such macules not a feature?

A. Neurofibromatosis
B. Ehlers–Danlos syndrome
C. Fanconi anaemia
D. McCune–Albright syndrome
E. Tuberous sclerosis

CASE 15

A 33-year-old lady with a history of regular sunny holidays presents with a changing pigmented lesion on her upper back. It has increased in size and become darker over the last six months and has bled on several occasions with no trauma. On examination of her upper back a 10 × 12 mm pigmented lesion is noted (see Figure 2.12).

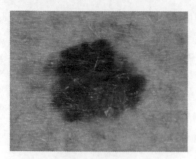

Figure 2.12

What is the most appropriate immediate management?

A. **Excision of the lesion with appropriate margins**

B. **Photograph and review in three months**

C. **Reassure and discharge with mole-watching advice**

D. **Cryotherapy**

E. **Perform an incisional biopsy of the darker portion of the lesion**

CASE 16

A 75-year-old lady presents with an 8-week history of a widespread itchy rash consisting of urticated patches with the recent onset of widespread tense blisters suspicious of bullous pemphigoid (see Figure 2.13). She has a history of a stroke, for which she takes regular medication.

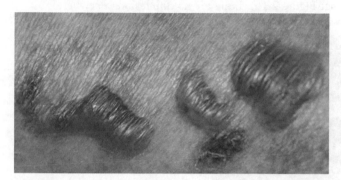

Figure 2.13

Which medication is most likely to have precipitated her bullous pemphigoid?

    A. **Furosemide**
    B. **Propanolol**
    C. **Aspirin**
    D. **Clopidogrel**
    E. **Ramipril**

CASE 17

A 63-year-old lady presents with an asymptomatic annular eruption on her anterior right thigh noted two weeks after returning from a hiking trip in the Lake District. She is not taking regular medication and is well on systematic questioning. On examination you note an annular, non-scaly erythematous patch on her anterior thigh (see Figure 2.14). There are no skin lesions elsewhere.

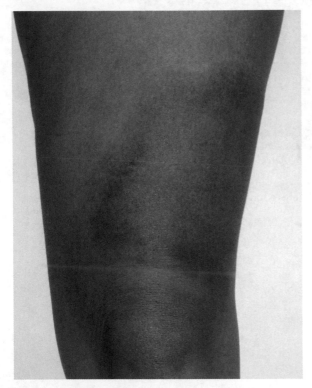

Figure 2.14

What is the most appropriate treatment for this patient?

    A. **Oral doxycycline**
    B. **Topical terbinafine**
    C. **Topical steroids**
    D. **Oral itraconazole**
    E. **Oral antihistamines**

CASE 18

A 23-year-old woman presents with a history of gradually enlarging asymptomatic papules affecting the dorsal aspect of her fingers. On examination, firm, skin-coloured, annular lesions with a smooth, papular edge are noted on the dorsal aspects of the fingers (see Figure 2.15).

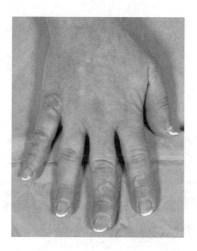

Figure 2.15

What is the most likely diagnosis?

A. **Granuloma annulare**
B. **Knuckle pads**
C. **Tuberous xanthoma**
D. **Tinea unguium**
E. **Viral warts**

CASE 19

A 13-year-old girl presents with velvety hyperpigmented plaques in the axilla and neck. She is systemically well and has no family history of similar lesions. On examination, she has a body mass index of 32 kg/m^2 and has evidence of velvety plaques in the axilla consistent with acanthosis nigricans.

What is the most likely cause of the acanthosis nigricans?

A. **Cushing syndrome**
B. **Familial**
C. **Normal variant**
D. **Obesity**
E. **Underlying malignancy**

CASE 20

A six-year-old girl is referred to a clinic because of the gradual onset of pigmentation around her lips. She has no significant past medical history. On closer examination there are discrete brown–black non-blanching macules on the buccal mucosa and lips only (see Figure 2.16). Her nails are normal. Her uncle has similar pigmentation of his lips and a history of intussusception.

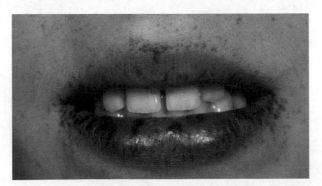

Figure 2.16

What is the most likely diagnosis?

A. **Addison's disease**
B. **Peutz–Jeghers syndrome**
C. **Laugier–Hunziker syndrome**
D. **Hereditary haemorrhagic telangiectasia**
E. **Carney complex**

CASE 21

A 28-year-old lady presents with the sudden onset of tender lumps on her anterior lower legs, associated with fever and arthralgia of her ankles and wrists. On examination, ill-defined, erythematous, tender, hot swellings are noted on her shins bilaterally, consistent with erythema nodosum. There is evidence of active synovitis of her wrists and ankles and a chest X-ray shows bihilar lymphadenopathy. See Figure 2.17.

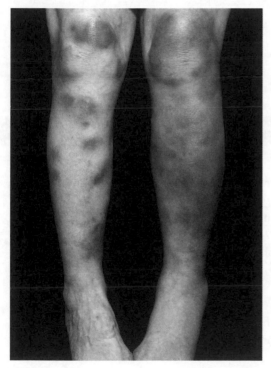

Figure 2.17

What is the prognosis of this condition?

  A. **100% likely to develop chronic arthritis**
  B. **100% likely to develop chronic lung disease**
  C. **No chance of chronic lung disease**
  D. **10% chance of complete resolution within near future**
  E. **90% chance of complete resolution within near future**

CASE 22

You are asked to review a 36-year-old woman who has a rash. On examination she has a widespread erythematous eruption with sheets of skin loss. Nikolsky's sign is positive. There is haemorrhagic oral crusting and conjunctivitis.

Which one of these drugs is most likely to be responsible?

A. **Phenytoin**
B. **Oral contraceptive pill**
C. **Paracetamol**
D. Codeine
E. **Enoxaparin**

CASE 23

A 48-year-old lady is referred with a history of intermittent flushing over the face and neck for a year, with progressive worsening. Over the last few months she has also developed copious diarrhoea for which she is under investigation with the gastroenterology team. On examination of the face, erythema with telangiectasia is noted. On examination of the precordium, a soft, systolic murmur is heard and a firm, irregular liver edge is palpable on abdominal examination.

What is the investigation of choice for this patient?

A. **Thyroid function tests**
B. **Urinary collection for 5-hydroxyindoleacetic acid (5-HIAA)**
C. **MRI scan of adrenal glands**
D. **Urinary metanephrines**
E. **Plasma metanephrines**

CASE 1

C: Henoch–Schönlein purpura (IgA vasculitis)

This young girl presented one to two weeks following a sore throat with a purpuric rash confined to the buttocks and lower limbs.

> ### Learning point
>
> The description of the rash, particularly the non-blanching purpura and the distribution as well as the history of a preceding sore throat, is typical of Henoch–Schönlein purpura (IgA vasculitis). This is an IgA-mediated systemic vasculitis of small blood vessels, the hallmarks of which are the tetrad of:
>
> ✦ non-thrombocytopenic purpura
>
> ✦ abdominal pain
>
> ✦ arthritis
>
> ✦ nephritis.

It is the most common type of vasculitis in children, presenting in the majority between 2 and 11 years of age. It is almost as common in boys as in girls. The prognosis is usually excellent and in the absence of renal disease episodes usually resolve in one month. The main differential diagnosis to consider in children presenting with purpura would be meningococcal septicaemia; however, this is not an option and the presence of petechiae or purpura in meningococcal septicaemia indicates rapidly progressive severe disease.

In measles, chickenpox, scarlet fever and rubella, the rash usually starts soon after a prodromal illness. Although measles can cause a transient non-thrombocytopenic purpura, the rash usually starts behind the ears and spreads cephalocaudally, typically consisting of red–brown blanching spots ranging from 1 to 10 mm, which often spare the palms and soles. Before the onset of the exanthem, white–blue spots develop in the mouth, known as Koplik's spots. These are characteristic of the disease.

Chickenpox is a very contagious disease caused by varicella zoster. It is largely a childhood disease but may occur in adults, particularly if immunocompromised. It is transmitted by airborne droplets, and presents following a short prodrome of approximately two days with an eruption of itchy papules, which progress into vesicles and subsequently crust. Although thrombocytopaenia and purpura may occur in healthy children as a complication of varicella, this is more often seen in immunocompromised children and adults. The rash

continued

of scarlet fever typically develops in children between 12 hours to 2 days following onset of a fever. It is caused by toxins released by a Group A streptococcal infection, eg pharyngitis. Again, the rash usually starts below the ears, neck, chest and groin before spreading to affect the whole body. As lesions progress, the skin may look 'sunburned' with goose pimples and a rough sand-like feel. Although purpura is not a feature, in the body folds, due to rupture of thin-walled capillaries, red streaks known as 'Pastia lines' can develop.

CASE 2

B: Calciphylaxis

Learning point

The development of non-inflammatory retiform purpura in a patient with high calcium phosphate product and chronic renal failure on haemodialysis is highly suggestive of calciphylaxis.

The absence of a recent lytic or arterial procedure or the recent addition of warfarin therapy (usually occurs within two months of starting therapy), as well as the normal eosinophil count, goes against the diagnosis of cholesterol embolisation. This is heralded by the sudden onset of livido reticularis, skin ulceration and eosinophilia in a patient with a history of one of the former interventions. The patient has low levels of anticardiolipin antibody, but these are present in up to 10% of the general population and are not diagnostic of the antiphospholipid antibody syndrome (APS). Transiently elevated levels of IgG or IgM anticardiolipin antibody, as well as a positive lupus anticoagulant test, can occur in otherwise normal individuals, and in the setting of viral or other infections. Confirmatory testing (> 12 weeks apart) is required to satisfy the laboratory criteria for APS. Coumarin necrosis (in the absence of heparin therapy) typically occurs within two to five days of starting warfarin therapy, coinciding with the expected early drop in protein C function. Thromboembolism from arteriovenous fistulae would not cause skin changes in the trunk and legs.

CASE 3

D: Oral steroids

Learning point

The history of a rapidly enlarging painful ulcer is typical of pyoderma gangrenosum, which is associated with an underlying systemic disease in approximately 50% of cases. Pyoderma gangrenosum can occur before, concurrent with or following the underlying associated diagnosis. Commonly associated systemic conditions include:

✦ inflammatory bowel disease (particularly Crohn's disease)

✦ haematologic disorders including leukaemia, monoclonal gammopathy (particularly IgA) and multiple myeloma

✦ inflammatory arthritis, particularly rheumatoid arthritis.

Less common associations include other immunologic diseases such as lupus erythematosus and hepatitis. The lesions of pyoderma may also occur peri-stomally in inflammatory bowel disease. The initial treatment of choice from the given answers is oral steroids. Alternative treatment options include topical or intralesional steroids or topical calcineurin inhibitors. Adjuvant therapy would include immunosuppressants (such as ciclosporin or mycophenolate mofetil), and in recalcitrant cases, tumour necrosis factor alpha inhibitors.

Regarding the other options, oral and topical antibiotics may be indicated if there are signs of secondary infection such as increasing erythema, pain, discharge etc; however, this is not an obvious problem in this scenario. Similarly, surgical debridement is relatively contraindicated owing to the risk of pathergy, a process whereby new ulcerations may occur after trauma or injury to the skin. This occurs in up to 30% of patients who already have pyoderma gangrenosum.

CASE 4

E: Lichen planus

In this case, the clinical history, appearance and distribution of the rash are characteristic.

> ### Learning point
>
>
> In lichen planus, the individual lesions are often described as purple or violacious flat-topped papules with white lines on the surface – so-called 'Wickham's striae'. Lichen planus tends to affect middle-aged adults, but may affect all ages. It tends to burn itself out in 12–18 months. Other sites that may be affected include genitalia, mucous membranes, nails and scalp. On the buccal mucosa, lichen planus can cause a white lace-like pattern of Wickham's striae. Lichenoid drug eruptions may also occur and are most often seen with antimalarials, captopril and gold.

To distinguish from the other differential diagnoses, pityriasis rosea usually presents as a 'herald patch' one to two weeks before the onset of an eruption, predominantly on the trunk along Langer's lines. The lesions are usually red/pink in colour and have a typical collarette of scale at their edge. The lesions of tinea corporis have an annular configuration and usually result in scaling. Tinea versicolor is usually asymptomatic and consists of brown/orange oval patches, typically in a seborrhoeic distribution on the chest and back with associated fine scaling. Guttate psoriasis typically presents in younger patients with the sudden onset of small, salmon-pink-coloured, scaly lesions on the trunk and limbs, most often following a streptococcal throat infection.

CASE 5

D: Dapsone

Learning point

The history of an extremely itchy vesicular rash on the extensor surfaces of the elbows, knees and buttocks resulting in excoriations, in the context of coeliac disease, is suggestive of dermatitis herpetiformis. This condition is associated with underlying gluten-sensitive enteropathy or coeliac disease. A patient presenting with such a rash should be investigated for coeliac disease and commenced on a gluten-free diet.

Although an important part in management, the option of a gluten-free diet is not given in this question. Therefore the most appropriate answer is dapsone. If the diagnosis of dermatitis herpetiformis is correct, the itch typically responds to treatment with dapsone within 24–48 hours. It can take months for the itch and rash to improve with a gluten-free diet only. An important side effect of dapsone is haemolytic anaemia, which is severe in patients with a history of glucose 6 phosphate dehydrogenase deficiency, but may also be idiosyncratic in some patients.

Dermatitis herpetiformis is a condition that is often refractory to topical steroids and, given the usual dramatic response to dapsone, oral steroids are not indicated. It is neither infectious nor contagious, so oral antibiotics or topical antifungals including terbinafine are not indicated.

CASE 6

B: Work-up for isotretinoin

This woman presents with persistent severe acne in her mid-twenties. It has not been responsive to two sequential oral antibiotics in combination with topical agents. In addition, she has had hormonal therapy with no demonstrable benefit. The next line in therapy would be isotretinoin, an oral retinoid. Isotretinoin is indicated for severe, cystic acne, or acne at risk of scarring that has not responded to previous conventional therapy with oral and topical antibiotics. Although the exact mechanism of action is still to be elucidated, the drug temporarily reduces sebaceous gland activity and appears also to have anti-inflammatory action.

Learning point

The most common side effects of isotretinoin are mucocutaneous, with drying of the lips and skin very common. Isotretinoin is highly teratogenic, so women of childbearing age must be established on two effective methods of contraception before, concurrently and for five weeks post therapy. Women also require monthly pregnancy testing. Mood disturbance and depression have also been reported. Patients should be aware of the association, and report any symptoms of depression or mood changes.

Isotretinoin therapy is successful in up to 80% of patients. Although another course of an oral antibiotic would not be contraindicated, it is unlikely to be of added benefit given the history of failure of two courses of oral antibiotics in the past.

CASE 7

B: Squamous cell carcinoma

Learning point

The history of a rapidly enlarging tender nodule on a chronically sun-exposed site (the ear in this case) is very suggestive of a squamous cell carcinoma. Risk factors for squamous cell carcinoma include:

+ chronic sun exposure
+ irradiation therapy
+ chronic scarring or inflammation, eg Marjolin's ulcer (squamous cell carcinoma arising in chronic leg ulcer)
+ smoking (particularly lesions of the lip)
+ arsenic exposure
+ immunosuppression, eg organ transplant recipients
+ human papilloma virus.

Basal cell carcinomas are slow-growing tumours of basal keratinocytes that may be subdivided into various types, including nodular, morphoeic, pigmented and superficial. They most often occur on the face of middle-aged and elderly patients and rarely metastasise. Nodular basal cell carcinomas appear as discrete, firm lesions typically with a pearly rolled edge, telangiectasia and central ulceration.

Epidermal cysts are benign skin appendage tumours consisting of fluctuant cystic lesions, usually with a central punctum. They may enlarge rapidly at times of acute inflammation, usually associated with erythema, pain and occasionally discharge.

Bowen's disease, or intraepidermal squamous cell carcinoma in situ, usually presents as an irregular erythematous scaly patch on chronic sun-damaged skin. Actinic keratosis also present on chronically sun-damaged skin as skin-coloured, or erythematous, rough scaly areas. Both of these lesions are slow-growing flat lesions on chronically exposed sites, compared with the rapidly enlarging nodule in this scenario. The most likely diagnosis here is squamous cell carcinoma and treatment is excision with appropriate margins.

CASE 8

A: Mycoplasma pneumonia

Mycoplasma pneumonia (caused by *Mycoplasma pneumoniae*) is the most likely diagnosis as the patient is suffering from a prodrome of upper respiratory tract symptoms associated with a dry cough and a targetoid rash in keeping with typical erythema multiforme (EM). *M. pneumoniae* is a common cause of community-acquired pneumonia in healthy patients under 40 years old. It causes an atypical pneumonia with a prodromal illness lasting approximately three weeks. Clinical suspicion of *M. pneumoniae* infection arises in a patient with a respiratory illness and any type of rash, but especially an EM-like eruption. Streptococcal pneumonia is typically of sudden onset and associated with pyrexia and pleuritic chest pain. Legionella is typically associated with multisystem pathology including gastrointestinal symptoms, biochemical abnormalities (eg abnormal liver function tests and hyponatraemia) or neurological involvement.

Learning point

Erythema multiforme is not associated with Legionella or any of the other options. It is a hypersensitivity reaction usually triggered by infection (in approximately 90% of cases), most commonly herpes simplex virus. Young adults (aged 20–40 years) are most often affected; however, *M. pneunomiae* is the next most common infectious trigger. EM associated with *M. pneumoniae* typically consists of raised, red target lesions with three distinct rings starting over the extremities and spreading to the trunk. Conjunctivitis, stomatitis and ulceration of the mouth and genitals are common.

Other infectious causes of EM include: parapox virus (orf), herpes zoster, cytomegalovirus, adenovirus and infectious mononucleosis. Drug causes represent less than 10% of cases. Triggers include: non-steroidal anti-inflammatory drugs, penicillins, sulfonamides, anticonvulsants and barbiturates. Treatment is usually supportive and aimed at the underlying cause if identified, eg antivirals for herpes simplex or oral antibiotics for *M. pneumoniae*. Offending drugs should be stopped.

CASE 9

D: Urinary porphyrins

Porphyrias are metabolic disorders of haem synthesis. There are eight recognised types of porphyria, which can be classified into acute/non-acute and cutaneous/non-cutaneous forms (Table 2.1). They can also be classified as hepatic or erythropoietic depending on whether the site of production/accumulation of pathway intermediate is in the liver or bone.

Acute	Non-acute
Cutaneous manifestations: ✦ Variegate porphyria ✦ Hereditary coproporphyria Non-cutaneous manifestations: ✦ Acute intermittent porphyria ✦ Aminolevulinic acid dehydratase deficiency porphyria	Cutaneous manifestations: ✦ Porphyria cutanea tarda ✦ Erythropoietic protoporphyria ✦ Congenital erythropoietic porphyria ✦ Hepatoerythropoietic porphyria

Table 2.1: Classification for recognised types of porphyria

Porphyria cutanea tarda (PCT) is the most common porphyria worldwide. Both acquired (80%) and hereditary (20%) forms exist. It results from decreased catalytic activity of uroporphrinogen decarboxylase, and the subsequent build up in the skin of unstable intermediates of the haem pathway. These undergo ultraviolet (UV)-induced degradation into free radicals, which damage surrounding cells. The cutaneous manifestations include photosensitivity, increased skin fragility, blistering and erosions, milia and scarring, hyperpigmentation, hypertrichosis, sclerodermoid and morphoeaform skin changes. The diagnosis is usually made with the demonstration of porphyrins in the blood, urine and faeces. Biochemical findings include elevated urinary excretion of uroporphyrin and coproporphyrins, increased excretion of isocoproporphyrin in the faeces (exclusive to PCT and hepatoerythropoietic porphyria). Triggering factors for PCT include: oestrogens, alcohol, hepatitis C, HIV and haemochromatosis.

Learning point

Importantly, variegate porphyria (VP) may present with similar clinical features and age of onset to PCT, and given the association with acute neurological attacks, it is important to perform further porphyrin screening of plasma and faeces once the initial urinary screen is found to be positive.

continued

Treatment includes avoidance of UV light exposure, sun-protective clothing and broad-spectrum sunscreens. Triggering factors should be avoided. In patients with iron overload, venesection should be commenced to reduce iron stores to low normal. In selected cases, hydroxychloroquine or chloroquine may be used.

CASE 10

A: Creatine kinase

This lady presents with a photodistributed rash associated with symptoms of a proximal myopathy and weight loss. The most appropriate initial investigation is therefore creatine kinase, which is likely to be raised. The violaceous oedematous periorbital rash is classical of the 'heliotrope' rash of dermatomyositis, with violaceous scaly papules over the interphalengeal joints characteristic of Gottron's papules. Dermatomyositis has a bimodal onset: juvenile disease is associated with cutaneous calcinosis, while adult onset disease is associated with underlying malignancy.

Learning point

Systemic manifestations of the disease include fever, arthralgia, malaise, Raynaud's phenomenon, cardiac disease and pulmonary fibrosis. Other cutaneous manifestations include:

✦ dilated nail-fold capillaries, prominent ragged cuticles and nail-fold infarcts

✦ periorbital oedema

✦ poikiloderma over the hips and shoulders ('holster' and 'shawl' signs, respectively)

✦ Gottron's sign: erythema over the elbows and knees.

Seborrhoeic dermatitis typically presents as an erythematous scaly rash affecting areas rich in sebaceous glands, particularly the eyebrows, nasolabial folds, chest, back and flexural areas. It is not associated with Gottron's papules or myopathy. Direct microscopy of skin scrapings would reveal *Malassezia* species on potassium hydroxide staining.

Regarding the other options in the scenario, urinalysis is unlikely to be helpful in the diagnosis of dermatomyositis, but may be useful in patients with systemic lupus erythematosus (SLE) to assess for renal disease. Regarding the facial rash in SLE, the classical 'butterfly rash' typically affects the malar area and nasal bridge, and spares the nasolabial folds (in this case the rash involves the nasolabial folds). Additionally, if present on the dorsal hands, typically the rash of SLE tends to affect the skin between the interphalangeal joints, helping distinguish the eruption from that of dermatomyositis. Air-borne contact dermatitis may affect both the face and the hands; however, it is typically eczematous in nature and is not directly associated with myopathy.

CASE 11

C: Guttate psoriasis

This young lady has developed an exanthem following a sore throat. The description of the rash including the colour, scaling and distribution is typical of guttate psoriasis, most often associated with streptococcal throat infections. Psoriasis is an inflammatory and proliferative polygenic disorder of the skin. The aetiology is unknown but genetic factors in combination with environmental factors are thought to be important. The risk of developing psoriasis if one parent has the disease is 20%, increasing if both parents are effected. Up to 30% of patients with psoriasis may have underlying psoriatic arthropathy, with several different forms including: distal interphalangeal joint disease, arthritis mutilans, asymmetric oligoarthritis, psoriatic spondylitis and sacroiliitis and symmetrical polyarthritis. Trigger factors for psoriasis include: drugs (eg β blockers, antimalarials, ACE inhibitors and lithium); infections including HIV and streptocococcal; psychological stress; alcohol; smoking; and trauma, ie the Koebner phenomenon whereby disease develops at areas of trauma.

Although pityriasis rosea and secondary syphilis are in the differential diagnosis of similar lesions in patients in this age group, these are not listed as possible answers. While Henoch–Schönlein purpura commonly presents following a streptococcal throat infection, the rash consists of purpuric (ie non-blanching) papules, which are not scaly and affect the legs and buttocks. This condition typically occurs in younger age groups (although it may occur in any age group). All other differential diagnoses would only follow a sore throat coincidentally. Atopic eczema typically affects flexural areas including the antecubital and popliteal fossae.

Lichen planus presents with violaceous flat-topped papules on the flexural aspects of the wrists, ankles and sacrum, which are not typically scaly. Pityriasis versicolor presents with hyperpigmented or hypopigmented macules, not papules, on the seborrhoeic areas of the chest and back. It is associated with overgrowth of the normal commensal yeast *Malassezia*.

CASE 12

D: Alopecia areata

The history of a sudden onset of an oval patch of hair loss is typical of alopecia areata (AA).

Learning point

When the alopecia affects the entire scalp it is known as alopecia totalis. AA is an autoimmune alopecia, which causes a lymphocytic infiltrate around the hair follicles and results in temporary hair loss. The prognosis is good where there is limited patchy AA, with up to 80% showing re-growth at one year. Poor prognostic features include marginal hairline involvement, an atopic history and a longer duration.

Telogen effluvium occurs approximately two to three months following a stressful episode, eg childbirth, illness (particularly if associated with a fever), stress or medications. It leads to increased hair shedding and patients often describe thinning of their hair. It is not associated with a single patch of hair loss, as in this case.

Tinea capitis commonly affects children. It typically causes an area of non-inflammatory alopecia with associated fine scaling or, when caused by zoophilic organisms (eg *Trichophyum tonsurans*), results in inflammatory alopecia which leads to an associated boggy swelling, otherwise known as a kerion. The history of sudden hair loss overnight and lack of scaling goes against this diagnosis; however, the scalp should be carefully examined in a child with this history. Trichotillomania is a condition characterised by the recurrent repetitive pulling of one's own hair, resulting in noticeable hair loss. Clues to the diagnosis may be hairs of varying length and unusual or bizarrely shaped patches of hair loss. It is much more common in children and most often affects the scalp, followed by eyebrows and eyelashes.

CASE 13

B: High-factor (SPF 50 with high UVA) sunscreen

Vitiligo is an acquired chronic pigmentation disorder of the skin. The history of symmetrical, depigmented, irregularly shaped patches on the distal limbs and perioral and periocular areas are typical of the condition. It is thought to be an autoimmune condition, which affects epidermal and follicular melanocytes, and may be associated with other autoimmune disorders, particularly autoimmune thyroid disease.

Learning point

Treatment options vary and include the short-term use of potent or super-potent topical steroids or calcineurin inhibitors. Other treatment options include narrow-band ultraviolet B (UVB) light treatment. In a patient with fair skin where the vitiligo is only noticeable if the surrounding skin is tanned, an appropriate treatment would include broad-spectrum sunscreen to protect the depigmented area and prevent the normal skin from becoming more tanned. These other options are not given in this scenario.

It is important to educate patients on the risk of sunburn in the depigmented areas, as the melanin found in melanocytes is photo protective. Therefore option D would not be appropriate. The other answers given are either topical or oral antifungal medications and could be used to treat pityriasis versicolor, one of the main differential diagnoses of vitiligo on the trunk. As mentioned previously, this superficial yeast infection results in pale and hypo-pigmented macules on the upper trunk in patients with darker skin, and an associated fine, dry, surface scale.

Wood's light is a useful test in patients presenting with a history of loss of pigment. In approximately one third of cases of pityriasis versicolor, yellow–green fluorescence will be detected. In contrast no fluoresence is detected with Wood's light in vitiligo.

CASE 14

B: Ehlers–Danlos syndrome

Café-au-lait macules (CALMs) are flat, round, well-circumscribed, light brown patches that are present at or soon after birth. Neurofibromatosis 1 (NF1) is an autosomal dominant condition resulting in a deletion or mutation in the gene on the long arm of chromosome 17, leading to a deficiency of the gene product neurofibromin, which acts as a tumour suppressor. The presenting sign of this condition is often the appearance of several CALMs which increase in size and number throughout childhood. The presence of more than five CALMs should prompt assessment for the condition. Axillary and inguinal freckles (Crowe's sign) occur in childhood and cutaneous neurofibromas also appear in later childhood and adolescence.

Learning point

Diagnosis of NF1 requires two from the following seven criteria:

✦ six or more CALMs or hyperpigmented patches > 5 mm in children or > 15 mm in adults

✦ the presence of axillary or inguinal freckling

✦ two or more neurofibromas or one plexiform neuroma

✦ two or more iris hamartomas (Lisch nodules) identified by slit lamp examination

✦ optic nerve glioma

✦ sphenoid dysplasia or typical long-bone abnormalities such as pseudarthrosis

✦ having a first degree relative with NF1.

NIH criteria consensus development conference 1988[1]

Associated conditions include hypertension (may be associated with phaeochromocytoma or renal artery stenosis secondary to fibromuscular dysplasia), learning difficulties, short stature and macrocephaly. In contrast with NF1, NF2 is associated with mainly central neurological abnormalities and a paucity of cutaneous features. It is also an autosomal dominant condition affecting the long arm of chromosome 22, affecting the coding of the cytoskeletal protein merlin.

Tuberous sclerosis (TSC) is a genodermatosis inherited in an autosomal dominant manner with two distinct chromosomal abnormalities. Abnormalities on chromosome 9 (also referred to as TSC1) or chromosome 16 (TSC2), which encode the tumour suppressor genes hamartin and tuberin, respectively, may cause the disease. Approximately three quarters of cases are the result of new genetic mutations.

> ## Learning point
>
> The cutaneous findings in TSC include the characteristic facial rash adenoma sebaceum, which usually appears at puberty in the centro-facial area. This consists of multiple angiofibromas, periungual fibromas, skin tags, CALMs, shagreen patches (connective tissue naevi on the back/neck) and ash-leaf macules (hypopigmented macules ranging from millimetres to several centimetres). Other features include:
>
> + cardiac rhabdomyoma
> + lung cysts
> + angiomyolipomas of kidneys, renal cysts and renal cell carcinoma
> + learning difficulties and seizures
> + cortical tubers, sub-ependymal nodules, intracranial calcification, hydrocephalus and giant cell astrocytoma.

McCune–Albright syndrome is a sporadic condition associated with CALMs; however, these are usually more irregular in shape and often do not cross the midline, unlike those in NF1. The condition is associated with polyostotic fibrous dysplasia of bone and endocrine abnormalities including precocious puberty.

Fanconi anaemia is one of the most frequently reported inherited bone marrow failure syndromes. The most common manifestation is bruising and petechiae in childhood associated with pigmentary abnormalities including CALMs. All of the listed disorders are associated with CALMs, with the exception of Ehlers–Danlos syndrome. Ehlers–Danlos syndrome is a genetic disorder resulting in a defect in collagen, which leads to fragile and hyper-elastic skin, hyper-extensible joints, and fragile tissue and blood vessels.

CASE 15

A: Excision of the lesion with appropriate margins

The lady is presenting with features suggestive of a superficial spreading malignant melanoma. In any patient presenting with pigmented lesions, a history of change should be sought. There are several criteria that can be used to help with the history. One of the more commonly used criteria is the Glasgow seven-point checklist (see Table 2.2). Using this scheme, any patient with a score of three or more, or where the suspicion is high, should be referred as a red flag (or within two weeks) to the dermatology service in secondary care. In this case, the patient has had a change in size and colour of their lesion. It has a diameter of > 7 mm and inflammation. It therefore scores six on the Glasgow scale checklist.

Major features	Minor features
✦ Change in size (2)	✦ Diameter > 7 mm (1)
✦ Irregular shape (2)	✦ Inflammation (1)
✦ Irregular colour (2)	✦ Oozing (1)
	✦ Change in sensation (1)

Table 2.2: Glasgow seven-point checklist[2]

Another commonly used tool for early detection of melanoma is the 'ABCDE' acronym (Asymmetry, Border irregularity, Colour variegation, Diameter > 6 mm and Evolution or history of change), which was introduced to alert patients and health professionals to the diagnosis of melanoma. This patient also has risk factors for melanoma, including a history of sunny holidays abroad.

The history and examination findings are highly suspicious for melanoma. The treatment of choice is complete excision with appropriate margins to determine the diagnosis and prognosis.

The Breslow depth is a millimetre measurement taken from the top of the granular layer of the skin to the deepest point of tumour involvement. It is a strong predictor of prognosis for the patient. The thicker the melanoma, the more likely it is to metastasise.

An incisional biopsy is only appropriate for more difficult cases (eg large lesions on the face) to confirm the diagnosis before surgical planning. Photography and reassurance could result in a poorer prognosis for the patient as the melanoma could become more invasive with a higher Breslow depth. Cryotherapy is not a treatment for melanocytic lesions, and in this case histological diagnosis is required to determine prognosis for the patient.

CASE 16

A: Furosemide

Bullous pemphigoid is the most common immunobullous disease. It presents in middle-aged and elderly patients with the development of tense, thick-walled blisters often with preceding or concurrent urticarial or eczematous patches and plaques. Mucous membrane involvement is uncommon compared with pemphigus vulgaris, an uncommon immunobullous disease often presenting in adults aged 50–60 years with mucous membrane blisters and superficial erosions and blisters of the skin (due to intraepidermal blister formation).

In bullous pemphigoid, autoantibodies are directed to components of the basement membrane, particularly the bullous pemphigoid (BP) antigens BP180 and BP230. In pemphigus vulgaris, autoantibodies are directed towards desmoglein 3.

Bullous pemphigoid is more prevalent in patients who have had neurological disease, particularly stroke, dementia and Parkinson's disease.

> **Learning point**
>
> Medications known to trigger bullous pemphigoid include:
> - furosemide
> - D-penicillamine
> - captopril
> - gold
> - potassium iodide.

Treatment depends on the severity of disease and the sites involved. It may include topical and oral steroids, dressings for denuded areas, antibiotics and immunosuppressants in more severe cases or those resistant to standard therapy.

CASE 17

A: Oral doxycycline

This lady presents with an asymptomatic, enlarging, annular patch on her posterior thigh several weeks following a hiking trip in an area endemic for Lyme disease. The rash is classical of erythema migrans and, along with the history given, should alert physicians to consider the diagnosis. The most appropriate management option is a 2-week course of oral doxycycline. Before this, serum should be sent for antibody testing for *Borrelia*.

Learning point

Lyme disease is the most common type of tick-borne disease in Europe and North America, and is caused by transmission of the spirochaetes of *Borrelia burgdorferi* from a tick bite. In Europe the main vector is *Ixodes ricinus*. The incubation period from bite to appearance of the rash is days to weeks. Often patients do not recall a tick bite, and so it is important to consider the diagnosis in returning travellers. Lyme disease may be associated with systemic symptoms including malaise, arthralgia and headache. Left untreated, it can lead to musculoskeletal, cardiac and nervous system complications.

Topical steroids would be appropriate treatment for either erythema annulare centrifugum (EAC) or granuloma annulare (GA). EAC is the main differential diagnosis in this case. It is classified as a figurate or gyrate erythema, the pathophysiology of which is unknown but thought to be a hypersensitivity reaction to various agents including infections, eg bacterial and fungal. It is characterised by a gradually enlarging papule over a period of weeks with a classic trailing scaly edge. There is no raised edge or trailing scale in this case.

Granuloma annulare usually consists of small, grouped, firm papules in an annular configuration, most often localised to the extremities. The lack of papules and the location makes this differential less likely here. A fixed drug eruption may be excluded in this case as the patient is not on any regular medication, and tinea corporis can be excluded as there is no evidence of any scaling of the rash. Urticaria is the final differential, which is characterised by the abrupt onset of itchy hives as well as fluctuation in lesions over days to weeks. Oral antihistamines would be an appropriate treatment.

CASE 18

A: Granuloma annulare

The history of gradually enlarging, asymptomatic, non-scaly papules on the dorsal aspect of the hands is very typical of granuloma annulare.

> ### Learning point
>
> Granuloma annulare is a very common benign condition characterised by the appearance of dermal papules and plaques, which are skin-coloured to erythematous in colour. Although the precise pathogenesis is unknown, the condition is thought to be a delayed hypersensitivity reaction to some component of the dermis resulting in palisading granulomatous inflammation. It is generally asymptomatic, but may occasionally be itchy. The patches usually disappear within months to years, but may recur. Granuloma annulare has been associated with type 1 diabetes, particularly if it is widespread.

The differential diagnosis includes other annular eruptions, particularly erythema annulare centrifugum (if on the trunk and limbs) and erythema elevatum dilutinum (a rare cause of vasculitis leading to the appearance of nodules and plaques on the extensor surfaces and sparing the trunk), neither of which is an option in this scenario. Although tinea manuum causes an annular rash, it is typically scaly and more superficial, and there is often evidence of tinea affecting other areas such as the nails. Viral warts are discrete lesions, often present on the hands, which typically have a warty or verrucous surface with tiny black dots on the surface corresponding to thrombosed capillaries.

Knuckle pads are benign, smooth, firm, skin-coloured papules, nodules or plaque-like lesions located over the interphalangeal joints. A history of repetitive trauma due to occupation or sports may be illicited. Tuberous xanthoma present as asymptomatic red–yellow nodules, which may coalesce, often affecting extensor surfaces or pressure areas, such as the knees. They are associated with hypercholesterolaemia, and can be familial, eg familial dysbetalipoproteinaemia and familial hypercholesterolaemia, or secondary to eg hypothyroidism. The latter differential diagnosis can be excluded by the lack of yellow discoloration on examination.

If there is any diagnostic doubt, a skin biopsy should always be performed, as each of these conditions has characteristic histopathological appearances.

CASE 19

D: Obesity

This teenager presents with a rash consistent with acanthosis nigricans (AN) (thickened hyperpigmented velvety patches that most often occur in skin folds, eg axilla, neck and groin). AN can be a normal variant (most common in patients with dark skin, particularly those of African American descent), or it can be inherited in an autosomal dominant fashion. Other associations include malignancy and endocrine disorders (Table 2.3).

+ Obesity
+ Genetic (autosomal dominant)
+ Normal variant (dark-skinned individuals)
+ Polycystic ovarian syndrome
+ Acromegaly
+ Insulin-resistant diabetes
+ Androgen-secreting tumours
+ Malignancy – particularly tumours of the gut and lung

Table 2.3: Causes of acanthosis nigricans

In this case, a diagnosis of Cushing syndrome is unlikely as the patient is asymptomatic. Similarly, there is no family history of note, which goes against familial AN (usually autosomal dominant inheritance). Paraneoplastic AN usually is of rapid onset, and is associated with mucosal and palmo-plantar velvety plaques. It is suggested by the rapid onset of the condition in a non-obese patient, and may precede or follow the diagnosis of cancer. Its appearance may also signify a relapse in patients with a prior history of cancer. This patient is obese with a BMI of 32 kg/m^2, so the most likely diagnosis is obesity-related AN. Dietary and exercise advice should be given, aimed at weight reduction.

CASE 20

B: Peutz–Jeghers syndrome

The description of the pigmented, non-blanching, melanocytic macules on the mouth, gums and buccal mucosa is typical of those described in Peutz–Jeghers syndrome (PJS). The main differential from the list given is Laugier–Hunziker syndrome, a sporadic condition in which middle-aged patients present with discrete, hyperpigmented macules on the lips and buccal mucosa, with associated longitudinal hyperpigmentation of the nails. It is not associated with systemic manifestations and is usually a diagnosis of exclusion. In this case, given the family history of similar melanocytic macules and intussusseption in an uncle, the diagnosis is most likely PJS. This is an autosomal dominant condition, most often caused by a germline mutation of the *STK11/LKB1* tumour suppressor gene on chromosome 19.

CHAPTER 2
ANSWERS

Learning point

In addition to the distinctive pigmented macules (which may also be found around the eyes, nostrils, fingers, palms and soles, and in the intestinal mucosa) patients may have gastrointestinal tract polyps (typically hamartomas). The pigmented macules tend to develop by the age of five years and often fade by puberty; however, buccal mucosa lesions may be more persistent. During the first three decades, intussusception (in up to 50% of patients), anaemia, rectal bleeding and obstruction are common complications. Patients with PJS have a 15-fold increased risk of developing intestinal cancer compared with the general population, as well as an increased risk of extra-intestinal malignancy, particularly gynaecologic cancers in women.

Addison's disease is unlikely as the patient is asymptomatic and the pigmentation in this condition is usually generalised with increasing pigment in areas of pressure and friction, eg palms, soles and flexural areas. Hereditary haemorrhagic telangiectasia (HHT) (or Osler–Rendu–Weber syndrome) is another autosomal dominant disorder where the most common presenting symptom is epistaxis. The onset of telangiectasia on the skin and mucous membranes tends to occur in the second decade. HHT has been classified into four types; however HHT1; are the most common types caused by endoglin mutations, and HHT2 caused by activin receptor-like kinase type 1 genes, found on chromosomes 9 and 12, respectively. The upper body is most commonly affected, eg face, mouth, nostrils, lips, ears, forearms, hands and fingers. The cutaneous telangiectasia should prompt an examination for telangiectasia in the gastrointestinal system and evidence of vascular abnormalities, particularly arteriovenous malformations in other organs.

continued

Carney complex is an autosomal dominant, inherited, multiple endocrine neoplasia syndrome characterised by spotty skin pigmentation (lentiginosis), cardiac and peripheral myxomas, schwannomas, and endocrine overactivity caused by an inactivating mutation of the tumour suppressor gene *PRKAR1A* on chromosome 17. The most common cutaneous features of Carney complex include lentigines, café-au-lait spots, freckling and blue naevi. The endocrine tumours associated with Carney complex include primary pigmented nodular adrenal cortical disease, growth-hormone-secreting pituitary adenomas, large-cell calcifying Sertoli cell tumours, Leydig cell tumours and thyroid neoplasms. Historically, cardiac myxomas have been reported to be responsible for more than 25% of the disease-specific mortality among patients with this condition.

CASE 21

E: 90% chance of complete resolution within near future

The rash described is typical of the initial phase of erythema nodosum. Erythema nodosum is a form of septal panniculitis that presents acutely in this manner with tender subcutaneous swellings on the lower legs. The lesions usually fade in one or two weeks to blue-purplish in colour, and eventually to a yellow colour reminiscent of a fading bruise. They can persist for up to six weeks. In this case, the history of synovitis affecting the ankles and wrists, hilar lymphadenopathy, fever and erythema nodosum is very suggestive of acute sarcoidosis or Löfgren syndrome. This presentation has an excellent prognosis, with complete resolution within several months in most patients. 90% of patients having a complete resolution within two years. There is a small risk of systemic disease including chronic lung disease.

Learning point

Erythema nodosum may be a manifestation of several diseases including tuberculosis, inflammatory bowel disease and streptococcal infection. Other causes include:

+ pregnancy
+ drugs, eg oral contraceptive pill, sulfonamides, penicillins
+ inflammatory bowel disease (most strongly associated with Crohn's disease)
+ Hodgkin's disease and lymphoma
+ sarcoidosis
+ Behçet's disease
+ infections:
    ◇ bacterial, eg streptococcal, tuberculosis, *Yersinia enterocolitica*, *Mycoplasma pneumoniae*, *Campylobacter*, *Salmonella*
    ◇ fungal, eg coccidioidomycosis, blastomycosis, histoplasmosis.

CASE 22

A: Phenytoin

The patient is suffering from toxic epidermal necrolysis (TEN), a potentially life-threatening dermatological emergency most often attributed to drug reactions.

Learning point

In TEN, there is full thickness epidermal necrosis due to widespread keratinocyte death leading to large areas of skin loss. There is often a prodromal illness consisting of fever and coryzal symptoms, with significant mucous membrane and eye involvement. There is a high mortality of up to 40%, with long-term morbidity among survivors – particularly ocular complications. Common causes include anticonvulsants, sulfonamides, non-steroidal anti-inflammatory drugs, beta-lactam antibiotics and allopurinol.

Stevens–Johnson syndrome (SJS) and TEN are thought to be on the spectrum of the same disorder. The main differences include the extent of skin and mucous membrane involvement. There is disagreement as to whether erythema multiforme is part of the SJS/TEN spectrum. In up to 50% of cases, SJS is idiopathic; however it may be caused by drug reactions, viral infections or malignancy. The rash is similar to that of erythema multiforme but with mucous membrane involvement. Treatment for both SJS and TEN is supportive; however, some dermatologists advocate intravenous immunoglobulins. Paracetamol and codeine may be used as analgesics for patients with TEN and deep venous thrombosis prophylaxis is very important in these patients, who are often immobile. The oral contraceptive pill is not associated with the development of TEN.

CASE 23

B: Urinary collection for 5-hydroxyindoleacetic acid (5-HIAA)

The constellation of clinical symptoms and signs including facial flushing, telangiectasia, weight loss and diarrhoea, and the associated findings of a palpable, craggy liver edge and cardiac murmur, are highly suggestive of carcinoid syndrome. Carcinoid tumours are neuroendocrine tumours that can metastasise. The symptoms and signs described above usually signify the presence of metastases as the vasoactive amines produced by the carcinoid tumour are not broken down by the liver and hence circulate via the hepatic veins into the systemic bloodstream causing symptoms. One hormone commonly implicated is serotonin, which is broken down into 5-hydroxyindoleacetic acid (5-HIAA) and excreted in urine. Hence, the investigation of choice in this case is a 24-hour urine collection for 5-HIAA.

Learning point

The main cutaneous feature in carcinoid syndrome is flushing, which occurs in up to 90% of cases. This can last for minutes to hours and lead to persistent skin changes including telangiectasia and plethora. Other causes of facial flushing include:

- ✦ physiological
- ✦ rosacea
- ✦ phaeochromocytoma
- ✦ hyperthyroidism
- ✦ systemic mastocytosis
- ✦ autonomic dysfunction
- ✦ neoplasms
- ✦ drugs, eg alcohol, calcium channel blockers, opioids, nitrates.

The measurement of metanephrines is useful in the diagnosis of phaeochromocytoma, which is suggested by episodic palpitations associated with headaches, sweating and severe hypertension. Phaeochromocytoma and hyperthyroidism do not cause persistent erythema or telangiectasia in the distribution of the flushing. Therefore, an MRI scan of the adrenal glands, measurement of serum and urinary metanephrines and testing of thyroid function would not be the next most appropriate investigation.

References

1. National Institutes of Health Consensus Development Conference Statement: Neurofibromatosis Arch Neurol Chicago. 1988. 45, 575–578

2. Northern Ireland Cancer Network (NICaN). 2007. Northern Ireland Referral Guidance for Suspected Cancer. www.cancerni.net/files/file/ReferralGuidanceMay2007.pdf

CHAPTER 3

Endocrinology and Metabolic Medicine

Paul McMullan

CASE 1

A 32-year-old woman is referred by her GP with a 3-month history of weight loss, heat intolerance, anxiety and tremor. She does not have a sore throat or fever. Her past medical history is otherwise unremarkable. Her eyes at times are dry and gritty but she reports no double vision. Her menstrual cycle has been irregular recently, but had previously been normal. She has two young children aged two and four. She does not take any exogenous iodine and is on no medications. On examination she has a moderate smooth goitre and moderate exopthalamos (see Figure 3.1). But no conjunctival injection or diplopia.

Blood tests reveal: Free thyroxine 36 pmol/litre, TSH < 0.01 mU/litre.

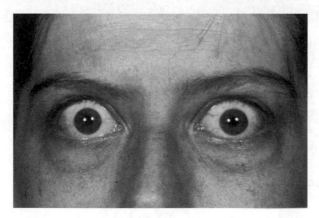

Figure 3.1

Which of the following would be the most appropriate treatment option?

- A. **Steroids**
- B. **Radioiodine therapy**
- C. **Observation**
- D. **Surgery**
- E. **Antithyroid medication eg carbimazole**

CASE 2

A 30-year-old lady presents to outpatients with nine months of gradual weight gain, lethargy and muscle weakness. Prior to this she had been well before this but was on sertraline 50 mg once daily. On further questioning her menstrual cycle was regular up until six months ago, but is now irregular. She bruises easily. On examination, blood pressure is 147/104 mmHg and abdominal striae are noted.

Investigations reveal: Urinary volume 1212 ml, Urine cortisol 260 nmol/24 h (< 210), Cortisol/creatinine ratio 35 (< 20).

Which of the following would be most appropriate to confirm the diagnosis?

A. **Androgen profile**
B. **High-dose dexamethasone suppression test**
C. **Random cortisol**
D. **CT scan of abdomen**
E. **Low-dose dexamethasone suppression test**

CASE 3

A middle-aged man is brought to the emergency department in a drowsy state. He had a witnessed seizure in the street, and an ambulance was called by a member of the public. On your initial assessment, you note the following: airway patent, respiratory rate 24 breaths/min, oxygen saturations 98% on a mask with oxygen reservoir bag, pulse rate 118 bpm and blood pressure 112/76 mmHg. The ambulance crew inform you that his seizure had stopped before their arrival and required no therapy. The Glasgow Coma Scale is 10/15 (E2 M5 V3). His capillary blood glucose is 5.8 mmol/litre. He is managed in the recovery position and kept in the emergency department for observation.

Blood tests reveal: Sodium 108 mmol/litre, Potassium 3.5 mmol/litre, Chloride 78 mmol/litre, Urea 5.7 mmol/litre, Creatinine 60 μmol/litre.

You are called back to the emergency department as he is having a further seizure. The seizure is of short duration, lasting two minutes. Which of the following is the most appropriate next stage in the patient's management?

A. **Administer chlordiazepoxide**
B. **Administer glucose**
C. **Administer hypertonic saline**
D. **Administer 0.9% saline**
E. **Arrange an urgent CT scan of brain**

CASE 4

A 26-year-old man is referred from the fertility clinic with oligospermia and hypogonadism. He and his wife have been trying for a child for over two years. He has had tiredness for many years but otherwise considers himself fit and well. He shaves every other day and has poor libido, but he feels erectile function including ejaculation is normal. On examination his left testis was small (6 ml), and the right was impalpable. He is tall and you note his appearance, as shown in Figure 3.2.

Biochemical testing revealed the following: Testosterone 4 nmol/litre, FSH 40 U/litre, LH 50 U/litre, Prolactin 300 mU/litre.

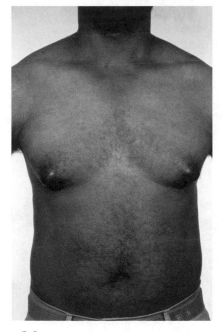

Figure 3.2

Which of the following is the most likely diagnosis?

   A. **Klinefelter's syndrome**
   B. **Kalmann syndrome**
   C. **Prader–Willi syndrome**
   D. **Lawrence–Moon–Biedel syndrome**
   E. **Exogenous steroid use**

CASE 5

A 57-year-old lady attends the rheumatology clinic for follow-up of inflammatory arthritis. Tests carried out show an elevated calcium level of 2.71 mmol/litre. She does not complain of any polyuria or polydipsia and she has no history of renal calculi. There is no family history of elevated calcium levels or renal calculi. Apart from the arthritis, which is controlled by methotrexate, her medical history includes hypertension and depression which is controlled on lisinopril, bendroflumethiazide and amlodipine. On examination she has no neck swellings and blood pressure is 114/56 mmHg.

Blood tests reveal: Sodium 135 mmol/litre, Potassium 4.0 mmol/litre, Urea 3.5 mmol/litre, Creatinine 70 μmol/litre, Calcium 2.71 mmol/litre, Adjusted calcium 2.68 mmol/litre, Phosphate 0.95 mmol/litre, ALP 58 U/litre.

Which of her medications is most likely contributing to the hypercalcaemia?

A. Methotrexate
B. Amlodipine
C. Lisinopril
D. Bendroflumethiazide
E. Fluoxetine

CASE 6

A 36-year-old gentleman is referred to clinic with hypertension. 24-hour ambulatory blood pressure monitoring carried out by his GP confirmed a high blood pressure with an average reading of 160/105 mmHg and he was commenced on amlodipine, lisinopril and atenolol. He consumes approximately ten units of alcohol per week and has cut down on salt intake. His blood pressure at clinic is 147/95 mmHg. You decide to screen him for secondary causes of hypertension.

Which of the following would not be considered an indication for testing for hyperaldosteronism?

A. Hypertension with hyperkalaemia
B. Resistant hypertension (taking three or more antihypertensive medications with poor blood pressure control)
C. Onset of hypertension at a young age (< 40 years)
D. Hypertension with a known adrenal mass
E. Severe hypertension (systolic > 160 mmHg, diastolic > 100 mmHg)

CASE 7

A 32-year-old lady who is currently 28 weeks' gestation is found to have an elevated random blood glucose level of 7.8 mmol/litre. This is her second pregnancy. She informs you that her boy in the previous pregnancy weighed 4.0 kg at birth but she was not diagnosed as having gestational diabetes. She has no other medical history but her father has type 2 diabetes. Her body mass index is 29 kg/m². An oral glucose tolerance resulted in the following glucose concentrations: 0 min, 5.4 mmol/litre; 120 min, 8.5 mmol/litre.

Which of the following is not considered an indication for screening for gestational diabetes?

    A. **Family origin from India**
    B. **Previous gestational diabetes**
    C. **Previous baby weighing 4 kg**
    D. **First degree relative with diabetes**
    E. **BMI > 30 kg/m²**

CASE 8

A 69-year-old is referred with an adrenal lesion. She had a total knee replacement recently carried out and while in hospital a CT pulmonary angiogram was done to investigate breathlessness. A left gland adrenal lesion was seen on the scan measuring 3.2 × 2.3 cm with a reported attenuation value of 6 Hounsfield units. She reports that she had been well before her surgery apart from joint pains. She has no headaches, palpitations, sweating or anxiety episodes. On examination there are no striae, and no proximal myopathy or evidence of bruising. Blood pressure was 124/78 mmHg.

Biochemical testing reveals: Sodium 138 mmol/litre, Potassium 4.4 mmol/litre, Urea 3.8 mmol/litre, Creatinine 66 μmol/litre, 24-h urinary catecholamines normal, 24-h urinary cortisol normal, Overnight dexamethasone suppression test normal (< 50 nmol/l).

Which of the following is the most appropriate follow-up for her?

    A. **Discharge**
    B. **Refer for surgery**
    C. **Commence on alpha blockade**
    D. **Commence on mitotane**
    E. **Repeat scan in three to six months**

CASE 9

A 49-year-old lady presents with nausea, polyuria, thirst and constipation. Her past medical history includes hypertension and depression managed on amlodipine and sertraline. She has no history of renal calculi. Her GP had sent some blood tests and advised her to attend the emergency department. Her blood pressure is mildly elevated but otherwise her examination was unremarkable.

Investigations reveal: Sodium 149 mmol/litre, Potassium 4.0 mmol/litre, Urea 8.2 mmol/litre, Creatinine 105 µmol/litre, Corrected calcium 3.5 mmol/litre, Alkaline phosphatise 130 U/litre, Plasma parathyroid hormone 17 pmol/litre.

Which of the following is the most appropriate initial therapy?

A. **Furosemide**
B. **Intravenous normal saline**
C. **Bisphosphonate therapy**
D. **Calcitionin**
E. **Cinacalcet**

CASE 10

A 30-year-old woman with type 1 diabetes presents to the emergency department. She had been drinking alcohol over the weekend and had started to vomit. As she was not eating she omitted her insulin therapy. Her airway is patent, respiratory rate is 28 breaths/min, oxygen saturations 95% breathing room air, pulse rate 120 bpm, blood pressure 104/72 mmHg.

Blood tests reveal: pH 7.24, Glucose 24 mmol/litre, Bicarbonate 16 mmol/litre, Sodium 134 mmol/litre, Potassium 4.4 mmol/litre.

She is initially treated with intravenous saline, potassium and insulin.

Six hours after commencement of the protocol, her results are as follows: Sodium 134 mmol/litre, Potassium 5.0 mmol/litre, Glucose 11 mmol/litre, Capillary ketones 3 mmol/litre, pH 7.28.

Which of the following treatment combinations is the most appropriate next step?

A. **10% dextrose/insulin/saline/potassium**
B. **Saline/potassium/insulin**
C. **Stop infusions and commence on subcutaneous insulin**
D. **10% dextrose/insulin/saline with no potassium**
E. **Saline with potassium only**

CASE 11

A 72-year-old man is referred by his cardiologist. He had a myocardial infarction ten years ago. He subsequently developed ventricular fibrillation from which he was successfully resuscitated. An implantable cardiac defibrillator was subsequently inserted. He is also maintained on amiodarone owing to the failure of alternative anti-arrhythmic drugs. Thyroid function tests had remained satisfactory until his last clinic visit when his free thyroxine level was noted to be 25 pmol/litre and TSH < 0.01 mU/litre. He does not have any palpitations, but the resting heart rate is elevated at 100 bpm. He is otherwise symptomatically euthyroid. Antithyroid peroxidase levels are normal and there is no uptake on a thyroid uptake scan.

Which of the following would be the preferred treatment option?

A. **Stop amiodarone**
B. **Steroid therapy**
C. **Antithyroid medication**
D. **Radioiodine therapy**
E. **Surgery**

CASE 12

A 27-year-old lady presents to the clinic stating she has not had a period in over eight months, since stopping the oral contraceptive pill (OCP). She has never been pregnant but is keen to start a family. Before the OCP she had regular menstrual cycles with menarche at the age of 12. She has no significant medical history, is on no regular medications and takes regular exercise. She reports no headaches. She has a body mass index of 18 kg/m² and has normal secondary sexual characteristics.

Biochemical tests reveal: Oestradiol< 50 pmol/litre, FSH 5.3 U/litre, LH 0.4 U/litre, Progesterone 1.9 nmol/litre, Prolactin 53 mU/litre, TSH 1.13 mU/litre, Free androgen index 0.5.

Which of the following is the most likely diagnosis?

A. **Polycystic ovarian syndrome**
B. **Prolactinoma**
C. **Hypothalamic amenorrhoea**
D. **Turner syndrome**
E. **Premature ovarian failure**

CASE 13

A 47-year-old gentleman presents to outpatients with palpitations and high blood pressure. Subsequent cardiology evaluation led to a diagnosis of mitral valve disease. He has known type 2 diabetes and is currently on metformin. During his consultation the appearance of his hands was noted to be as shown in Figure 3.3.

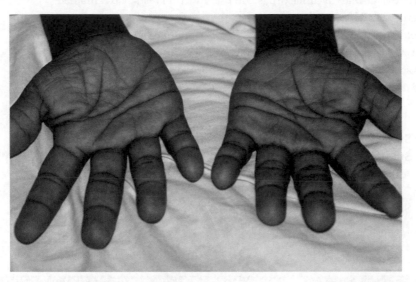

Figure 3.3

Which of the following biochemical tests would be most useful to confirm the most likely diagnosis?

    A. IGF1 level

    B. Random growth hormone level

    C. Oral glucose tolerance test

    D. Prolactin level

    E. MRI scan of the pituitary gland

CASE 14

A 15½-year-old boy attends clinic with his mother. They are concerned that his growth and development is behind other boys at school. His height is 165.5 cm (below 25th centile) and weight 80 kg (above 95th centile). His voice has not broken and he has no hair growth on his face. He admits that this has affected his mental health and his mother feels that his school work has declined. His father is 178 cm tall and his mother 168 cm, and there has been no delayed puberty in his three older siblings. On examination, his testes measure 6 ml and Tanner score is two. He does not have proximal myopathy, striae or easy bruising. He has no headaches, and visual fields are full to confrontation.

Biochemical testing reveals: Testosterone 0.6 nmol/litre, FSH 3.7 mU/litre, LH 1.0 U/litre, Prolactin 203 mU/litre.

Which of the following would be helpful in determining the most likely cause?

A. **X-ray of left hand and wrist**
B. **MRI scan of pituitary**
C. **Ultrasound scan of testes**
D. **Karyotyping**
E. **Vitamin B12 and folate levels**

CASE 15

A 53-year-old lady presents with a right thyroid swelling. She has no cold/heat intolerance or palpitations. On examination, she has a smooth nodule on the right side of her thyroid gland measuring approximately 1.0 × 1.5 cm. There is no lymphadenopathy. Subsequent fine needle biopsy reveals a medullary thyroid carcinoma. She is fit and well but does have a family history of heart disease. Her sister was also diagnosed with medullary thyroid carcinoma and her younger brother suffered sudden death at the age of 35 years.

Investigations reveal: Free thyroxine 15 pmol/litre, TSH 1.8 mU/litre, Calcium 2.5 mmol/litre.

Before surgical consideration what is the most appropriate step?

A. **Genetic testing**
B. **24-hour urine collection for catecholamines**
C. **Parathyroid hormone level**
D. **Radioiodine therapy**
E. **External beam radiation**

CASE 16

You are asked to see a 32-year-old lady on the ENT ward. She underwent a parathyroid gland excision two days ago and has developed tingling and paraesthesiae around her mouth. Chvostek's and Trousseau's signs are positive.

Investigations reveal: Haemoglobin 120 g/litre, White cells 6×10^9/litre, Platelets 300×10^9/litre, Sodium 142 mmol/litre, Potassium 4.2 mmol/litre, Urea 4.8 mmol/litre, Creatinine 85 μmol/litre, Corrected calcium 1.50 mmol/litre.

Following intravenous calcium therapy what is the most appropriate additional therapy?

- A. **Bisphosphonates**
- B. **Phosphate supplementation**
- C. **Intravenous fluids**
- D. **Vitamin D**
- E. **Magnesium supplementation**

CASE 17

A 52-year-old gentleman is brought to the emergency department with a 4-day history of headache. This started suddenly in the occipital area and gradually increased in severity. On arrival his airway is patent, respiratory rate is 24 breaths/min, blood pressure is 90/60 mmHg, remaining low despite two litres of intravenous crystalloid. He is drowsy with a Glasgow Coma Scale of 13/15 (E3 M6 V4). There are no other neurological features and visual fields appear intact. From his medical notes you see he has been under follow-up for a non-functioning pituitary adenoma.

Blood tests reveal: Sodium 132 mmol/litre, Potassium 5.6 mmol/litre, Urea 5.4 mmol/litre, Creatinine 56 μmol/litre, Glucose 3.5 mmol/litre, Free thyroxine 8.8 pmol/litre, TSH 0.8 mU/litre.

Which of the following is the most appropriate next stage in the patient's management?

- A. **Corticosteroid administration**
- B. **Thyroxine administration**
- C. **Urgent pituitary surgery**
- D. **MRI scan of brain**
- E. **Full pituitary hormone profile**

CASE 18

A 24-year-old lady is referred to clinic with secondary amenorrhoea. She had a normal menarche at the age of 12 years, and her periods were regular until three years ago. She has hirsutism which she tells you has been of gradual onset over the last year but has not required any treatment to date. On examination she is overweight with a BMI of 29 kg/m². On examination she has the appearance shown in Figure 3.4.

Biochemical testing reveals: Oestradiol 214 pmol/litre, LH 6.2 U/litre, FSH 3.5 U/litre, Sex hormone binding globulin 12 nmol/litre, Prolactin 238 mU/litre, Testosterone 1.8 nmol/litre, Dehydroepiandrosterone sulfate 8.1 μmol/litre, Free androgen index 15.0, 17-OH progesterone 3.7 nmol/litre.

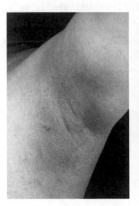 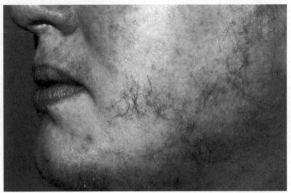

Figure 3.4

What is the most likely diagnosis?

    A. **Prolactinoma**
    B. **Premature ovarian failure**
    C. **Congenital adrenal hyperplasia**
    D. **Polycystic ovarian syndrome**
    E. **Androgen-producing ovarian tumour**

CASE 19

A 45-year-old lady is referred following the incidental finding of a left adrenal adenoma that was detected during the investigation of lower back pain. On further questioning she appears to have had palpitations, sweating, flushing and anxiety for over two years, and these symptoms have progressively got worse. Her past medical history includes psoriasis, coeliac disease and diverticulitis. On examination her blood pressure is 150/85 mmHg and pulse rate 110 bpm.

Investigations reveal:

- ✦ 24-hour urinary catecholamines: volume 1790 ml; noradrenaline 3224 nmol/24 hours; adrenaline 50 nmol/24 hours; dopamine 2782 nmol/24 hours.

- ✦ 24-hour urinary cortisol: volume 1590 ml; urinary free cortisol 125 nmol/24 hours.

- ✦ CT scan of adrenals: the left-sided adrenal lesion measures 4 cm (Hounsfield units 60).

Which of the following would be the most suitable for the management of her high blood pressure?

A. **Diltiazem**
B. **Phenoxybenzamine**
C. **Lisinopril**
D. **Labetolol**
E. **Atenolol**

CASE 20

A 24-year-old lady with known hypothyroidism contacts the ward. She has been on thyroxine since the age of 14 years, and stable on a daily dose of 100 μg. She is now pregnant and currently eight weeks' gestation. She remembered that during her last pregnancy she had her thyroxine adjusted and asks whether this is required. She assures you that she is compliant with her thyroxine.

Thyroid function tests are as follows: Free thyroxine 14.0 pmol/litre, TSH 4.2 mU/litre.

Which of the following is appropriate?

A. **Continue on current dose**
B. **Increase thyroxine dose**
C. **Decrease thyroxine dose**
D. **Switch to triiodothyronine (T$_3$) therapy**
E. **Daily administration of thyroxine under supervision**

CASE 21

A 17-year-old girl presents to clinic. She has had type 1 diabetes for nine years, but control has been somewhat suboptimal over the last two to three years with her haemoglobin A_{1c} ranging from 76 to 91 mmol/mol. She was switched from twice daily analogue insulin to a basal bolus regimen two years ago. She has at least two hypoglycaemic episodes per week, and has had one third-party-assisted hypoglycaemic episode in the last six months. She does not smoke or drink alcohol. She is worried about her diabetes affecting her school work, and is keen to discuss treatment options. Her current insulin regimen comprises: aspart insulin 7 units with breakfast and lunch, 9 units with dinner and glargine 14 units at 10pm.

Investigations reveal: Haemoglobin A_{1c} 69 mmol/mol, Free thyroxine 14.6 pmol/litre, TSH 2.0 mU/litre; Coeliac screen: normal.

Which of the following is the most appropriate next step in management?

A. **Switch glargine to twice daily isophane insulin**
B. **Structured education, eg carbohydrate counting**
C. **Insulin pump therapy**
D. **Refer for islet transplantation**
E. **Continuous glucose monitoring system**

CASE 22

A 53-year-old gentleman presents with erectile dysfunction. This has been a problem for around a year, and he has had both difficulty achieving and sustaining erections. He shaves on alternate days, and this has not changed in frequency. He is not aware of any change in body hair. Energy levels are reasonable, but he does admit to poor mood. He has a background of type 2 diabetes diagnosed 15 years ago. This was initially treated with dietary modification, but he is now on metformin. He had a myocardial infarction five years ago and also suffers from hypertension. He is a non-smoker and drinks approximately 12 units of alcohol per week. On examination, he is obese with a body mass index of 38 kg/m^2. His blood pressure is 148/86 mmHg. He has no proximal muscle weakness or evidence of bruising. His testes are approximately 20 ml in volume. Cardiovascular, respiratory and abdominal examinations are otherwise unremarkable.

Blood testing reveals: Haemoglobin 144 g/litre, White cells 7.0 × 10^9/litre, Platelets 230 × 10^9/litre, Sodium 145 mmol/litre, Potassium 4.4 mmol/litre, Testosterone 9.0 nmol/litre, LH 3.0 U/litre, FSH 2.7 U/litre.

Which of the following is the most appropriate test to perform next?

A. **Sex hormone binding globulin**
B. **MRI scan of pituitary**
C. **Ultrasound scan of testes**
D. **Ferritin**
E. **Repeat early morning testosterone**

CASE 23

A 28-year-old woman is brought to the emergency department with acute abdominal pain. She is taken to theatre and undergoes an appendicectomy. Post-operatively she remains well. Histology reveals a 25 × 15 × 9 mm carcinoid tumour with serosal invasion. At review, she reports no flushing or diarrhoea, and a repeat CT scan of abdomen is otherwise unremarkable. She is otherwise fit and well.

Post-operative investigations reveal: Chromogranin A = 11 U/litre, Neurokinin A = 9 ng/litre, 24 hour 5-HIAA urinary collection: volume 1670 ml, 5-HIAA output 12.4 μmol/24 hours (10–47).

Which of the following is the most appropriate next step in her management?

A. **Reassure and discharge**
B. **Repeat the scan in three to six months**
C. **Discuss right hemicolectomy**
D. **Commence on sandostatin analogue**
E. **Refer for chemotherapy**

CASE 24

A 24-year-old lady presents to outpatients with galactorrhoea. This started after a miscarriage two years ago. After this, her menstrual cycle became irregular, occurring approximately every four to eight weeks, but over the last 12 weeks she has not had any periods. She reports an occasional headache but no visual disturbance. She takes no regular medications. On further questioning, she is planning a further pregnancy.

Biochemical testing reveals: Oestradiol 63 pmol/litre, FSH 1.2 U/litre, LH < 0.2 U/litre, Prolactin 1642 mU/litre, TSH 1.2 mU/litre.

An MRI scan of the pituitary gland shows a 0.8 × 0.7 mm pituitary adenoma.

Which of the following would be the most appropriate therapy?

A. **Thyroxine**
B. **Oral contraceptive pill**
C. **Dopamine agonist (eg bromocriptine)**
D. **Clomifene citrate**
E. **In vitro fertilisation treatment**

CASE 25

A 38-year-old lady is referred to clinic following the detection of high serum calcium (2.83 mmol/litre) on blood tests carried out by her GP. These had been done as part of a health check for a new job. She has no thirst or polyuria. There is no history of renal calculi. She is not on any medications, and her only history is of an appendicectomy carried out 18 years ago. Her brother has also been found to have a high calcium level but has not had surgery. On examination, her blood pressure is 138/78 mmHg. There are no palpable neck masses. Cardiovascular, respiratory and abdominal examinations are unremarkable.

Biochemical testing reveals: Sodium 136 mmol/litre, Potassium 4.0 mmol/litre, Urea 4.0 mmol/litre, Creatinine 77 μmol/litre, Adjusted calcium 2.86 mmol/litre, Phosphate 0.83 mmol/litre, Urinary calcium 1 mmol/litre (normal 3–9 mmol/litre), Urinary calcium:creatinine ratio 0.0079, Parathyroid hormone 48 pmol/litre, TSH 2.1 mU/litre.

Which of the following is the most likely diagnosis?

A. Malignancy
B. Hyperthyroidism
C. Vitamin D intoxication
D. Familial hypocalciuric hypercalcaemia
E. Primary hyperparathyroidism

CASE 26

A 72-year-old lady is referred back to clinic for management of hypothyroidism. She was diagnosed over 20 years ago and had been stable until the last six months when, despite dose titration of levothyroxine to 250 µg daily, her TSH level remains elevated at 7 mU/litre. She feels more tired and her skin is dry with brittle hair. She had a stroke nine months ago and is currently on the following medications: aspirin 75 mg, ramipril 2.5 mg, amlodipine 10 mg, simvastatin 40 mg and omeprazole 40 mg daily. On examination, she has no palpable thyroid gland but does appear hypothyroid in appearance.

Blood tests reveal: Free thyroxine 22 pmol/litre, TSH 6 mU/litre.

Which of the following medications may interfere with the absorption of her thyroxine?

- A. **Aspirin**
- B. **Ramipril**
- C. **Amlopdine**
- D. **Simvastatin**
- E. **Omeprazole**

CASE 27

A 52-year-old gentleman with a history of type 2 diabetes for over 20 years attends for review. He was admitted three months ago with a myocardial infarction with subsequent mild congestive cardiac failure. Following this, he has been looking after himself better, attending a rehabilitation exercise scheme and maintaining a reasonable diet. His current medications include metformin 500 mg twice daily and gliclazide 160 mg twice daily. He is also on ramipril 5 mg, bisoprolol 10 mg, atorvastatin 40 mg and bumetanide 2 mg daily. He has developed mild renal impairment but renal function has remained stable over the last six months. He is an ex-smoker and consumes less than eight units of alcohol per week. His body mass index is 28 m/kg^2.

Investigations reveal: Haemoglobin A$_{1c}$ 74 mmol/mol, Urinary albumin:creatinine ratio 5, Cholesterol 3.7 mmol/litre, Low-density lipoprotein cholesterol 1.8 mmol/litre, High-density lipoprotein cholesterol 1.2 mmol/litre, Urea 5.7 mmol/litre, Creatinine 147 µmol/litre, eGFR 40 mL/min per 1.73 m^2.

Which of the following agents would be most suitable for improving glycaemic control in this patient?

    A. **Sodium/glucose co-transporter 2 inhibitor**

    B. **Glucagon-like peptide-1 agonist**

    C. **Insulin**

    D. **Acarbose**

    E. **Pioglitazone**

CASE 28

A 30-year-old gentleman is admitted to hospital with lethargy, weight loss, nausea, light-headedness and general aches and pains. He has coeliac disease but otherwise has no significant medical history. On examination, he has a dark complexion and postural hypotension.

Biochemical testing reveals: Sodium 125 mmol/litre, Potassium 5.4 mmol/litre, Chloride 86 mmol/litre, Glucose 3.3 mmol/litre, Bicarbonate 32 mmol/litre, Urea 9.9 mmol/litre, Creatinine 104 µmol/litre, Free thyroxine 13.7 pmol/litre, TSH 3.88 mU/litre.

Which test is likely to confirm the most likely diagnosis?

    A. **Short Synacthen® test**
    B. **Adrenal antibodies**
    C. **Random cortisol**
    D. **Urinary sodium and osmolality**
    E. **Thyroid function tests**

CASE 29

A 58-year-old gentleman is referred with bilateral gynaecomastia. This has developed gradually over the last six months and he is quite concerned about it. He has known hypertension and had a myocardial infarction with subsequent heart failure approximately ten years ago. He is a non-smoker and drinks approximately ten units of alcohol per week. He has two children aged seven and ten years. His libido and erectile function are normal. On examination, he is overweight with a BMI of 26.0 kg/m². Both breasts are enlarged, with rubbery glandular tissue palpable beneath the areolae measuring 2.5 cm on both sides.

Which of the following medications is most commonly associated with this condition?

    A. **Atenolol**
    B. **Spironolactone**
    C. **Furosemide**
    D. **Ramipril**
    E. **Bendroflumethiazide**

CASE 30

A 72-year-old lady presents to the acute medical ward with malaise. Her dietary intake has been limited, but she has been drinking plenty of fluid. She has a history of a meningioma with surgery carried out ten years ago. Following the surgery she developed hypopituitarism and is currently on hydrocortisone 15 mg 8 am with 5 mg at 5 pm, levothyroxine 100 µg daily and desmopressin two puffs twice daily (10 µg per puff). She has not missed any of her medications. On examination, she has a blood pressure of 120/77 mmHg and is euvolemic.

Initial tests are as follows: Sodium 124 mmol/litre, Potassium 3.8 mmol/litre, Glucose 4 mmol/litre, Urea 2.4 mmol/litre, Creatinine 77 µmol/litre, TSH 1.8 mU/litre

Which of the following should be the next most appropriate step?

A. **Give an intravenous dose of hydrocortisone**

B. **Reduce desmopressin dose**

C. **Intravenous saline**

D. **Increase dose of levothyroxine**

E. **Arrange an urgent CT scan of brain**

CASE 31

A 52-year-old gentleman is referred with a seizure in the setting of a recorded blood glucose concentration of 1.8 mmol/litre. He is treated with intravenous 10% glucose, but on cessation of this, he becomes symptomatic of hypoglycaemia and requires further intravenous glucose. On further questioning, he has been having episodes of syncope, sweating and feeling hungry over the last six months, relieved by taking Lucozade®. He informs you that three months ago he was investigated for a dry cough and was found to have a large right-sided lung mass measuring 19 × 12 cm. He is due to see the thoracic surgeons regarding this mass. His past medical history is otherwise unremarkable. On examination, he has multiple bruises on his limbs which he blames on a number of collapse episodes. His blood pressure is 120/68 mmHg and pulse rate 78 bpm. His body mass index is 20 kg/m².

Investigations reveal: Glucose 1.8 mmol/litre, Beta hydroxybutyrate 0.22 mmol/litre, Insulin < 3.0 mU/litre, C-peptide < 0.1 ug/litre, Cortisol level 30 minutes following Synacthen® 885 nmol/litre.

What is the likely diagnosis?

- A. **Insulinoma**
- B. **Factitious hypoglycaemia due to insulin therapy**
- C. **Factitious hypoglycaemia due to sulfonylurea treatment**
- D. **Non-islet cell tumour**
- E. **Glycogen storage disorder**

CASE 1

E: Antithyroid medication eg carbimazole

This is primary hyperthyroidism, most likely Graves' disease since there is eye involvement. First-line management is generally antithyroid medication either as a dose titration or a 'block and replace' regimen. Steroids, although not currently indicated in this case, may be used in thyroid storm, active thyroid eye disease and in cases of thyroiditis.

Radioiodine therapy may be considered as a first-line therapy, but in view of the potential eye involvement and two young children, it would not be the preferred option in this case. Observation may be adopted in cases of thyroiditis. However, it has been over a year since she was pregnant and there is no suggestion of thyroid tenderness, making this diagnosis less likely. Although surgery may be considered, it is not the preferred option for primary hyperthyroidism unless the goitre is significant in size causing compression, or for cosmetic reasons.

Learning point

Antithyroid drugs have common side effects including nausea, joint pains and rash. A rare (1 in 500 cases) but dangerous side effect causes severe reduction in white cell number (agranulocytosis). Patients starting these medications should be advised to watch out for signs of sore throat, unexplained fever or mouth ulcers, and if these develop to make an urgent appointment with their doctor to get their blood count checked.

CASE 2

E: Low-dose dexamethasone suppression test

The most likely diagnosis here is Cushing syndrome. Although exogenous steroid use remains the most frequent cause of this condition, it can also be caused by excess endogenous glucocorticoids secreted from a pituitary adenoma (Cushing's disease), adrenal adenoma, adrenal hyperplasia, ectopic secretion (eg small cell lung cancer) and adrenal carcinoma.

Although polycystic ovarian syndrome can present with similar symptoms, features that best discriminate Cushing syndrome (most do not have a high sensitivity):

- easy bruising
- facial plethora
- proximal myopathy (or proximal muscle weakness)
- striae (especially if reddish purple and > 1 cm wide)
- in children, weight gain with decreasing growth velocity)

Other associated features include hypertension, diabetes, depression, obesity, osteoporosis and menstrual irregularity.

High-dose dexamethasone testing is used for the localisation of cortisol secretion. It differentiates ACTH-dependent Cushing syndrome from ectopic secretion. Although this may well be carried out in due course, the first step to confirm the diagnosis is by a second screening test. As cortisol is secreted in a circadian rhythm, a random measurement will not be helpful. A CT scan of the abdomen may be considered if ACTH-independent Cushing syndrome is diagnosed.

CHAPTER 3
ANSWERS

Learning point

Suitable screening tests for Cushing syndrome include: urinary free cortisol (at least two samples, as levels are variable), a late-night salivary cortisol level, a 1 mg overnight dexamethasone suppression test and a low-dose dexamethasone suppression test (2 mg/d over 48 h). In a low-dose dexamethasone suppression test, a normal response is for cortisol levels to suppress to less than 50 nmol/litre. It is important to ensure that women have not been taking the oral contraceptive pill in the six weeks before testing as oestrogen increases cortisol binding globulin resulting in a high false positive rate (> 50%). For further reading, see reference.[1]

CASE 3

C: Administer hypertonic saline

This gentleman has likely had a seizure due to the profound hyponatraemia. Serum sodium levels are severely low. Other causes such as alcohol withdrawal, intracranial bleeding etc are also possible but the initial management should be to stabilise the patient with the treatment of his severe hyponatraemia before sending for a CT scan of the brain. Any use of hypertonic saline must be closely monitored, ideally in a high-dependency unit. Over-rapid correction can lead to central pontine myelinolysis and serum sodium levels need to be monitored after 20 min and at least every two to four hours. In first 24 hours there should be a rise of no more than 10 mmol/litre of serum sodium in 24 hours, and an additional 8 mmol/litre during every 24 hours thereafter until the serum concentration reaches 130 mmol/litre.

His glucose level is satisfactory and administration of glucose is not necessary. Repeat blood tests are required, but as he has symptomatic severe hyponatraemia the correct action would be to administer hypertonic saline.

CHAPTER 3
ANSWERS

Learning point

Classification of severe hyponatraemia[2]

Moderately severe

- ✦ nausea without vomiting
- ✦ confusion
- ✦ headache

Severe

- ✦ vomiting
- ✦ cardiorespiratory distress
- ✦ abnormal and deep somnolence
- ✦ coma (GCS < 8)

CASE 4

A: Klinefelter's syndrome

This is most likely Klinefelter's syndrome. This results from the failure of development of Leydig cells and seminiferous tubules and carries the karyotype XXY.

Learning point

This syndrome is the most common cause of primary hypogonadism occurring in approximately 1/1000 live births. Patients are typically tall, lacking secondary sexual characteristics and have gynaecomastia. They are often infertile, but most have normal erectile function and ejaculation. Semen may not contain spermatozoa.

Kalmann syndrome often presents with failure of puberty and is due to hypogonadotrophic hypogonadism (low FSH and LH). It is often associated with a lack of smell. Prader–Willi syndrome is a chromosomal disorder which presents with delayed puberty and is associated with hyperphagia and weight gain. Lawrence–Moon–Biedel syndrome is a rare autosomal recessive condition that is often associated with hypogonadism, retinitis pigmentosa, spastic paraplegia and extra digits. Exogenous steroid use generally causes hypogonadotrophic hypogonadism.

CHAPTER 3 ANSWERS

CASE 5

D: Bendroflumethiazide

This lady has asymptomatic hypercalcaemia. Thiazide diuretics can result in mild hypercalcaemia. They reduce calcium excretion in the urine and therefore increase calcium levels in the blood. If possible, they should be stopped in cases of hypercalcaemia and alternative antihypertensive therapy used if required.

Other medications associated with hypercalcaemia include: lithium (increases release of parathyroid hormone), calcium-containing antacids, and vitamin A or D intoxication.

CASE 6

A: Hypertension with hyperkalaemia

Conn syndrome (primary hyperaldosteronism) is due to inappropriate aldosterone production. This is non-suppressible by sodium loading. It results in suppressed renin levels, hypertension, sodium retention and potassium excretion with subsequent hypokalaemia (9–37% of patients). It is often caused by an adrenal adenoma, but can also be caused by adrenal hyperplasia and glucocorticoid remediable aldosteronism (GRA).

Learning point

Indications for case detection of primary aldosteronism:[3]

- ✦ hypertension with spontaneous hypokalaemia
- ✦ resistant hypertension (three or more antihypertensive therapies with poor blood pressure control)
- ✦ severe hypertension (systolic > 160 mmHg, diastolic > 100 mmHg)
- ✦ hypertension with adrenal mass
- ✦ onset of hypertension at a young age (< 40).

CASE 7

C: Previous baby weighing 4 kg

Gestational diabetes is glucose intolerance of any degree with the onset or first recognition in pregnancy. An estimated 85% pregnancies complicated by diabetes are due to gestational diabetes. The condition usually responds to changes in diet and exercise, but insulin or oral hypoglycaemic agents such as metformin may be needed if glucose remains uncontrolled.

Learning point

Risk factors for screening for gestational diabetes include:

+ a body mass index > 30 kg/m²
+ a previous macrosomic baby weighing 4.5 kg or above
+ previous gestational diabetes
+ minority ethnic family origin from a region with a high prevalence of diabetes (South Asian, Black Caribbean and Middle Eastern).

Nice Guidelines for diagnosis of gestational diabetes[4]

+ a fasting plasma glucose level of 5.6 mmol/l or above, or
+ a 2 hour plasma glucose level of 7.8 mmol/l or above.

This lady therefore would be classified as having gestational diabetes.

CASE 8

E: Repeat scan in three to six months

This is a case of a typical adrenal incidentaloma. This is the term used if an unsuspected adrenal lesion is detected on radiologic imaging. The prevalence is approximately 3.4–4.4%. A homogeneous adrenal mass with a smooth border and an attenuation value < 10 Hounsfield units on unenhanced CT is very likely to be benign.

The clinical features and biochemical testing are in keeping with a non-functioning adenoma, although 10–15% of adrenal incidentalomas secrete excess amounts of hormones necessitating functional testing. The structure of the gland should be reassessed after three to six months. If the adenoma remains stable on two imaging studies carried out at least six months apart and does not exhibit hormonal hypersecretion after four years, further follow-up may not be warranted.

Learning point

Indications for surgery include: evidence of a syndrome of hormonal excess attributable to the adrenal mass, biochemical evidence of a phaeochromocytoma, mass diameter > 4 cm on CT scanning, and an indeterminate or malignant lesion on imaging.

This lesion is not suspicious of a phaeochromocytoma and therefore alpha blockade is not warranted. Mitotane is a drug used in adrenocortical carcinoma. For further reading, see reference.[5]

CASE 9

B: Intravenous normal saline

This lady has severe hypercalcaemia and needs emergency treatment. Intravenous saline is the most appropriate initial therapy, 4–6 l in 24 hours . This not only corrects volume depletion but may enhance clearance of urinary calcium. Although intravenous fluids are unlikely to normalise calcium levels here, adequate hydration is required before initiation of other therapies. Furosemide may be used to increase calciuresis but only after adequate hydration, eg zoledronic acid 4 mg over 15 min. Large doses with aggressive hydration are often needed, necessitating close monitoring of all electrolytes. Bisphosphonate therapy may also be used, but only after adequate hydration. These agents inhibit calcium release by interfering with osteoclast-mediated bone resorption but they can take several days to reduce levels. Bisphosphonates are nephrotoxic and may cause further complications in a dehydrated patient. Calcitionin can be used for severe hypercalcaemia, but its effects are usually transient. It increases renal calcium excretion and decreases bone resorption. It is usually reserved if there has been a poor response to biophosphates.[6]

CASE 10

A: 10% dextrose/insulin/saline/potassium

Diabetic ketoacidosis is a medical emergency and needs high-level care. Specific initial therapies are fluids, insulin and potassium. In this case, the patient initially responded well, but glucose has now fallen below 12 mmol/litre and significant ketones still persist. A fixed-weight insulin infusion is continued until resolution of the ketosis, but without the addition of glucose, hypoglycaemia would be inevitable. Therefore, 10% glucose is required to be added to reverse ketosis and restore normal glucose/insulin metabolism.

Reducing or stopping intravenous insulin should be avoided until ketosis is resolved, unless following senior advice for the management of hypokalaemia.[7]

Learning point

Insulin moves extracellular potassium into the cells: hence serum potassium levels will fall. This is the reason for the inclusion of 40 mmol of potassiumin in every litre (except the initial litre) of intravenous fluid when the serum potassium level is between 3.5 and 5.5 mmol/litre.

CHAPTER 3 ANSWERS

CASE 11

B: Steroid therapy

This is a case of type two amiodarone-induced thyroiditis (AIT). Amiodarone induced thyrotoxicosis occurrs in up to 6% of patients taking this medication in iodine sufficient areas of the world and in up to 10% in iodine deficient areas. Amiodarone has a very high concentration of iodine (37% by molecular weight) and therefore patients on this therapy require monitoring of their thyroid function. The reduced uptake on the scan and negative antibody levels are in keeping with this diagnosis. Type 2 AIT is due to direct destructive effect of aminodarone on thyrocytes. Steroid therapy would be the mainstay of treatment, initially starting at 40–60 mg daily and tapering as the gland settles. There is a risk of hypothyroidism, so thyroid function needs to be monitored closely.

This gentleman has an implantable defibrillator and is maintained on amiodarone for control of ventricular arrhythmias. Only under the advice of a cardiologist should the amiodarone be discontinued. Antithyroid medication may be considered in cases when type one amiodarone-induced thyroiditis is suspected, or if it is not clear which type is present. Radioactive iodone is not an option until the iodine load has been cleared, which can take several months. As amiodarone has a high concentration of iodine, the uptake of radioiodine by the thyroid gland is likely to be poor. Surgery would only be considered if no alternative treatment existed or if there was significant compression by the gland on other structures.[8]

CASE 12

C: Hypothalamic amenorrhoea

This is a case of secondary amenorrhoea, ie the cessation of established, regular menstruation for six months or longer.

> ### Learning point
>
> The most common cause is hypothalamic amenorrhoea (34%) and the biochemical tests listed with low oestradiol and inappropriately low gonadotrophins would be in keeping with this. A thorough history should include eating habits, exercise and recent stressful events, as all these factors have been associated with hypothalamic hypogonadism. Unrecognised weight loss while taking the OCP can result in amenorrhoea when it is stopped.

Primary ovarian failure would present with elevated gonadotrophin levels. Elevated prolactin levels would be associated with prolactinoma-induced amenorrhoea. Headaches and visual field changes can be associated. Turner syndrome (45XO) often presents with primary amenorrhoea. This is the failure to start menses by the age of 16 years. Physical features include short stature, a webbed neck, lack of breast development and scanty axillary hair. Polycystic ovarian syndrome has biochemical and/or physical signs of hyperandrogenism. The free androgen index is often raised and sex hormone binding globulin is suppressed.

CASE 13

C: Oral glucose tolerance test

This is a case of suspected acromegaly. This is an uncommon disorder affecting three to four people per million per year. Its clinical features are due to the excess exposure of growth hormone (GH) on tissues. Typical features include increased frontal bossing, coarse facial features, wide nasal bridge, protruding jaw, large hand size, dental malocclusion, carpal tunnel syndrome, hypertension (up to 30% of patients), diabetes mellitus, sleep apnoea, joint pains and increased sweating. Hypertension may lead to cardiac hypertrophy or cardiomyopathy as in this case. Acromegaly has an insidious onset, typically over 5–10 years, and in over 95% of cases it is due to a pituitary somatotroph adenoma.

Learning point

Growth hormone secretion is pulsatile. Approximately 30% of patients with acromegaly will have a GH level in the reference range when tested. This makes random GH levels unsuitable for confirmation of diagnosis. Insulin-like growth factor-1 (IGF1) mediates virtually all actions of GH. Lack of standardisation of the assay and variations with nutrition, renal impairment, poorly controlled diabetes etc make it unsuitable on its own for diagnosis.

An oral glucose tolerance test would be the recommended screening test to confirm acromegaly. A non-suppressed GH level is suspicious of acromegaly following a 75 g oral glucose load. The current cut-off value of 1 ng/ml (0.3 mU/litre) is used for diagnosis. Other screening tests could include a 24-hour GH profile (a mean value of > 1 ng/ml would be in keeping with a diagnosis of acromegaly).

Prolactin can often be elevated owing to co-secretion of this hormone by the adenoma or owing to pressure effects within the pituitary gland. However, it is not used in confirming acromegaly. An MRI scan of the pituitary gland may be required in due course, but initial biochemical screening tests should be carried out first. MRI scans may miss small pituitary microadenomas. For further reading, see reference.[9]

CASE 14

A: X-ray of left hand and wrist

This is a case of delayed puberty. The first sign of puberty in boys is testicular enlargement, followed by penile and scrotal changes. Delayed puberty is defined as failure to progress into puberty by greater than two standard deviations later than the average, ie no testicular enlargement by 14 years in boys. In this case, the testes are small and testosterone levels low. Gonadotrophin levels are low normal.

> **Learning point**
>
> First-line investigations of delayed puberty include gonadotrophin levels and plain radiography of the wrist to assess bone age. This correlates well with stage of maturation, better than chronological age. Constitutional delay is likely if puberty progresses with pubertal bone age. If it does not, then gonadotrophin deficiency is likely.

An MRI scan of the pituitary may be considered if there is gonadotrophin deficiency or if symptoms such as headache or visual disturbance are present. Vitamin B12 and folate levels might help to rule out malabsorption, eg due to coeliac disease. Although this may be considered in cases of delayed puberty, in this case weight is higher than predicted, making malabsorption less likely.

Both testes are palpable and therefore ultrasound is unlikely to be helpful in his initial screening. If gonadotrophin levels had been elevated, karotyping may have been considered.

CHAPTER 3 ANSWERS

CASE 15

B: 24-hour urine collection for catecholamines

Medullary thyroid carcinomas are rare, representing 3% of thyroid cancers in adults; 25% of cases are familial. In familial cases, assessments of other endocrine organ functions are needed. The sudden death of her younger brother may have been related to a phaeochromocytoma. This needs to be excluded in patients, as even minor surgery can precipitate a phaeochromocytoma crisis in an undiagnosed patient.

Although genetic testing may be considered, it is not the most appropriate next step. RET mutation analysis should be performed even in the absence of a positive family history in medullary thyroid carcinoma. Parathyroid hormone assessment may be required during follow-up of these patients but the normal calcium levels essentially exclude hyperparathyroidism. Radioiodine therapy and external beam radiotherapy is not generally required for treatment of medullary thyroid carcinoma. For further reading, see reference.[10]

CASE 16

D: Vitamin D

Severe hypocalcaemia (< 1.9 mmol/l and/or symptomatic at any level below reference range) is a medical emergency. Administer IV calcium gluconate (10–20 ml 10% calcium gluconate in 50–100 ml of 5% dextrose IV over 10 min with ECG monitoring. Treatment of post operative hydrocal hypocalcaemia consists of 1-alfa calcidol or calcitriol therapy. Starting doses should be approximately 0.25–0.5 mcg per day.[11]

Learning point

This lady likely has hungry bone syndrome. This occurs following parathyroid surgery for primary hyperparathyroidism when parathyroid hormone levels dramatically decrease. This causes an abrupt cessation of osteoclast activity; however, osteoblast mineralisation continues to occur leading to hypocalcaemia.

There is some evidence that bisphosphonate therapy before surgery may reduce the risk of hungry bone syndrome, but its effectiveness in the post-operative stage has not been proven. Vitamin D increases calcium in the extracellular fluid, and improves calcium absorption in the GI tract. High-dose vitamin D along with calcium restores normal bone turnover. Although adequate phosphate and magnesium levels are required, the most appropriate therapies are calcium and vitamin D. Intravenous saline is not likely to improve calcium levels.

CASE 17

A: Corticosteroid administration

Learning point

This is a case of pituitary apoplexy. This is a medical emergency and rapid treatment with hydrocortisone may be lifesaving. It is characterised by the sudden onset of headache, visual disturbance, vomiting and decreased consciousness caused by haemorrhage into the pituitary gland. All patients with a pituitary tumour should be warned of the features of apoplexy and advised to seek urgent medical attention should they develop any of these symptoms or signs.

In adults, 100–200 mg hydrocortisone as an intravenous bolus is appropriate, followed by 50–100 mg six-hourly by intramuscular injection. Indications for empirical steroid therapy include haemodynamic instability, altered consciousness level, reduced visual acuity and severe visual field defects.

Although secondary hypothyroidism is suggested by the above results, commencing thyroxine before steroids may precipitate an adrenal crisis. Pituitary surgical consultation is required, but steroid administration is the immediate priority. Surgery will require an adequate steroid response and this would be best achieved by exogenous steroid administration in this case. MR imaging of the pituitary gland and full pituitary biochemical testing may be requested but should not delay initiation of steroids. For further reading, see reference.[12]

CASE 18

D: Polycystic ovarian syndrome

The likely diagnosis here is polycystic ovarian syndrome. This is the diagnosis in up to 30% of women presenting with secondary amenorrhoea. The overall prevalence is 6.5–8%. The condition should be suspected if there is biochemical or clinical evidence of androgen excess, ovulatory dysfunction or polycystic ovaries on imaging. Biochemical testing usually shows a high testosterone level, raised free androgen index, a high LH:FSH ratio, low sex hormone binding globulin level and normal dehydroepiandrosterone. Weight loss is the mainstay of treatment. Prolactinomas are associated with hypogonadism but not androgen excess. Congenital adrenal hyperplasia usually presents with virilisation. 17-OH progesterone levels are high. Androgen-secreting ovarian tumours typically present with acute onset hirsutism and virilisation. Testosterone levels are often much higher (ie > 5 nmol/litre).[13]

CASE 19

B: Phenoxybenzamine

This is a case of a phaeochromocytoma. This is a tumour arising from adrenomedullary chromaffin cells that produce catecholamines. The overall prevalence is approximately 0.01–0.1% and it is typically found in between 0.2 and 0.6% of patients attending outpatient clinics with hypertension. Hounsfield units > 60 (less lipid) on CT imaging would be in keeping with a phaeochromocytoma, but could also represent adrenal cortical carcinoma, metastatic disease or a lipid poor adenoma. Phaeochromocytomas are typically large adrenal lesions (> 4 cm in size), and if left untreated carry a high cardiovascular morbidity and mortality. Up to a third of patients have a germline mutation. Indications for genetic testing include: bilateral phaeochromocytoma, unilateral phaeochromocytoma with a family history, unilateral phaeochromocytoma< 30 years of age.

CHAPTER 3 ANSWERS

Learning point

Alpha blockers, eg phenoxybenzamine, are the first-line therapy for phaeochromocytoma-induced hypertension and prevention of hypertensive crises. Pre-operative medical treatment is generally required for 7–14 days to allow adequate time to normalise blood pressure and heart rate. Beta blockers should be avoided until after the establishment of alpha blockade, since unopposed stimulation of alpha adrenergic receptors can induce a hypertensive crisis. Calcium channel blockers are the most often used add-on drugs to further improve blood pressure control in patients already treated with an α blocker. Labetolol has more potent beta than alpha antagonistic activities and can result in paradoxical hypertension or even a hypertensive crisis. For further reading, see reference.[14]

CASE 20

B: Increase thyroxine dose

Learning point

Hypothyroidism in pregnancy has been associated with poor outcomes for both mother and her offspring. Thyroxine is especially important for nerve and brain development in the fetus, particularly in the early stages of pregnancy. The fetus only starts to produce thyroxine from approximately 12 to 16 weeks' gestation. Current guidance recommends a target TSH level of < 2.5 mU/litre, and therefore the correct answer is to increase the thyroxine dose (usually by 25–30%).

Reducing the thyroxine dose will decrease the maternal supply and may affect fetal development. T_3 is the active hormone but has a short half-life. Evidence for its safety is limited and it therefore should not be recommended without specialist input. This lady states that she takes her thyroxine therapy. The increase in demand during pregnancy has increased TSH levels. Therefore, supervised administration is unlikely to be helpful. For further reading, see reference.[15]

CASE 21

B: Structured education, eg carbohydrate counting

A basal bolus regimen is flexible and suited to most young, active people. Glycaemic control is clearly not good in this case, with a suboptimal Haemoglobin A_{1c} and hypoglycaemia. The first step is to ensure that she has undergone structured education such as DAFNE. She can then calculate her insulin doses based on carbohydrate intake, as well as adjusting for activity, sickness and stress.

Although twice daily isophane insulin may suit some individuals, it may carry a higher risk of hypoglycaemia and would not be the most suitable option here. Insulin pump therapy would be considered in someone with a suboptimal Haemoglobin A_{1c} and frequent hypoglycaemia, but patients should have undergone structured education before consideration for pump therapy. Possible indications for islet cell transplantation are:

✦ two or more episodes of severe hypoglycaemia (requiring other people to help) within the last two years

✦ impaired awareness of hypoglycaemia

✦ severe hypoglycaemia/impaired awareness in patients with a functioning kidney transplant.

A continuous glucose monitoring system may give information regarding insulin adjustment and can therefore be a useful tool; however, structured education would remain the priority.[16]

CASE 22

E: Repeat early morning testosterone

This is a case of hypogonadotrophic hypogonadism with a low testosterone level and inappropriately normal LH/FSH. It would be important to repeat the testosterone level test, as 30% of men may have a normal testosterone level on repeat measurement. Testosterone levels also vary significantly as a result of circadian and circannual rhythms, episodic secretion and measurement variations.

Bioactive testosterone includes free testosterone and also testosterone weakly bound to albumin and is calculated from total testosterone, free testosterone and albumin levels. If hypogonadotrophic hypogonadism is confirmed, an MRI scan of the pituitary would be indicated to ensure that there are no structural lesions. An ultrasound scan of the testes would be unlikely to be helpful here as this picture is in keeping with secondary hypogonadism. Haemochromatosis with a raised serum ferritin could cause the same picture, but we would expect to see abnormal liver function tests and pigmentation.

Learning point

Conditions associated with alterations in SHBG concentrations:

Decreased SHBG:

- ✦ moderate obesity
- ✦ nephrotic syndrome
- ✦ hypothyroidism
- ✦ use of glucocortciods, progestins and androgenic steroids
- ✦ acromegaly
- ✦ diabetes mellitus

CASE 23

C: Discuss right hemicolectomy

Learning point

Most patients presenting with emergency appendicitis due to carcinoid tumours will have sufficient surgery. More radical surgery such as a right hemicolectomy is considered when a carcinoid of the appendix has been removed which is over 2 cm in diameter, despite the absence of obvious malignant features.

Tumours sized 1–2 cm or those invading the serosal surface may require further resection, particularly if atypical with goblet cell or adenocarcinoid features. Further intervention should also be considered if tumours are located at the base of the appendix, or if histology shows mesoappendiceal and/or vascular invasion.

The recommended follow-up time for uncomplicated appendiceal carcinoid would be five years. If there were symptoms of carcinoid syndrome, medical therapies such as sandostatin analogues may be considered. The role of chemotherapy is less certain, but appears to be of benefit with carcinoid tumours that are less well differentiated and anaplastic. Although repeat imaging is reasonable, given the size of the carcinoid tumour along with the serosal invasion, hemicolectomy should be discussed with the patient.[18]

CHAPTER 3
ANSWERS

CASE 24

C: Dopamine agonist (eg bromocriptine)

This is a case of a microprolactinoma. Prolactinomas account for over 40% of all pituitary tumours. Typical features of hyperprolactinaemia are infertility, hypogonadism and galactorrhoea, but many are asymptomatic.

Dopamine agonist therapy should be considered. Prolactinomas are sensitive to oral therapy and are the preferred option. Resolution of hyperprolactinaemia-induced infertility occurs in approximately 78% of patients treated with this therapy. Women not wishing to have a baby on this therapy should be advised about additional contraception. On confirmation of pregnancy, dopamine agonist therapy should be stopped; however, if there is a large macroadenoma this should be discussed further with a specialist.

Hypothyroidism can cause hyperprolactinaemia but here the TSH is normal and therefore thyroxine therapy is not indicated. Although oestrogen therapy can be considered for bone protection, it is not appropriate in this case as she is keen to have a baby. Clomifene citrate and in vitro fertilisation treatment may be options for the treatment of infertility; however, these would not be first-line therapies in this case.[19]

CASE 25

D: Familial hypocalciuric hypercalcaemia

> **Learning point**
>
> This is a case of familial hypocalciuric hypercalcaemia. This is a benign disorder affecting the regulation of calcium metabolism. It is an autosomal dominant genetic disease with almost 100% penetrance. It is caused by an inactivating mutation in the *CASR* gene, which encodes for the calcium-sensing receptor. Index cases are usually picked up incidentally as the condition is often asymptomatic. The clues in this case are the lack of symptoms, the family history and the low urinary calcium:creatinine ratio.

Malignancy would often be associated with weight loss. The most common cancers associated with hypercalcaemia include breast, lung, renal tumours and multiple myeloma. Parathyroid hormone levels are usually suppressed.

Although hyperthyroidism can be associated with hypercalcaemia, the lack of symptoms and normal TSH effectively rules this out. Primary hyperparathyroidism is often symptomatic with polyuria, polydipsia, abdominal pain and constipation. Calcium levels are often elevated in the urine also, with an expected calcium:creatinine ratio> 0.01. Vitamin D intoxication suppresses parathyroid hormone levels. Short courses of steroid therapy have been useful in the treatment of vitamin-D-induced hypercalcaemia.

CASE 26

E: Omeprazole

Inappropriately elevated TSH in patients with previously controlled hypothyroidism normally reflects non-compliance with treatment. Excluding this, one would next need to exclude malabsorption. Certain medications can affect the absorption of thyroxine. These include proton pump inhibitors, iron therapy, calcium-containing therapies, ie antacids, cholestyramine and sucralfate. General advice would be to take these medications at least four hours after thyroxine therapy. Thyroxine therapy is best absorbed 1 hr prior to breakfast or 3 hrs after a meal.

CASE 27

C: Insulin

From studies including UKPDS and ADVANCE, the target Haemoglobin A_{1c} should be 58 mmol/mol or less to reduce cardiovascular risk. Although his metformin dose is only 500 mg twice daily (half the full dose), in view of his renal function, this may be difficult to titrate up further.

Sodium-glucose co-transporter 2 inhibitors work by inhibiting glucose resorption in the kidney. There is a slight risk of increased urinary complications, mainly genito-urinary infections, with these agents.

A glucagon-like peptide-1 (GLP-1) agonist is indicated when the body mass index (BMI) is elevated. NICE recommends their use as third-line agents if BMI is > 35 kg/m^2, or if BMI < 30 kg/m^2 if weight loss would benefit other co-morbidities. Impaired renal function at this level would generally exclude GLP-1 agonist therapy and SGLT2 ihibitor therapies. Acarbose prevents glucose absorption in the gastrointestinal tract. It can be difficult to tolerate, and will be less likely to achieve an adequate Haemoglobin A_{1c} when compared to insulin. Pioglitazone would be contraindicated in the presence of heart failure.[20]

CASE 28

A: Short Synacthen® test

This is a typical presentation of Addison's disease. This condition results in glucocorticoid and mineralocorticoid deficiency. It is usually of insidious onset, although it can present as a crisis. Pigmentation is typically seen in the buccal mucosa, skin creases and scars. A short Synacthen® test is used to confirm the diagnosis. After 250 μg of synthetic ACTH administration, a 30-minute cortisol level of over 550 nmol/litre excludes the diagnosis. Adrenal antibodies may be useful in determining the aetiology of confirmed adrenal insufficiency. Cortisol levels peak in the morning and fall progressively during the day. Random measurements should therefore be interpreted with caution. Urinary sodium and osmolality may be used for investigation of hyponatraemia. Addison's disease and hypothyroidism induced hyponatraemia is often associated with a high urinary sodium level and a high urinary osmolality.

CASE 29

B: Spironolactone

Gynaecomastia is a benign proliferation of the glandular tissue of the male breast. It may be unilateral or bilateral, and drugs represent the cause in approximately 10–15% of cases.

> **Learning point**
>
> The following drugs are often associated: oestrogens, spironolactone (androgen receptor antagonist), cimetidine (androgen receptor antagonist), digitoxin (oestrogen-like activity), ketoconazole (decreases testosterone by Leydig cell damage or inhibition), metoclopramide (increases prolactin) and proton pump inhibitors (mechanism uncertain).

CASE 30

B: Reduce desmopressin dose

This lady has symptomatic hyponatraemia. The most likely cause in this case is water excess due to combination of increased water intake and excess desmopressin. Reducing her desmopressin will allow free water excretion and correction of the hyponatraemia. It should only be done, however, under specialist supervision. This requires careful monitoring of her sodium levels.

The features in this case are not suggestive of an adrenal crisis. If she was unable to keep her tablets down, then intravenous or intramuscular hydrocortisone should be considered. Otherwise she should be safe to continue oral hydrocortisone, with a doubling of her maintenance dose if she is clinically unwell. She is normovolaemic and therefore intravenous fluids may not be appropriate. TSH levels are adequate and therefore no dose adjustment to the thyroxine is required. An urgent CT scan of her brain is not required, but if there was a deterioration in her central nervous system observations, this may be considered.

CHAPTER 3 ANSWERS

CASE 31

D: Non-islet cell tumour

Evaluation of hypoglycaemia is recommended if Whipple's triad is documented – symptoms, signs or both consistent with hypoglycaemia, a low plasma glucose concentration, and resolution of those symptoms or signs after the plasma glucose is raised.

The answer is one of exclusion. Insulin and C-peptide levels are appropriately low, ruling out most of the answers. An insulinoma would have non-suppressed levels of both insulin and C-peptide during hypoglycaemic episodes. Factitious hypoglycaemia due to insulin administration would have non-suppressed insulin levels but low C-peptide levels. Sulfonylurea therapy would produce non-suppressed insulin levels and C-peptide during hypoglycaemic episodes. Glycogen storage disorders are likely to present in childhood with delayed growth and development.[21]

Learning point

The most likely cause here is IGF2-mediated non-islet cell tumour hypoglycaemia. IGF2 is likely being produced by the lung mass, as this phenomenon is usually associated with large, clinically apparent, mesenchymal tumours. Endogenous insulin secretion is suppressed appropriately in non-islet cell tumour hypoglycaemia.

References

1. Nieman L et al. 2008. The diagnosis of Cushing's syndrome: An Endocrine Society clinical practice guideline. Journal of Clinical Endocrinology & Metabolism, 93, 1526–1540

2. Spasovski G et al. 2014. Clinical practice guideline on diagnosis and treatment of hyponatraemia. European Journal of Endocrinology, 170, G1–G47

3. Funder J et al. 2008. Case detection, diagnosis, and treatment of patients with primary aldosteronism: An Endocrine Society clinical practice guideline. Journal of Clinical Endocrinology & Metabolism, 93, 3266–3281

4. NICE. 2008. Diabetes in pregnancy: Management of diabetes and its complications from conception to the postnatal period. NICE clinical guideline 63. www.nice.org.uk/guidance/cg63

5. Zeiger M et al. 2009. American Association of Clinical Endocrinologists and American Association of Endocrine Surgeons Medical Guidelines for the Management of Adrenal Incidentalomas. Endocrine Practice, 15, Supplement 1, 1–20

6. Society for Endocrinology. 2013. Acute hypercalcaemia. www.endocrinology.org/policy/docs/ 13-02_EmergencyGuidance-AcuteHypercalcaemia.pdf

7. Savage et al. 2011. Joint British Diabetes Societies guideline for the management of diabetic ketoacidosis. Diabetic Medicine, 28, 508–515

8. Bahn et al. 2011. Hyperthyroidism and other causes of thyrotoxicosis: management guidelines of the American Thyroid Association and American Association of Clinical Endocrinologists. Endocrine Practice, 17, 456–520

9. Katznelson L et al. 2011. American Association of Clinical Endocrinologists medical guidelines for clinical practice for the diagnosis and treatment of acromegaly – 2011 update. Endocrine Practice, 17, Supplement 4, 1–44

10. Colley P et al. 2014. British Thyroid Association guidelines for the management of thyroid cancer. Clinical Endocrinology, 81, Supplement 1, i–122

11. Society for Endocrinology. 2013. Acute hypocalcaemia. www.endocrinology.org/policy/docs/ 13-02_EmergencyGuidance-AcuteHypocalcaemia_(inAdults).pdf

12. Rajasekaran S. 2011. UK guidelines for the management of pituitary apoplexy. Clinical Endocrinology, 74, 9–20

13. Legro R et al. 2013. Diagnosis and treatment of polycystic ovary syndrome: an Endocrine Society clinical practice guideline. Journal of Clinical Endocrinology & Metabolism, 98, 4565–4592

14. Lenders J et al. 2014. Phaeochromocytoma and paraganglioma: An Endocrine Society clinical practice guideline. Journal of Clinical Endocrinology & Metabolism, 99, 1915–1942

15. De Groot et al. 2012. Management of thyroid dysfunction during pregnancy and postpartum: an Endocrine Society clinical practice guideline. Journal of Clinical Endocrinology & Metabolism, 97, 2543–2565

16. NICE. 2004. Type 1 diabetes: Diagnosis and Management of type 1 diabetes in children, young people and adults. NICE clinical guideline 15. www.nice.org.uk/guidance/cg15

17. Bhasin S et al. 2010. Testosterone therapy in men with androgen deficiency syndromes: an Endocrine Society clinical practice guideline. Journal of Clinical Endocrinology & Metabolism, 95, 2536–2559

18. Ramage J et al. 2005. Guidelines for the management of gastroenteropancreatic neuroendocrine (including carcinoid) tumours. Gut, 54, Supplement 4, 1–16

19. Melmed S et al. 2011. Diagnosis and treatment of hyperprolactinemia: An Endocrine Society clinical practice guideline. Journal of Clinical Endocrinology & Metabolism, 96, 273–288

20. NICE. 2009. Type 2 diabetes: The management of type 2 diabetes. NICE clinical guideline 87. www.nice.org.uk/guidance/cg87

21. Cryer P et al. 2009. Evaluation and management of adult hypoglycemic disorders: an Endocrine Society Clinical Practice Guideline. Journal of Clinical Endocrinology & Metabolism, 94, 709–728

CASE 1

A 50-year-old man is admitted to the emergency department following a large-volume fresh haematemesis. He has no co-morbidities and does not take any regular medication. He has, however, been taking over-the-counter diclofenac for back pain for the past two weeks. On initial assessment, he is alert with a heart-rate of 120 bpm and blood pressure 90/50 mmHg.

His blood test results show: Haemoglobin 80 g/litre, White cells 10×10^9/litre, Platelets 200×10^9/litre, Coagulation screen: normal, Urea 15 mmol/litre, Creatinine 100 μmol/litre.

What is the next most important management step?

- A. **Gastroscopy**
- B. **Aggressive resuscitation with fluids and blood products**
- C. **Administration of a proton pump inhibitor**
- D. *Helicobacter pylori* **eradication therapy**
- E. **Stopping diclofenac**

CASE 2

A 75-year-old lady presents to the gastrointestinal clinic with a several-month history of dysphagia, mainly to solids. She describes a sensation of food sticking at the cricoid level and would regurgitate undigested food that she has eaten earlier. She also complains of borborygmus in her throat when she eats or drinks.

What is the most likely diagnosis?

- A. **Pharyngeal pouch**
- B. **Goitre**
- C. **Oesophageal malignancy**
- D. **Gastro-oesophageal reflux disease**
- E. **Oropharyngeal dysphagia from a stroke**

CASE 3

A 65-year-old lady is referred after she is noted to have the following blood results. Apart from lethargy, she denies any gastrointestinal symptoms.

Blood tests reveal: Haemoglobin 92 g/litre, MCV 76 fl, MCH 26 pg, White cells 4.0×10^9/litre, Platelets 164×10^9/litre, Ferritin 10 µg/litre.

Which of the following tests would not be recommended as part of her investigations?

A. **Anti-transglutaminase antibodies**
B. **Urinalysis**
C. **Gastroscopy**
D. **Colonoscopy**
E. **Faecal occult blood testing**

CASE 4

A 42-year-old lady is seen at the gastroenterology clinic with chronic watery diarrhoea which started following her laparoscopic cholecystectomy two years previously. The diarrhoea is associated with bloating, urgency and sometimes faecal incontinence. She is now afraid to go out because of her 'accidents' when she could not locate a toilet in time.

What would be her treatment of choice?

A. **Loperamide**
B. **Probiotics**
C. **Colestyramine**
D. **Codeine phosphate**
E. **Mebeverine**

CASE 5

A 35-year-old lady is admitted to the hospital following a non-accidental overdose of paracetamol. She took the overdose on impulse after an argument with her boyfriend. She is commenced on N-acetylcysteine. Later that day, nursing staff report that she has become more drowsy.

Repeat blood testing reveals the following: Urea 15 mmol/litre, Creatinine 100 μmol/litre, Total bilirubin 40 μμmol/litre, ALT 2350 U/litre, ALP 150 U/litre, INR 3.5 s, pH 7.20, Lactate 3.0 mmol/litre.

What is the most appropriate next step in this lady's management?

A. **Arrange CT scanning of the brain**
B. **Refer to a liver unit**
C. **Give vitamin K**
D. **Administer more intravenous fluids**
E. **Give fresh frozen plasma**

CASE 6

A 50-year-old gentleman is referred for an open access OGD because of persistent dyspepsia. His OGD shows an ulcerating, friable mass in the gastric antrum. Biopsies confirm a well-differentiated adenocarcinoma.

What is the next most appropriate investigation?

A. **Transabdominal ultrasound scan**
B. **CT scan of chest, abdomen and pelvis**
C. **Endoscopic ultrasound (EUS)**
D. **Diagnostic laparoscopy**
E. **Positron emission tomography (PET)**

CASE 7

A 66-year-old lady presents to the colorectal clinic with a 6-month history of loose, frequent motions, associated with urgency and weight loss. She has type 2 diabetes and takes metformin. She undergoes a colonoscopy, which is normal. Serial colonic biopsies and were reported as showing a thick, subepithelial collagen band and inflammatory cell infiltrate in the epithelium and lamina propria.

What is the diagnosis?

    A. **Irritable bowel syndrome**
    B. **Ulcerative colitis**
    C. **Metformin-induced diarrhoea**
    D. **Collagenous colitis**
    E. **Crohn's colitis**

CASE 8

A 56-year-old gentleman, who has a history of gastro-oesophageal reflux disease, underwent an OGD to investigate his intermittent dysphagia. He is a heavy smoker and drinks a moderate amount of alcohol. He does not take any medication. His OGD shows a 4 cm segment of non-dysplastic Barrett's oesophagus, which is confirmed histologically.

What is the most appropriate recommendation for this gentleman?

    A. **Surveillance OGD and proton pump inhibitor therapy**
    B. **Nissen fundoplication**
    C. **Expectant treatment**
    D. **Surveillance OGD**
    E. **Radiofrequency ablation**

CASE 9

A 40-year-old obese man who has type 2 diabetes attends the emergency department with acute severe epigastric pain radiating to the back, associated with nausea and vomiting. He denies alcohol consumption. His only medications are metformin and insulin. On initial assessment, he is slightly tachycardic but apyrexic. The abdomen is tender in the epigastrium but there is no sign of peritonism.

Blood results reveal: Liver function tests: normal, Serum lipase 2300 U/litre, HbA1c 9.4 mmol/mol, Ultrasound scan of abdomen: fatty liver, normal gall bladder and biliary tree. Pancreas obscured by overlying bowel gas.

X-ray and CT scan of abdomen: see Figures 4.1 and 4.2.

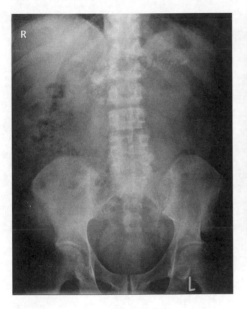 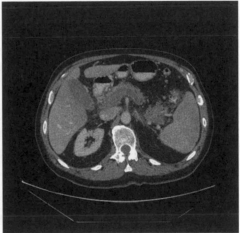

CHAPTER 4 QUESTIONS

Figure 4.1   **Figure 4.2**

What is the most likely cause for this man's clinical diagnosis?

 A. **Microlithiasis**
 B. **Hypertriglyceridaemia**
 C. **Adverse drug reaction**
 D. **Trauma**
 E. **Autoimmune disease**

CASE 10

A 23-year-old woman presents to the emergency department with a 3-week history of abdominal pain and swelling. She has no significant past medical history and the only notable medication she is on is an oral contraceptive pill. Abdominal examination revealed tender hepatomegaly and ascites.

What is the best diagnostic test for her?

A. **Liver function tests**
B. **Transabdominal ultrasound scan**
C. **Paracentesis**
D. **Serumascites albumin gradient (SAAG)**
E. **Doppler ultrasound scan of liver**

CASE 11

A 31-year-old woman is referred to the gastroenterology clinic because of dysphagia to both solids and liquids, regurgitation, chest pain and weight loss. She is fearful to have OGD, therefore a barium swallow is performed (see Figure 4.3).

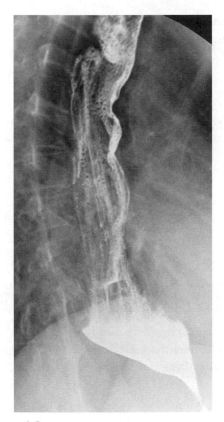

Figure 4.3

What is the most likely diagnosis?

    A. **Gastro-oesophageal reflux disease**
    B. **Hypertensive lower oesophageal sphincter**
    C. **Benign oesophageal stricture**
    D. **Achalasia**
    E. **Oesophageal malignancy**

CASE 12

A 41-year-old lady was admitted with a 3-day history of recurrent epigastric and right upper quadrant pain radiating to her back. The pain was associated with nausea. She then started noticing that she was passing dark urine and her husband commented that she looked yellow.

Blood results reveal: Bilirubin 128 μμmol/litre, ALP 208 U/litre, ALT 440 U/litre, Albumin 43 g/litre, Amylase 34 U/litre, C-reactive protein < 3 mg/litre, White cells 4.55×10^9/litre.

An ultrasound of abdomen revealed a thin-walled gall bladder without calculi, normal bile ducts and pancreas.

What is the next appropriate investigation for her?

A. **MR cholangiopancreatography**
B. **CT scan of abdomen and pelvis**
C. **ERCP**
D. **Endoscopic ultrasound**
E. **Liver biopsy**

CASE 13

A 25-year-old man attends the gastroenterology clinic with lethargy and abdominal bloating that has continued for a few months. He has intermittent episodes of loose motions but no rectal bleeding. There is no unintentional weight loss.

Blood results reveal: Haemoglobin 130 g/litre, White cells 4.64×10^9/litre, Platelets 197×10^9/litre, Ferritin 130 μg/litre, Folate 6.2 μg/litre, Vitamin B12 429 ng/litre.

OGD normal. Duodenal biopsies taken.

Histology is reported as showing partial villous atrophy with hypertrophy of the crypts of Lieberkühn.

What is the diagnosis?

A. **Irritable bowel syndrome**
B. **Lactose intolerance**
C. **Coeliac disease**
D. **Crohn's disease**
E. **Small bowel bacterial overgrowth**

CASE 14

A 70-year-old lady is admitted with a 2-day history of persistent vomiting, abdominal cramping pain and constipation. She had a hysterectomy many years ago. Abdominal examination revealed a distended, tender abdomen with scanty bowel sounds.

Investigations reveal: Haemoglobin 120 g/litre, White cells 13 × 10⁹/litre, Platelets 200 × 10⁹/litre, Urea 15 mmol/litre, Creatinine 135 µmol/litre.

Abdominal X-ray: see Figure 4.4.

CT scan of abdomen: see Figure 4.5.

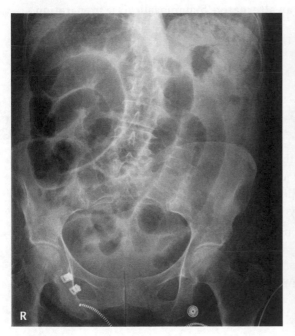

Figure 4.4

What is the most likely diagnosis?

- A. **Colonic tumour**
- B. **Gallstone ileus**
- C. **Intussuception**
- D. **Pseudo-obstruction**
- E. **Adhesions-related intestinal obstruction**

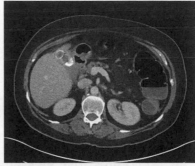

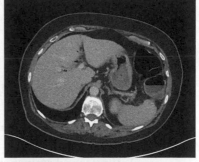

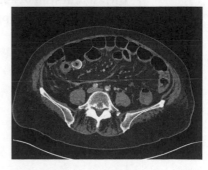

Figure 4.5

CASE 15

A 25-year-old man is seen at the colitis clinic. He was diagnosed with distal ulcerative colitis two years previously, and he was commenced on mesalazine at the time of his diagnosis. Over the past eight months, he has required two courses of prednisolone for relapses of his colitis despite taking maximal doses of mesalazine. His recent flexible sigmoidoscopy shows ongoing active colitis.

What is the next appropriate management step?

A. **Start azathioprine**
B. **Give a course of antibiotics**
C. **Switch mesalazine to an alternative 5-aminosalicylate preparation**
D. **Start probiotics**
E. **Send stool cultures**

CASE 16

A 75-year-old lady presents to the emergency department with pyrexia and severe left iliac fossa pain. She has frequent bowel movements (three or four times a day), and her stools are fairly soft. She denies rectal bleeding. On examination, she was tachycardic with a low-grade pyrexia. She was tender in the left iliac fossa.

Blood results reveal: Haemoglobin 135 g/litre, White cells 14×10^9/litre, Platelets 200×10^9/litre.

What is the next appropriate investigation?

A. **Barium enema**
B. **Plain abdominal X-ray**
C. **CT scan of abdomen**
D. **Ultrasound scan of abdomen**
E. **Flexible sigmoidoscopy**

CASE 17

A 23-year-old woman, who is 32 weeks in gestation, was admitted with intense pruritus, particularly in her palms and soles. The pruritus is worse at night. Examination revealed excoriation marks from scratching and a gravid uterus.

Blood results reveal: Haemoglobin 108 g/litre, White cells 8.7 × 10⁹/litre, Platelets 146 × 10⁹/litre, Bilirubin 8 μmol/litre, ALP 216 U/litre, ALT 200 U/litre, Albumin 37 g/litre, Bile acids 115 μmol/litre.

What is the most likely diagnosis?

- A. **Viral hepatitis**
- B. **Primary biliary cirrhosis**
- C. **HELLP syndrome**
- D. **Intrahepatic cholestasis of pregnancy**
- E. **Primary sclerosing cholangitis**

CASE 18

A 50-year-old man is admitted with chronic diarrhoea and some unintentional weight loss. He has been complaining of epigastric pain for a few months but has not sought advice from his GP. Further questioning reveals that he consumes at least 40 units of alcohol per week. An image from his CT scan is shown in Figure 4.6.

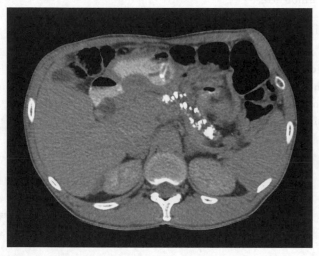

Figure 4.6

Which test is most likely to provide an explanation for his diarrhoea?

    A. **Coeliac serology**

    B. **Stool culture**

    C. **Faecal elastase**

    D. **Colonoscopy**

    E. **CT scan of abdomen**

CASE 19

A 45-year-old woman presents to the gastroenterology clinic with a several-month history of dyspepsia but no other associated symptoms. She has a background history of type 1 diabetes and hypothyrodisim. Her OGD shows chronic diffuse atrophic gastritis in the fundus confirmed on histology.

What test would best help in this woman's diagnosis?

A. **Anti-parietal cell and anti-intrinsic factor antibodies**
B. **Vitamin B level**
C. **Urea breath test**
D. *Helicobacter pylori* **serology**
E. **Anti-transglutaminase antibody**

CASE 20

A 42-year-old man presents to his GP with intermittent arthralgia. He has recently been diagnosed with diabetes. On examination, he has a bronze discoloration of his skin, spider naevi in his upper chest and mild ascites.

Blood tests reveal: Bilirubin 20 μmol/litre, ALP 98 U/litre, ALT 56 U/litre, Albumin 28 g/litre, Prothrombin time 13.5 s.

What is the most likely cause for this man's chronic liver disease?

A. **Alcohol**
B. **Non-alcoholic fatty liver disease**
C. **Primary sclerosing cholangitis**
D. **Chronic hepatitis C infection**
E. **Haemochromatosis**

CASE 21

An 80-year-old lady was admitted feeling acutely unwell with pruritus, lethargy, anorexia and jaundice. Two weeks before this admission, she was prescribed co-amoxiclav by her GP to treat suspected diverticulitis. She is otherwise fit and healthy and does not take regular medication.

Blood results reveal: Bilirubin 142 µmol/litre, ALP 617 U/litre, ALT 337 U/litre, Albumin 42 g/litre, Prothrombin time 10.5 s.

What is the most likely diagnosis in the lady?

A. **Co-amoxiclav-induced cholestasis**
B. **Primary biliary cirrhosis**
C. **Autoimmune hepatitis**
D. **Pancreatic malignancy**
E. **Viral hepatitis**

CASE 22

A 21-year-old lady is seen by her GP with a 4-week history of epigastric pain associated with nausea. She denies any vomiting, anorexia or weight loss. She does not take any medication and does not have any significant past medical history. Her routine blood tests are unremarkable.

What would be the next appropriate step in her management?

A. **Refer her for open access gastroscopy**
B. **Treat her empirically with a month's course of proton pump inhibitor**
C. **Request an ultrasound scan of abdomen**
D. **Refer her to a gastroenterologist**
E. **Treat her with metoclopromide**

CASE 23

A 65-year-old lady is admitted with a 2-month history of vomiting, nausea, abdominal bloating and weight loss. She has had type 2 diabetes for 25 years. Her OGD shows a moderate amount of gastric residue without evidence of gastric outlet obstruction. Her CT scan of abdomen was normal. A diagnosis of diabetic gastroparesis is made. Despite attempts with medical intervention, her oral intake remains poor and it is decided that she needs long-term enteral nutritional support.

Which type of enteral feeding is the most appropriate for her?

A. **Nasogastric tube**
B. **Percutaneous endoscopic gastrostomy**
C. **Surgical jejunostomy**
D. **Percutaneous endoscopic gastrostomy with a jejunal tube extension**
E. **Nasojejunal tube**

CASE 24

A 36-year-old gentleman presents to the emergency department in the early hours of the morning with an acute onset of non-bloody diarrhoea and abdominal cramps. He had some Chinese takeaway for dinner the night before.

What is the likely diagnosis?

A. **Salmonella gastroenteritis**
B. *Bacillus cereus* **food poisoning**
C. **Campylobacter enteritis**
D. **Shigella infection**
E. **Yersinia enterocolitis**

CASE 25

A 27-year-old gentleman is referred to the outpatient clinic with a 2-month history of central abdominal cramps associated with nausea and weight loss. He has also started passing loose, frequent stools. There is no rectal bleeding.

His investigations reveal: Haemoglobin 116 g/litre, White cells 9.1 × 10⁹/litre, Platelets 511 × 10⁹/litre, MCV 100 fl, C-reactive protein 151 mg/litre.

See Figure 4.7.

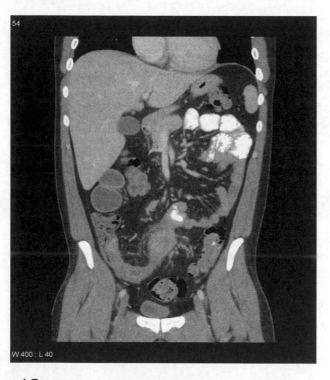

Figure 4.7

What is the most likely cause for his anaemia?

    A. **Vitamin B12 deficiency**

    B. **Thiamine deficiency**

    C. **Folic acid deficiency**

    D. **Iron deficiency**

    E. **Zinc deficiency**

CASE 26

A 69-year-old lady, with a known history of metastatic ovarian carcinoma, is admitted with painless jaundice.

Her investigations reveal: Bilirubin 157 µmol/litre, ALP 1051 U/litre, ALT 363 U/litre, Albumin 39 g/litre.

Ultrasound scan of abdomen: intrahepatic duct dilatation with a large lymph node at the porta hepatis.

What would be the most appropriate next management plan for this lady?

A. **Antibiotic prophylaxis**
B. **Biliary stenting**
C. **Palliative chemotherapy**
D. **Palliative care**
E. **Lymph node biopsy**

CASE 27

A 25-year-old man with a history of HIV is admitted with a several-day history of non-bloody diarrhoea, vomiting and nausea. His last CD4 count was 89/mm^3 and he has not been very compliant with his highly active antiretroviral medications.

What is the most likely cause for his diarrhoea?

A. **Campylobacter**
B. **Salmonella**
C. **Shigella**
D. **Microsporidium**
E. *Escherichia coli*

CASE 28

An 86-year-old gentleman is referred for an OGD because of progressive dysphagia and weight loss. He is quite frail and he has a past medical history of ischaemic heart disease and stroke. He is currently not able to tolerate any solids. His OGD shows a malignant stricture in the distal oesophagus and biopsies confirm this to be an adenocarcinoma.

What is the next most appropriate plan in this gentleman's further management?

A. Staging CT scan of his chest, abdomen and pelvis
B. Endoscopic ultrasound scan of oesophagus
C. Palliative oesophageal stenting
D. Referral to palliative care team
E. Referral for palliative chemotherapy

CASE 29

A 21-year-old man is admitted to hospital with a 1-week history of pyrexia, malaise, anorexia and sore throat. On examination, his temperature is 38.5 °C. He has an infected pharynx and cervical lymphadenopathy. The tip of the spleen is palpable.

Blood results reveal: Bilirubin 15 μmol/litre, ALP 90 U/litre, ALT 363 U/litre, AST 300 U/litre, Albumin 39 g/litre.

What is the most likely cause for his presentation?

A. Hepatitis A virus infection
B. Cytomegalovirus infection
C. Epstein–Barr virus infection
D. Hepatitis B virus infection
E. Herpes simplex virus infection

CASE 30

A 35-year-old woman is seen at the colitis clinic. She was diagnosed with ulcerative colitis a year ago, but for the past eight months she has had several relapses requiring steroid therapy. In view of her steroid-dependent colitis, the consultant decides to start her on azathioprine. Three weeks later, she contacts the advice helpline because of epigastric pain.

Blood tests reveal: Haemoglobin 12 g/litre, White cells 11.5×10^9/litre, Platelets 200×10^9/litre, Urea 8 mmol/litre, Creatinine 90 µmol/litre, Bilirubin 10 µmol/litre, ALP 80 U/litre, ALT 15 U/litre, Albumin 43 g/litre, Amylase 350 U/litre.

What is the next most appropriate step in her management?

- A. **Admit her to hospital**
- B. **Check her calcium level**
- C. **Stop her azathioprine**
- D. **Arrange an ultrasound scan of abdomen**
- E. **Repeat her amylase**

CASE 31

A 42-year-old gentleman, with a history of ulcerative colitis, was noted to have mildly deranged liver function tests on routine blood tests. The liver enzyme abnormalities persisted on repeat testing. He takes mesalazine to control his colitis.

Investigations reveal: Bilirubin 12 µmol/litre, ALP 300 U/litre, ALT 35 U/litre, AST 30 U/litre, Albumin 43 g/litre.

Ultrasound scan of abdomen: normal.

What is the next most appropriate test to investigate his deranged liver function tests?

- A. **MR cholangiopancreatography**
- B. **Liver biopsy**
- C. **Anti-mitochondrial antibody**
- D. **CT scan of abdomen**
- E. **ANCA**

CASE 32

A 30-year-old man is referred to the gastroenterology clinic with chronic diarrhoea and a rash. He is known to have alcohol dependence but no other significant past medical history. On examination, he has a perioral dermatitis.

What is the likely diagnosis?

A. **Vitamin B12 deficiency**
B. **Zinc deficiency**
C. **Selenium deficiency**
D. **Vitamin C deficiency**
E. **Thiamine deficiency**

CASE 33

A 30-year-old man is brought to the emergency department with haematemesis. He has a history of alcohol dependence and was drinking heavily the night before. Before the haematemesis, he was vomiting bile at home.

What is the most likely cause for his haematemesis?

A. **Mallory–Weiss tear**
B. **Oesophageal varices**
C. **Severe gastritis**
D. **Peptic ulcer disease**
E. **Gastric varices**

CASE 34

A 42-year-old gentleman is referred to the liver clinic with abnormal liver function tests. He has hypertension, type 2 diabetes and hypercholesterolaemia. On examination, he is obese and he does not have any stigmata of chronic liver disease.

Blood tests reveal: Bilirubin 10 μmol/litre, ALP 45 U/litre, ALT 110 U/litre, AST 100 U/litre, Albumin 43 g/litre.

What is the diagnostic modality of choice to differentiate steatosis from steatohepatitis?

    A. **CT scan of abdomen**
    B. **Ultrasound scan of abdomen**
    C. **Liver biopsy**
    D. **MRI scan of liver**
    E. **CT-PET scan of abdomen**

CASE 35

An 18-year-old lady presents to the emergency department with an acute onset of retrosternal chest pain, dysphagia and odynophagia. She has no history of oesophageal disorders or other medical illnesses. Drug history revealed that she has been prescribed doxycycline for her acne a week ago and started taking this medication two days before the onset of her symptoms.

What is the likely cause for her symptoms?

    A. **Reflux oesophagitis**
    B. **Doxycycline-induced oesophagitis**
    C. **Herpes simplex oesophagitis**
    D. **Diffuse oesophageal spasm**
    E. **Oesophageal candidiasis**

CASE 36

An 82-year-old lady is admitted to hospital with a 5-day history of non-bloody diarrhoea and abdominal cramps. She lives in a residential home and has been treated with a course of antibiotics for a suspected urinary tract infection in the community recently. She has hypertension and a previous history of peptic ulcer disease. She takes amlodipine, bendroflumethiazide and omeprazole. On examination, she is pyrexic and there is mild generalised abdominal tenderness without guarding or rebound tenderness.

Blood tests reveal: Haemoglobin 12 g/litre, White cells 22.5×10^9/litre, Platelets 400×10^9/litre, Sodium 134 mmol/litre, Potassium 3.7 mmol/litre, Urea 16 mmol/litre, Creatinine 135 μmol/litre, C-reactive protein 350 mg/litre.

Abdominal X-ray: non-specific mild dilatation of the large bowel.

What is the likely diagnosis for this lady?

- A. **Ischaemic colitis**
- B. **Ulcerative colitis**
- C. **Diverticulitis**
- D. *Clostridium difficile* **colitis**
- E. **Campylobacter enteritis**

CASE 37

A 55-year-old man is admitted with a 4-week history of progressive abdominal distension and dyspnoea. On abdominal examination, he has shifting dullness, and subsequent ultrasound examination of his abdomen confirms ascites. A diagnostic paracentesis is performed. A serum sample for albumin is taken at the same time.

Results are shown: Serum albumin 3.2 g/dl, Ascites fluid albumin 2.0 g/dl, Ascites fluid protein 18 g/dl.

What is the most likely cause for this man's ascites?

- A. **Nephrotic syndrome**
- B. **Pancreatitis**
- C. **Peritoneal malignant deposits**
- D. **Cirrhosis**
- E. **Intestinal infarction**

CASE 38

A 30-year-old woman was diagnosed with ulcerative colitis about a year ago and she was commenced on high-dose mesalazine. Colonoscopy at the time showed active pancolitis. Her colitis was reasonably well controlled until a week ago when her symptoms started to flare with frequent bloody diarrhoea and abdominal pain. Both her white cells and C-reactive protein are elevated. She is already taking mesalazine at the maximum dose.

What would be the next most appropriate treatment for her colitis exacerbation?

A. **Steroid enema**
B. **Tapering course of prednisolone**
C. **Mesalazine enema**
D. **Azathioprine**
E. **Switch to an alternative mesalazine preparation**

CASE 39

A 60-year-old gentleman is seen at the gastroenterology clinic with a 10-week history of progressive dysphagia to solids. He is only managing a liquid diet at the moment. He has also lost some weight. He denies reflux symptoms. His GP has started him on a trial of a proton pump inhibitor without significant improvement in his dysphagia. His blood tests are unremarkable.

What is the next most appropriate test to investigate this man's dysphagia?

A. **OGD**
B. **Barium swallow**
C. **CT scan of chest and abdomen**
D. **Videofluoroscopy**
E. **Oesophageal manometry**

CASE 40

A 47-year-old lady is referred for percutaneous endoscopic gastrostomy (PEG) placement. She has a background history of multiple sclerosis and a recent assessment revealed that she has a poor swallow and is at risk of aspiration. After discussing the benefits and risks of PEG feeding with the patient and her family, she is listed for the procedure.

Which of the following is the most common complication of PEG tube placement?

A. **PEG tube leakage**
B. **Bleeding**
C. **Peg site infection**
D. **Buried bumper syndrome**
E. **Peritonitis**

CASE 41

A 42-year-old gentleman is admitted with jaundice and right upper quadrant pain. He is known to have alcohol dependence and he has been drinking quite heavily the preceding two days. On examination, he is jaundiced but there are no stigmata of chronic liver disease. His abdomen is mildly distended with ascites and he has a tender hepatomegaly.

Blood tests reveal: Haemoglobin 91 g/litre, White cells 21.5×10^9/litre, Platelets 91×10^9/litre, Sodium 129 mmol/litre, Potassium 4.9 mmol/litre, Urea 10.9 mmol/litre, Creatinine 140 µmol/litre, Bilirubin 312 µmol/litre, ALP 141 U/litre, ALT 116 U/litre, Albumin 35 g/litre, Prothrombin time 18.5 s, C-reactive protein 36 mg/litre.

Ultrasound scan of abdomen: enlarged liver with increased echogenicity. Small volume of ascites. Spleen size normal.

What is the most likely diagnosis?

A. **Budd–Chiari syndrome**
B. **Acute hepatitis B**
C. **Alcoholic hepatitis**
D. **Acute hepatitis C**
E. **Infectious mononucleosis**

CASE 42

A 35-year-old gentleman is seen at the clinic with a 3-month history of intermittent dysphagia to mostly solids. An OGD is carried out and shows a ring-like narrowing at the distal oesophagus and this is moderately tight.

How would this patient's symptoms be best managed?

A. Reassurance and observation
B. Oesophageal dilatation
C. High-dose proton pump inhibitor
D. Surgery
E. Advice on eating slowly and chewing food properly

CASE 43

A 30-year-old woman is referred for an OGD because of a several-month history of dyspepsia associated with anorexia, weight loss and vomiting. Her OGD reveals a gastric ulcer and a rapid urease test is found to be positive.

Which of the following is the most appropriate follow-up plan for this lady?

A. Long-term maintenance dose of proton pump inhibitor
B. Avoid non-steroidal anti-inflammatory drugs in the future
C. Confirm eradication of *Helicobacter pylori* with serology
D. Repeat OGD in eight weeks and confirm eradication of *Helicobacter pylori* with a urease breath test
E. Repeat OGD in four weeks and confirm eradication of *Helicobacter pylori* with a urease breath test

CASE 44

A 62-year-old lady, who has cirrhosis secondary to primary biliary cirrhosis, presents with ascites and encephalopathy. Her ascites has proved refractory to dietary salt restriction and aggressive diuretic treatment. She has no other significant co-morbidity.

What is the next most appropriate step in this lady's management?

A. **Perform regular therapeutic paracentesis**
B. **Prescribe prophylactic antibiotics to prevent spontaneous bacterial peritonitis**
C. **Refer for liver transplant assessment**
D. **Insert transjugular intrahepatic portosystemic shunt**
E. **Insert a peritoneovenous (LeVeen) shunt**

CASE 45

A 25-year-old man is admitted with an acute onset of left-sided, crampy, abdominal pain, diarrhoea and rectal bleeding. He has no prior medical history but has a history of recreational drug use, using cocaine on a regular basis. On examination, he is tender over the left iliac fossa.

Blood tests reveal: Haemoglobin 14 g/litre, White cells 14×10^9/litre, Platelets 400×10^9/litre, Sodium 135 mmol/litre, Potassium 3.7 mmol/litre, Urea 8.0 mmol/litre, Creatinine 119 μmol/litre, C-reactive protein 65 mg/litre.

An abdominal X-ray is shown in Figure 4.8.

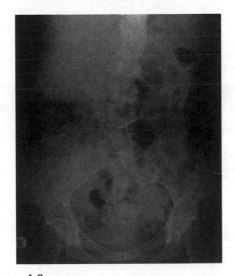

Figure 4.8

Sigmoidoscopy showed mucosal erythema, superficial ulceration and congestion with haemorrhagic nodules in the sigmoid colon.

What is the most likely diagnosis for this man's symptoms?

    A. **Ulcerative colitis**
    B. **Ischaemic colitis**
    C. *Escherichia coli* **enteritis**
    D. **Crohn's colitis**
    E. **Campylobacter enteritis**

CASE 46

A 40-year-old man presents to his local emergency department because of acute severe abdominal pain. On examination, the expected hepatic dullness on percussion is absent.

What is the most likely cause for the absent hepatic dullness?

A. **Pseudomyxoma peritonei**
B. **Hepatic abscess**
C. **Perforated duodenal ulcer**
D. **Hepatic malignancy**
E. **Ruptured hepatic cyst**

CASE 47

A 45-year-old gentleman is referred to the liver clinic because he tested positive for hepatitis C virus (HCV) when he consulted his GP and was found to have mildly abnormal transaminases. His risk factor for HCV infection is intravenous drug use when he was in his twenties. He is otherwise well and physical examination is unremarkable.

Which of the following tests is most helpful in estimating his prognosis from chronic HCV infection?

A. **HCV genotype**
B. **Liver biopsy**
C. **Viral load**
D. **ALT level**
E. **AST level**

CASE 48

A 25-year-old man, who has a background history of ulcerative colitis, is admitted with an acute severe relapse. He normally takes mesalazine 2.4 g daily. He is given intravenous prednisolone for the relapse and daily bloods are taken to monitor his biochemical response.

Blood tests on day three reveal: Haemoglobin 10.5 g/litre, White cells 14×10^9/litre, Platelets 495×10^9/litre, Sodium 135 mmol/litre, Potassium 3.5 mmol/litre, Urea 8.0 mmol/litre, Creatinine 110 μmol/litre, C-reactive protein 65 mg/litre.

He is still passing loose, bloody motions at least ten times per day at this stage.

What would be his next most appropriate management step?

A. **Continue with intravenous prednisolone for a total of one week**
B. **Commence him on azathioprine**
C. **Increase the mesalazine to 2.4 g twice daily**
D. **Consider infliximab infusion**
E. **Switch intravenous prednisolone to methylprednisolone**

CASE 49

A 25-year-old lady is seen at the gastroenterology clinic with a year's history of recurrent vomiting, chest pain and dysphagia. She has recently lost weight, which prompted the referral. Her OGD shows a small volume of food debris in her oesophagus but is otherwise normal. She also has a barium swallow which is unremarkable. Oesophageal manometry is subsequently performed and this shows aperistalsis and failure of the lower oesophageal sphincter (LES) to relax.

What is the most appropriate treatment for her?

A. **Heller myotomy**
B. **Calcium channel blocker**
C. **Botulinum toxin injection into the lower oesophageal sphincter**
D. **Nitrates**
E. **Oesophageal dilatation with a rigid dilator**

CASE 50

A 30-year-old man, who has HIV infection and a current CD4 count of 100/mm^3, is admitted with a 1-week history of bloody diarrhoea, fever and abdominal cramps. Stool cultures are negative for enteric organisms, *Clostridium difficile*, ova and parasites.

What is the next appropriate investigation for this man?

A. **CT scan of abdomen**

B. **OGD and duodenal biopsies**

C. **Mesenteric angiogram**

D. **Flexible sigmoidoscopy and colonic biopsies**

E. **MRI scan of abdomen**

CASE 51

A 40-year-old gentleman has recently been diagnosed with chronic hepatitis C infection and is referred to the hepatitis clinic for evaluation for treatment.

Blood tests reveal: Bilirubin 10 μmol/litre, ALP 80 U/litre, ALT 100 U/litre, Albumin 40 g/litre, Prothrombin time 10.0 Vs, HCV genotype: genotype two, HCV viral load: 2.5 million IU/ml.

Which of the following treatments should be offered next?

A. **Pegylated interferon alpha and ribavirin for 48 weeks**

B. **Pegylated interferon alpha and ribavirin for 24 weeks**

C. **Standard interferon and ribavirin for 24 weeks**

D. **Pegylated interferon alone for 48 weeks**

E. **Ribavirin alone for 48 weeks**

CASE 52

A 45-year-old woman, with a history of primary biliary cirrhosis, presents with fatigue, weight loss, easy bruising and diarrhoea. Stool studies show the presence of faecal fat. Her prothrombin time is prolonged.

What would be the next most appropriate plan for this woman?

A. **Pancreatic enzyme replacement**
B. **OGD and duodenal biopsies**
C. **Fat-soluble vitamin replacement**
D. **Colonoscopy and biopsies**
E. **CT scan of abdomen**

CASE 53

A 25-year-old lady presents with a 1-year history of daily abdominal pain, particulary in the right iliac fossa, associated with periods of loose motions alternating with constipation. The abdominal pain is usually relieved by defaecation and can be exacerbated before menstruation. She also complains of postprandial bloating but no weight loss. Her routine blood tests are normal. Coeliac screen is negative.

What is the next most appropriate test which would help support the clinical diagnosis for this lady?

A. **Flexible sigmoidoscopy and biopsies**
B. **Ultrasound scan of abdomen and pelvis**
C. **Colonoscopy**
D. **Faecal calprotectin**
E. **CT scan of abdomen**

CASE 1

B: Aggressive resuscitation with fluids and blood products

This gentleman has an upper gastrointestinal (GI) bleed, most likely secondary to non-steroidal anti-inflammatory drugs. He is in hypovolaemic shock and aggressive fluid and blood resuscitation is paramount in improving outcome. Oesophago-gastro-duodenoscopy (OGD) will be crucial in diagnosing the cause of his GI bleed but this should not be attempted before stabilising the patient. Proton pump inhibitor therapy can be administered before OGD, but active resuscitation of the patient remains key in the management of upper GI bleeds. Stopping his diclofenac seems sensible. Not all patients with GI bleeding require *Helicobacter pylori* eradication.

CASE 2

A: Pharyngeal pouch

The symptoms described in this case are classical for a pharyngeal pouch or Zenker's diverticulum.

Learning point

This condition tends to occur in the elderly. Other symptoms of a pharyngeal pouch could include chronic cough, aspiration pneumonia, halitosis and weight loss. The diagnosis is readily established on barium swallow. Treatment is either expectant (usually reserved for frail patients) or surgery (open neck surgery or endoscopic). Endoscopic stapling of pouches is gaining popularity as it is less invasive, allows for a shorter hospital stay and more rapid recovery.

CASE 3

E: Faecal occult blood testing

All patients with iron deficiency anaemia (IDA) should be screened for coeliac disease. Postmenopausal women and men of all age groups should have both OGD and colonoscopy to investigate IDA unless they have significant overt non-GI blood loss. Urinalysis to look for haematuria is important to rule out a renal cause. Faecal occult blood testing is of no benefit in the investigation of IDA. These recommendations are outlined in the British Society of Gastroenterology guidelines.[1]

CASE 4

C: Colestyramine

This is a case of bile acid diarrhoea or bile acid malabsorption. The presence of bile acids in the colon stimulates the secretion of water and electrolytes, hence producing a secretory-type diarrhoea. They also increase colonic motility, resulting in urgency. The mainstay of treatment for bile acid malabsorption is bile acid sequestrants such as colestyramine (widely used), colestipol and the newer agent, colesevelam.

CASE 5

B: Refer to a liver unit

This patient has paracetamol-induced acute liver failure with encephalopathy and coagulopathy. The only effective therapeutic intervention for acute liver failure is emergency liver transplantation. It is therefore important to refer such patients to a liver transplant unit without delay, especially when they are potential transplant candidates.

Learning point

There are different prognostic indicators studied, but the most widely used are the King's College Hospital criteria. These criteria include: arterial pH < 7.3 (irrespective of encephalopathy grade) after volume resuscitation, or the combination of encephalopathy grade III or above, INR > 6.5 (or prothrombin time > 100 s) and creatinine > 300 μmol/litre. It is important to manage these patients in an intensive care unit to maximise support while awaiting transfer to a liver transplant unit.

CASE 6

B: CT scan of chest, abdomen and pelvis

Once a histological diagnosis of gastric carcinoma has been made, the next step is to exclude distant metastases by performing a staging CT scan of chest, abdomen and pelvis. If the staging CT is inconclusive, or if there is uncertainty as to whether a lesion or nodule is a metastasis or not, a PET scan is usually performed. EUS is not necessary if there are distant metastases. It is, however, useful for local staging (ie for assessing depth of tumour involvement) of early gastric cancer and when endoscopic resection for early cancer is being considered.

CASE 7

D: Collagenous colitis

These histological findings are characteristic for collagenous colitis. Collagenous colitis is a type of inflammatory bowel disease termed microscopic colitis. It commonly affects middle-aged (fifth and sixth decade) women. It has a benign natural history. Certain drugs, such as omeprazole and simvastatin, have been implicated in microscopic colitis and stopping these drugs can lead to symptom resolution. Most patients do not require any treatment as they resolve spontaneously, but if they remain symptomatic, drug treatment including anti-diarrhoeal medication, steroids, 5-aminosalicylates and immunosuppression can be given.

CASE 8

A: Surveillance OGD and proton pump inhibitor therapy

Barrett's oesophagus is associated with a small risk of oesophageal carcinoma. This risk is further increased by smoking and alcohol consumption, as in this gentleman. The British Society of Gastroenterology guidelines generally recommend surveillance OGD and biopsies to detect dysplasia and early stage oesophageal cancer.[2] The interval for surveillance OGD depends on the length of the Barrett's segment and the presence of dysplasia. Continuous acid suppression with a proton pump inhibitor is advocated to control reflux symptoms and to prevent recurrent oesophagitis.

CASE 9

B: Hypertriglyceridaemia

This man has acute pancreatitis and he has risk factors for hypertriglyceridaemia (obesity and poorly controlled diabetes). Hypertriglyceridaemia is an uncommon but well-recognised cause of pancreatitis, following alcohol and gallstones. Treatment of the pancreatitis is similar, regardless of aetiology, and in this case, the hypertriglyceridaemia must be managed with optimal diabetic control and triglyceride-lowering drugs to prevent pancreatitis recurrence.

CASE 10

E: Doppler ultrasound scan of liver

The clinical presentation here is consistent with Budd–Chiari syndrome, which is due to hepatic venous outflow obstruction. It is usually caused by hypercoagulable states, either hereditary or acquired (such as the oral contraceptive pill, as in this case), and less commonly tumour invasion (eg hepatoma) or idiopathic. Doppler ultrasound is the test of choice when Budd–Chiari syndrome is suspected. Liver function tests are abnormal and the SAAG is raised in Budd–Chiari, but these are not diagnostic, only supportive.

CASE 11

D: Achalasia

The barium swallow shows a dilated oesophagus and the 'bird's beak sign', which are classical radiological features of achalasia. Barium swallow imaging can also demonstrate aperistalsis of the oesophagus and poor emptying of barium.

Learning point

Achalasia is a primary oesophageal dysmotility disorder characterised by impaired relaxation of the lower oesophageal sphincter and aperistalsis of the oesophagus. Diagnosis is confirmed on oesophageal manometry when either or both OGD and barium swallow show suggestive features.

Pseudoachalasia, caused by tumours of the gastro-oesophageal junction and gastric cardia, can have similar manometric and radiological features to primary achalasia. It is therefore important to rule these conditions out by performing an OGD.

CASE 12

A: MR cholangiopancreatography

This lady has biliary colic and obstructive jaundice, and the commonest cause is choledocholithiasis. An ultrasound scan of abdomen is usually the first investigation to investigate the gall bladder and biliary tree. However, it has only average sensitivity for detecting biliary stones. Routine contrast CT scanning of the abdomen is moderately sensitive. MR cholangiopancreatography (MRCP) is the gold standard investigation for diagnosing choledocholithiasis and it has replaced ERCP, which has become largely therapeutic. Endoscopic ultrasound (EUS) is another modality with high diagnostic performance like MRCP, and can be used as an alternative. However, the utility of EUS depends on resource availability and expertise.

CASE 13

C: Coeliac disease

All the conditions listed above could be potential causes accounting for the symptoms, but coeliac disease is the diagnosis here as indicated by the villous atrophy on duodenal biopsies. Duodenal biopsies remain the gold standard diagnostic investigation for coeliac disease. Patients with coeliac disease can present with irritable bowel-type symptoms, therefore it is always important to bear this diagnosis in mind.

CASE 14

B: Gallstone ileus

The abdominal x-ray shows small bowel obstruction. The CT scan images show portal venous gas, stones in the gall bladder with an eroded gall bladder wall, and a stone in the bowel with small bowel obstruction. These are classic images of gallstone ileus. Gallstone ileus is an uncommon cause of small bowel obstruction, but should be suspected in elderly women who present with episodic subacute small bowel obstruction. Other diagnostic imaging includes ultrasound and CT scanning of the abdomen. The treatment of choice is surgery (enterolithotomy and stone removal) to relieve the intestinal obstruction.

CASE 15

A: Start azathioprine

This man has steroid-dependent ulcerative colitis and treatment with an immunomodulator such as azathioprine or mercaptopurine is the next step-up therapy. Thiopurines are more effective than mesalazine in inducing clinical remission and are effective maintenance therapy for steroid-dependent patients. Alternatively, patients can have potentially curative surgery if they are not keen on the long-term complications of thiopurines. There is no role in switching mesalazine unless there are compliance issues or drug intolerance. Probiotics and antibiotics have limited role in chronic active ulcerative colitis.

CASE 16

C: CT scan of abdomen

Severe left iliac fossa pain associated with pyrexia strongly favours a diagnosis of diverticulitis. A CT scan of the abdomen is the investigation of choice in confirming the diagnosis. It also helps to exclude a diverticular abscess or perforation.

CASE 17

D: Intrahepatic cholestasis of pregnancy

The presentation of pruritus, particularly in the palms and soles and worse at night, and elevated bile acids are very suggestive of intrahepatic cholestasis of pregnancy.

Learning point

It is usually seen in the second and third trimesters of pregnancy. Treatment is aimed at relieving the pruritus. Early delivery may be required to reduce fetal complications. Pruritus usually disappears within days of delivery, with normalisation of serum bile acids and liver enzymes.

CASE 18

C: Faecal elastase

The image shows pancreatic calcification suggestive of chronic pancreatitis, most likely secondary to heavy alcohol consumption. The diarrhoea (typically steatorrhoea) and weight loss are most likely due to pancreatic insufficiency from his chronic pancreatitis. The most widely used non-invasive pancreatic function test is faecal elastase. It is an excellent indicator for pancreatic insufficiency, with low levels correlating with impaired pancreatic exocrine function.

CASE 19

A: Anti-parietal cell and anti-intrinsic factor antibodies

This is a case of autoimmune atrophic gastritis. Patients with this condition produce antibodies to gastric parietal cells and intrinsic factor, leading to hypo- or achlorhydria with subsequent vitamin B12 deficiency and pernicious anaemia. Serum gastrin is usually elevated due to uninhibited gastrin secretion on account of achlorhydria. The condition may be associated with other autoimmune disorders such as type 1 diabetes. Autoimmune atrophic gastritis tends to affect the fundus and body of the stomach, whereas *Helicobacter pylori*-associated gastritis predominantly affects the gastric antrum.

CASE 20

E: Haemochromatosis

The combination of arthralgia, diabetes and cirrhosis should raise the clinical suspicion of haemochromatosis. It is an autosomal recessive disorder where mutations in the *HFE* gene cause increased intestinal iron absorption leading to iron deposition in tissues, particularly the liver, heart and pancreas.

Learning point

Patients can present with liver disease, arthralgia, skin pigmentation, cardiomyopathy, diabetes and impotence in men. Diagnosis is confirmed by iron studies (typically, raised serum ferritin > 500 μg/litre and transferrin saturation > 50%) and genetic tests (*HFE* gene mutation). Treatment is with regular venesection.

CASE 21

A: Co-amoxiclav-induced cholestasis

Drug-induced liver injury should always be considered in patients presenting with liver disease. The diagnosis is based on the clinical course and pattern of liver test abnormalities. Amoxicillin rarely causes hepatotoxicity; it is the combination with clavulanic acid or the clavulanic acid itself that causes the liver injury.

Learning point

Cholestasis is the predominant feature of co-amoxiclav-induced hepatotoxicity but a hepatitis or even a combination of hepatitis and cholestasis picture can be seen. Symptoms can present at the end of treatment and up to seven weeks post treatment. Prognosis is generally good, and cholestasis resolves with drug discontinuation, although it can take up to 16 weeks for complete recovery. Cholestyramine can be used to treat the pruritus; ursodeoxycholic acid has also been used.

continued

Primary biliary cirrhosis is unlikely because patients generally have a more chronic presentation and they do not present with jaundice until their liver disease decompensates. Pancreatic malignancy has an insidious presentation. The clinical presentation and liver abnormalities are more cholestatic than hepatitic, and this would make both viral and autoimmune hepatitis unlikely.

CASE 22

B: Treat her empirically with a month's course of proton pump inhibitor

Learning point

The NICE guideline on dyspepsia (2004) recommends that either empirical treatment with a proton pump inhibitor for a month, or a 'test and treat' approach for *Helicobacter pylori* infection, should be offered first to young patients with uncomplicated dyspepsia.[3] Gastroscopy in young patients with uncomplicated dyspepsia offers a very low diagnostic yield and is therefore not necessary. Patients who are > 55 years old, on the other hand, who present with new onset dyspepsia should be offered gastroscopy.

CASE 23

C: Surgical jejunostomy

Direct feeding into the jejunum is the most appropriate type of enteral feeding because of the gastroparesis. Therefore both nasogastric tube and percutaneous endoscopic gastrostomy feeding are excluded. Options C, D and E provide direct jejunal feeding. Given the need for long-term enteral feeding, options D and E are not appropriate because these tubes are easily blocked and displaced.

CHAPTER 4
ANSWERS

CASE 24

B: *Bacillus cereus* food poisoning

Bacillus cereus is an anaerobic, spore-forming, gram-positive bacteria, which is usually found in rice dishes. It can cause both vomiting and diarrhoeal illnesses, the latter associated with a longer incubation period (8–16 hours). The diarrhoea is usually non-bloody and can be profuse. *Bacillus cereus* food poisoning is self-limiting and symptoms usually disappear within 24 hours.

CASE 25

A: Vitamin B12 deficiency

Vitamin B12 deficiency is the most likely cause because of the expected impaired vitamin B12 absorption at the inflamed terminal ileum. Patients with inflammatory bowel disease can have iron deficiency anaemia but usually this is in the setting of active colitis with persistent blood loss.

CASE 26

B: Biliary stenting

The priority for this lady is biliary decompression with a biliary stent to reduce the risk of cholangitis. Biliary stenting is purely palliative in this case, given the metastatic nature of her disease. Palliative chemotherapy should be discussed, but this would only be given once her jaundice has improved. There is no role for antibiotic prophylaxis or lymph node biopsy.

CASE 27

D: Microsporidium

Microsporidium are spore-forming parasites and can cause opportunistic intestinal infections in immunocompromised hosts such as patients with HIV or transplant patients. Microsporidiosis usually occurs when CD4 counts fall below $100/mm^3$. Typical symptoms include non-bloody diarrhoea, nausea, vomiting, abdominal pain and weight loss.

CASE 28

C: Palliative oesophageal stenting

Given his frailty, co-morbidities and age, palliative care would be the mainstay of his management. Palliative care includes palliation of his dysphagia (which is his main concern) with an oesophageal stent, and therefore should be the next most appropriate plan. Further staging investigations are not particularly useful here as they are not going to influence his management.

CASE 29

C: Epstein–Barr virus infection

Epstein–Barr virus (EBV) is the causative agent for infectious mononucleosis, which is characterised by the classical triad of pyrexia, oropharyngitis and lymphadenopathy. In the acute phase of the illness, hepatitis with resultant elevated transaminases is common and it is usually mild and self-limiting. Very rarely it can lead to fulminant hepatitis and liver failure. Diagnosis of infectious mononucleosis is made by a combination of clinical and laboratory findings, positive EBV IgM antibody and a positive heterophile antibody. Treatment is generally supportive as it is a self-limiting illness.

CHAPTER 4
ANSWERS

CASE 30

C: Stop her azathioprine

This patient has acute pancreatitis. The most likely cause for her pancreatitis is the azathioprine. It is prudent to advise the patient to stop the azathioprine immediately. Gallstone pancreatitis is another possibility and performing an ultrasound of abdomen is appropriate, but the decision to stop her azathioprine first is the key advice. If the patient is reasonably well, hospital admission is not usually required. The amylase concentration can be repeated to ensure that the pancreatitis is resolving. Azathioprine-induced pancreatitis is not uncommon, and patients must be advised to report any abdominal pain while they are taking azathioprine.

CASE 31

A: MR cholangiopancreatography

The likely diagnosis here is primary sclerosing cholangitis (PSC). PSC can complicate inflammatory bowel disease, with a higher incidence in ulcerative colitis.

Learning point

When PSC is suspected, imaging of the biliary tract must be considered and this could be either with MR cholangiopancreatography (MRCP) or ERCP. MRCP is being increasingly used because it is non-invasive and does not utilise ionising radiation. MRCP findings include focal or multiple biliary strictures and dilatation, and these can sometimes give rise to a beaded appearance of the biliary tract. Liver biopsy is rarely used in the diagnosis, but it can confer the stage and prognosis of the disease.

CASE 32

B: Zinc deficiency

Zinc deficiency can result in dermatitis (usually perioral and acral), diarrhoea, impaired taste, alopecia, anorexia, impaired wound healing and depression. The likely cause for the zinc deficiency in this case is poor dietary intake as a result of the alcohol dependence.

CASE 33

A: Mallory–Weiss tear

These are all plausible causes of haematemesis, but Mallory–Weiss tear is the diagnosis and this is suggested by the history of vomiting before the onset of haematemesis. Mallory–Weiss tears are usually associated with forceful retching, and tears are located in the distal oesophagus and proximal stomach. Most patients have a history of heavy alcohol drinking leading to vomiting. OGD is the diagnostic modality of choice to demonstrate the presence of a gastro-oesophageal tear and it is also a therapeutic modality to achieve haemostasis.

CASE 34

C: Liver biopsy

Although all these imaging modalities can demonstrate fatty liver, the only test that can reliably differentiate simple steatosis from steatohepatitis is a liver biopsy.

CASE 35

B: Doxycycline-induced oesophagitis

The temporal relationship between the onset of the oesophageal symptoms and the ingestion of doxycycline makes drug-induced oesophagitis very likely. Drug-induced oesophagitis is not uncommon but is perhaps under-recognised. Doxycycline is one of the more common antibiotics that can cause oesophagitis. This is a self-limiting condition; symptoms resolve with drug discontinuation. It can be diagnosed based on the history and clinical presentation. OGD is the diagnostic tool of choice and can be considered in patients who have severe or atypical symptoms.

CASE 36

D: *Clostridium difficile* colitis

Learning point

This lady has all the risk factors for *Clostridium difficile*-associated diarrhoea/colitis, which include advanced age, being a residential home resident, recent antibiotic use and long-term use of proton pump inhibitor. *Clostridium difficile* colitis should be suspected in patients who have received antibiotic treatment in the previous three months, those who have recently been hospitalised or who have developed diarrhoea at least 48 hours after hospitalisation. *Clostridium difficile* diarrhoea is usually mild to moderate but it can lead to fulminant colitis with toxic megacolon. The remaining listed causes tend to produce a bloody diarrhoea.

CASE 37

D: Cirrhosis

The serum ascites albumin gradient (SAAG) has largely replaced the transudate/exudate concept in the classification of ascites.

Learning point

SAAG can be calculated by subtracting the ascites fluid albumin from the serum albumin. SAAG correlates with portal pressure with good accuracy. A SAAG of 1.1 g/dl or greater reflects portal hypertension.

Causes of high SAAG ascites include cirrhosis, alcoholic hepatitis, vascular occlusion, massive hepatic metastases and congestive cardiac failure.

CASE 38

B: Tapering course of prednisolone

This acute exacerbation needs to be treated aggressively, and treatment is escalated to high-dose prednisolone, which is gradually reduced over the course of several weeks. If she had not been taking mesalazine at the maximum dose, increasing the dose in the first instance may have been appropriate, but with a low threshold to start prednisolone if the patient did not improve. Changing from one mesalazine preparation to another does not usually help in treating exacerbations. As the extent of involvement is pan-colonic, topical treatment is of limited benefit. Azathioprine has a delayed onset of action (about 2–3 months), hence it does not have a role in the treatment of acute exacerbations.

CASE 39

A: OGD

This gentleman has worrying symptoms of progressive dysphagia and weight loss, and a malignant stricture of the oesophagus needs to be excluded. The best diagnostic tool here is an OGD, which not only allows direct mucosal visualisation but also enables tissue sampling for histological confirmation. Barium swallow and oesophageal manometry are useful in cases of suspected oesophageal dysmotility. A CT scan may show oesophageal thickening but an OGD will still be required. A CT scan of the chest, abdomen and pelvis is indicated for staging purposes if a malignancy is diagnosed. Videofluoroscopy has a limited role in the investigation of oesophageal dysphagia.

CASE 40

C: Peg site infection

These are all complications associated with PEG tube placement, with buried bumper syndrome being an uncommon delayed complication. PEG site infection is the commonest complication, with a reported incidence as high as 30%. Patient factors that can predispose to a higher rate of infection include a history of diabetes and poor nutritional status. The risk of PEG site infection can be reduced by giving prophylactic antibiotics 30 minutes before the PEG placement, and by vigilant PEG tube and site care post placement.

CASE 41

C: Alcoholic hepatitis

This is a classic case of alcoholic hepatitis. Patients with alcoholic hepatitis typically have a long history of daily excessive alcohol consumption. Clinically, they have jaundice, anorexia, right upper quadrant/epigastric pain (due to tender hepatomegaly) and fever. They can also present with ascites, encephalopathy and malnutrition. Characteristically, their blood tests reveal neutrophilia, transaminitis (enzyme levels typically less than 300 U/litre with an elevated AST/ALT ratio ≥ 2), raised prothrombin time and hyperbilirubinaemia.

CASE 42

B: Oesophageal dilatation

A Schatzki's ring of the distal oesophagus is a common cause of intermittent, non-progressive dysphagia to mainly solids. Treatment depends on how symptomatic the patient is and the degree of oesophageal narrowing. In this case, the ring is moderately tight, which means that treatment other than simple advice is indicated. Oesophageal dilatation, either with a bougie dilator or balloon dilator, is the treatment of choice. It is effective, although repeat dilatation may be required if there is recurrence of dysphagia. It is advisable to treat any co-existing reflux symptoms with a proton pump inhibitor. Surgery for Schatzki's ring is rarely required.

CASE 43

D: Repeat OGD in eight weeks and confirm eradication of *Helicobacter pylori* with a urease breath test

The British Society of Gastroenterology recommends repeating an OGD in six to eight weeks in patients diagnosed with gastric ulcers to ensure complete ulcer healing.[3] Confirmation of *H. pylori* eradication is important, and confirmatory tests should be carried out at least two weeks post proton pump inhibitor treatment or four weeks post antibiotic treatment, as these drugs can suppress the bacteria and result in false negative results. Long-term proton pump inhibitor therapy is not necessary once ulcer healing has been confirmed, unless there is an indication, such as recurrent ulcers, to continue with maintenance acid suppression.

CASE 44

C: Refer for liver transplant assessment

This patient has signs of decompensated cirrhosis and, with the development of ascites, she has an expected two-year survival rate of only 50%. Therefore, this presentation should prompt a referral to a liver unit for liver transplantation assessment, especially if the patient is fit and has no other co-morbidities which preclude surgery. There is no role for prophylactic antibiotics to prevent spontaneous bacterial peritonitis. Encephalopathy is a contraindication to portosystemic shunting.

CASE 45

B: Ischaemic colitis

> **Learning point**
>
> Although ischaemic colitis is commonly seen in older patients, young patients who have certain risk factors, such as the use of illicit drugs like cocaine (as in this case), vasculitis and long-distance running, can develop ischaemic colitis. Symptoms are usually acute and self-limiting. The rectal bleeding seen in ischaemic colitis is usually mild. If colitis is severe, transmural infarction can result in peritonism.

The sigmoid colon and splenic flexure are the regions most often affected because they are the so-called 'watershed areas'. Endoscopic findings vary depending on the severity of ischaemia, but haemorrhagic nodules are fairly typical. Treatment depends on the acuteness and severity of the clinical presentation. In most cases, no specific therapy is required because the condition is transient and symptoms resolve spontaneously.

CASE 46

C: Perforated duodenal ulcer

The absence of hepatic dullness on percussion is suggestive of free air in the peritoneal cavity and the most likely cause is a perforated viscus.

CASE 47

B: Liver biopsy

Liver biopsy is the best test for prognosticating patients with HCV infection. Key histological indicators for progression to cirrhosis include the degree of inflammation, fibrosis and steatosis. Patients with mild inflammation and no/minimal fibrosis have a low risk of progressing to cirrhosis. ALT has been used to predict liver inflammation and fibrosis but at any one point in time; ALT correlates poorly with liver histology. Viral load is useful in monitoring response to antiviral treatment.

CASE 48

D: Consider infliximab infusion

CHAPTER 4
ANSWERS

> **Learning point**
>
> It is important to assess the response to intravenous steroids early in the management of patients with acute severe ulcerative colitis, as failure to respond to steroids predicts a colectomy rate of 85% during that admission. If patients continue to have frequent, loose motions (> 8 per day), C-reactive protein is > 45 mg/litre and stool frequency is between three and eight per day (the Travis criteria), patients are considered as steroid non-responders, as in this case. At this juncture, colectomy or medical salvage therapy either with infliximab or ciclosporin must be considered and discussed with the patient. Switching to an alternative steroid or maximising mesalazine treatment is not effective. Azathioprine takes a few weeks to work, hence there is no role in the treatment of acute severe colitis.

CASE 49

A: Heller myotomy

This is a case of achalasia with characteristic manometric findings. Graded pneumatic dilatation or Heller myotomy with partial fundoplication (to reduce risk of reflux) remains the first-line treatment for young patients, patients who are fit and willing to consider surgery. Botulinum toxin injection is usually reserved for patients who are not suitable for either dilatation or surgery, and the therapeutic effect is quite short-lasting (about six months). Dilatation using standard rigid dilators (bougies) or balloon dilators is not sufficiently effective in disrupting the muscles of the lower oesophageal sphincter to provide clinical relief. Drugs are the least effective treatment modality, and their use is commonly limited by side effects.

CASE 50

D: Flexible sigmoidoscopy and colonic biopsies

Cytomegalovirus (CMV) colitis is a frequent cause of bloody diarrhoea in immunocompromised patients in whom other infective causes have been ruled out. Flexible sigmoidoscopy usually shows mucosal inflammation with ulcerations and erosions. Staining of colonic biopsies with haematoxylin and eosin reveals giant cells with inclusion bodies (owl's eyes), which are characteristic for CMV colitis. Biopsies can also be sent for PCR testing to identify the CMV. CT and MRI scans of abdomen will show colitis but cannot determine aetiology. Mesenteric angiography is useful if mesenteric ischaemia is suspected, but this is unlikely in this young patient. Gluten-sensitive enteropathy does not cause bloody diarrhoea, hence duodenal biopsies would be unhelpful in this case.

CASE 51

B: Pegylated interferon alpha and ribavirin for 24 weeks

The current recommendation for chronic HCV treatment is a combination treatment with pegylated interferon and ribavirin. The duration of treatment depends on the virus genotype. Patients with genotypes two and three are treated for 24 weeks, whereas genotype one patients require 48 weeks of treatment.

CASE 52

C: Fat-soluble vitamin replacement

Learning point

Patients with primary biliary cirrhosis are at risk of developing fat malabsorption and consequently fat-soluble vitamin deficiencies, in this case vitamin K deficiency. This is due to impaired bile acid flow into the intestinal lumen and subsequently reduced amounts of micelles required for fat absorption. Replacement of fat-soluble vitamins is crucial in preventing or correcting complications caused by the deficiencies. A fat-restricted diet is usually necessary; patients should consume alternative calorie-providing substitutes. A medium-chain triglyceride diet is another alternative.

Options A and B are also reasonable answers, especially in cases where weight loss and steatorrhoea are prominent.

CHAPTER 4
ANSWERS

CASE 53

D: Faecal calprotectin

Learning point

This lady has symptoms which fulfil the Rome III criteria for irritable bowel syndrome (IBS): recurrent abdominal pain for at least three days/month for the preceding three months, associated with two or more of the following: 1. pain that improves with defaecation; 2. onset associated with a change in stool frequency; and 3. onset associated with a change in stool form.

The diagnosis of IBS is usually made on the clinical history and is supported by normal blood tests. However, in some patients, distinguishing IBS from inflammatory bowel disease (IBD) may not be that clear cut. NICE recommends the use of faecal calprotectin in distinguishing between IBS and IBD. Calprotectin is a protein found in the cytosol of neutrophils and faecal calprotectin is a sensitive marker for detecting intestinal inflammation. Hence, if the test is negative, this would support IBS and avoid unnecessary invasive procedures.

References

1. Goddard A et al. 2011. Guidelines for the Management of Iron Deficiency Anaemia. Gut, 60, 1309–1316

2. Fitzgerald R et al. 2014. British Society of Gastroenterology guidelines on the diagnosis and management of Barrett's oesophagus. Gut, 63, 7–42

3. NICE. 2014. Dyspepsia and gastro-oesophageal reflux disease: Investigation and management of dyspepsia, symptoms suggestive of gastro-oesophageal reflux disease, or both. NICE clinical guideline 184. www.nice.org.uk/guidance/cg184

Geriatric Medicine

Ciarán Trolan

CASE 1

A 92-year-old lady is admitted from her care home with a 3-day history of having taken nothing orally, including her medications. She has a history of Alzheimer's disease, type 2 diabetes (on metformin and saxagliptin), and has been treated by her GP for several urinary tract infections. Normally she mobilises independently with a Zimmer rollator and requires assistance of one person with personal care and toileting due to macular degeneration. History taking is impaired by hypoactive delirium. There is no evidence of a systemic inflammatory response. A chest X-ray is normal and a 12-lead ECG shows sinus rhythm. Urinalysis could not be reliably obtained due to newly acquired double incontinence.

Her bloods tests are as follows: Sodium 169 mmol/litre, Potassium 3.9 mmol/litre, CO_2 22 mmol/litre, Urea 18.7 mmol/litre, Creatinine 210 µmol/litre, Glucose 42 mmol/litre, Ketones 0.2 mmol/litre, C-reactive protein 16 mg/litre, Haemoglobin 98 g/dl, MCV 94 fl, White cells 9.8×10^9/litre.

Which of the following would be the most appropriate course of action?

- A. **Commence on intravenous co-amoxiclav**
- B. **Obtain urine for urinalysis and/or culture with an 'in and out' catheter**
- C. **Discuss with the next of kin about palliative care**
- D. **Pass a nasogastric tube to facilitate use of metformin**
- E. **Commence on an intravenous insulin infusion and fluid replacement**

CASE 2

A 92-year-old man is admitted from his nursing home with reduced oral intake over several days. He has had vascular dementia for approximately eight years. He is nursed in bed and requires assistance with feeding. He has no significant communication. He takes thickened fluids and a pureed diet but unfortunately has had four hospitalisations in the last six months with aspiration pneumonitis. He has a history of ischaemic heart disease, a previous partial anterior circulation infarct and type 2 diabetes. His medications are glimepiride, liraglutide, perindopril, aspirin and fenofibrate. He is detected to be in atrial fibrillation for the first time during this hospitalisation. Capillary blood glucose is 7.1 mmol/litre.

What would be an appropriate course of action regarding his medications?

A. **Commence a statin**
B. **Commence an oral anticoagulant**
C. **Stop glimepiride and liraglutide, and give rapid-acting insulin**
D. **Titrate perindopril to achieve a target blood pressure of < 125/70 mmHg**
E. **Switch glimepiride to metformin**

CASE 3

You are in a memory clinic. A 61-year-old barrister attends for the second time. He previously attended 12 months ago after he found it difficult to speak publicly. In the interim, he has now noticed some problems with anterograde recall and he can no longer follow conversations with more than one person. The Addenbrooke's cognitive examination score was 76/100. You note multiple syntax errors and marked loss of verbal fluency. His past medical history includes hypertension and hazardous use of alcohol. He has a 20 pack year smoking history. Investigations undertaken since his previous appointment include a normal indices for urea and electrolytes profile, vitamin B12, folate, full blood picture and thyroid function. His ECG showed sinus rhythm. An MRI scan of the brain showed minor cerebral atrophy only.

Which is the most likely dementia subtype?

A. **Posterior cortical atrophy**
B. **Semantic (logopenic) dementia**
C. **Dementia with Lewy bodies**
D. **Vascular dementia**
E. **Fronto-temporal lobe dementia**

CASE 4

You are fast-bleeped to the emergency department following an ambulance service pre-alert about a 'FAST-positive' patient currently in transit. You establish that the she is an 85-year-old lady with a history of atrial fibrillation for which she receives warfarin. Her INR was last checked two weeks ago and was 1.9. Other past medical history includes hypertension, heart failure, type 2 diabetes and hyperlipidaemia. She has no known allergies.

On arrival you find moderate expressive and receptive aphasia, right upper and lower limb drift to bed and a lower right facial droop. She is right-hand dominant. Her husband witnessed the onset of her symptoms 62 minutes ago.

An unenhanced CT scan of the brain is reported as 'No intracranial haemorrhage'. Her point-of-care INR is 1.4. Blood glucose is 5.6 mmol/litre and blood pressure is 152/60 mmHg.

The patient is unable to consent but her husband assents to 'whatever treatment you think is right'.

What would be the most appropriate treatment?

A. **Give aspirin 300 mg**
B. **Give aspirin 75 mg and clopidogrel 75 mg**
C. **Give apixaban 2.5 mg**
D. **Give intravenous tissue plasminogen activator (tPA)**
E. **Refer to local interventional neuroradiologist for clot removal and give IV tPA**

CASE 5

You are in the neurovascular rapid access clinic where you assess a 52-year-old, right-hand dominant, taxi driver. He smokes 25 g of roll-up tobacco a week. Two days ago, he describes a transient left monocular visual loss of sudden onset and gradual offset lasting 15 minutes. Peripheral and central nervous system examinations detect lifelong strabismus only. Blood pressure was 158/94 mmHg. His GP commenced aspirin 300 mg and simvastatin 40 mg on the day of referral.

An MRI scan of brain at the clinic reveals no infarction or haemorrhage. A Doppler ultrasound carotid examination reveals a 60% stenosis of the left internal carotid artery and a 70% stenosis of right internal carotid artery. The resting 12-lead ECG was in sinus rhythm.

What is the priority for management?

A. Arrange left carotid endarterectomy
B. Arrange right carotid endarterectomy
C. Arrange a CT-angiogram of his aortic arch to the circle of Willis
D. Arrange 24-hour ambulatory blood pressure monitoring
E. Commence perindopril 2 mg daily and titrate against his blood pressure

CASE 6

It is 0200 h, and you are the medical registrar on-call in a district general hospital. You are fast-bleeped to the resuscitation room and upon your arrival you find a 50-year-old woman with a Glasgow Coma Scale of 13/15. She is severely aphasic and has a right homonymous hemianopia. There appears to be right hemi-attention. The onset of her symptoms was witnessed by her husband at 0010 h. There was no trauma. Her blood pressure is 245/105 mmHg and her heart rate is 88 bpm on the monitor. She is taking no regular medications. She begins to vomit en route to the CT scanner. A CT scan of brain is reported as showing a subcortical, left parietal haematoma approximately 2 × 2.2 cm in size. There is very minimal surrounding oedema.

Which is the most appropriate immediate management option?

- A. **Aggressively lower systolic blood pressure to a target of 130–150 mmHg**
- B. **Lower systolic blood pressure to a target of < 180 mmHg**
- C. **Give prothrombin complex concentrate**
- D. **Place intermittent pneumatic compression hosiery**
- E. **Recommend an extraventricular drain to the neurosurgical team**

CASE 7

You assess an octogenarian man at the multidisciplinary falls clinic. His Barthel index is 19/20. His 'timed get up and go' is 4.3 seconds. The Berg balance score was 42/45. When you delve into his history, he tells you that he has suffered three episodes of transient loss of consciousness in the last four months that had resulted in his falls, including one that occurred when sitting over the sink in his barber's. In addition, he has experienced multiple near falls and is now reluctant to leave the home.

Past medical history includes mild cognitive impairment, hyperlipidaemia and poliomyelitis resulting in a left lower limb monoparesis.

Chest auscultation was normal. His monoparesis is effectively addressed with an ankle–foot orthosis. There was no reproducible orthostatic hypotension at 0, 1 and 3 minutes but his heart rate rose from 75 bpm on lying to 95 bpm on standing.

The resting 12-lead ECG showed normal sinus rhythm. Right-sided carotid sinus massage is performed in the semi-recumbent position with verbal consent. He has jerking of all four limbs for approximately 10 seconds. The rhythm strip is shown in Figure 5.1.

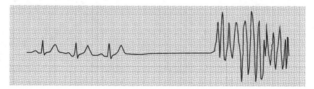

Figure 5.1

His medications are simvastatin, tamsulosin and bendroflumethiazide.

What is the diagnosis?

- A. **Dysautonomic syncope**
- B. **Partial motor seizures**
- C. **Carotid body hypersensitivity**
- D. **Postural orthostatic tachycardia syndrome**
- E. **Posterior circulation transient ischaemic attacks**

CASE 8

A 71-year-old woman with a history of osteoporosis and coeliac disease is reviewed at the falls clinic. She had an L3 vertebral fracture and a Colles' fracture a decade ago. Her menopause occurred at 32 years. She has been taking bisphosphonates for eight years. Since her last attendance two years ago she has lost height. You review her serial dual-energy X-ray absorptiometry (DEXA) scan results.

Site	T-score	
	2013	2015
L1	−2.8	−2.9
L2	−2.7	−2.6
L3	−0.5	−0.9
L4	−3.0	−1.4
Left neck of femur	−2.8	−3.1

Table 5.1: Bone mineral density results

What is the most likely explanation of the above findings?

    A. **New fracture of lumbar vertebra**
    B. **Osteoblastic activity up-regulation by alendronate**
    C. **Osteoclastic activity down regulation by alendronate**
    D. **Poor adherence to alendronate**
    E. **Malpositioning of the patient in the scanner**

CASE 9

A previously active 77-year-old woman is reviewed at the bone health clinic giving a 6-week history of back pain. It is markedly impairing her functional status. An MRI scan undertaken two weeks following her initial presentation to the emergency department reveals a 40% loss of vertebral height at T10. She is tender over T10. She has no known active cancer. She finds her COPD and exercise tolerance is worse since the onset of pain. Her pain is refractory to oxycodone 125 mg BD and paracetamol 1 g QDS. She was intolerant of gabapentin and pregabalin. She has declined a back brace.

What is the next most appropriate step?

A. **Refer to chronic pain service**
B. **Admit for a period of spinal traction**
C. **Increase oxycodone dose**
D. **Refer for vertebroplasty**
E. **Give subcutaneous calcitonin at the clinic**

CASE 10

A 65-year-old obstetrician fell off her mountain bike sustaining a fractured neck of femur. She is the carer for her partner who has multiple sclerosis. The orthopaedic surgeon suggested a general anaesthetic (GA); however, she previously had awareness under GA for a Caesarean section. A subsequent Caesarean section was uneventful when spinal anaesthesia was used. She asks you about the risk of post-operative cognitive dysfunction.

What is the likely incidence of long-term (over one year) post-operative cognitive dysfunction in her situation?

A. **0–9%**
B. **10–29%**
C. **30–49%**
D. **50–69%**
E. **70–89%**

CASE 11

What is the implantable device shown in Figure 5.2?

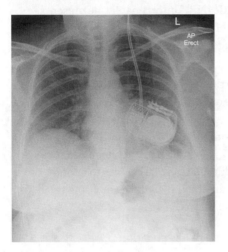

Figure 5.2

    A. Permanent pacemaker
    B. Cardiac resynchronisation therapy defibrillator
    C. Spinal cord stimulator device
    D. Deep brain stimulator device
    E. Implantable loop recorder

CASE 12

A 73-year-old man who has atrial fibrillation presents with an acute motor lacunar syndrome in the setting of a sub-therapeutic INR. Unfortunately, he presents outside the thrombolysis window. He rehabilitates well and is discharged three days later with the early supported discharge scheme. Warfarin is switched to rivaroxaban.

He re-presents three weeks later with a further stroke in the same vascular territory. There had been no witnessed seizure activity and he cannot provide history due to new moderate aphasia. A CT scan of brain reveals no acute changes and rivaroxaban is continued. Again he makes a substantial recovery within 24 hours. However, over the next 72 hours, he has further episodes of deterioration in power without recovery. Cumulatively he evolves to a total anterior circulation syndrome. Serial CT scan of brain confirms multiple small areas of newly acquired, subcortical cerebral infarct.

What would be the most appropriate next line of investigation?

A. **Doppler carotid ultrasound**
B. **CT angiography of the craniocervical vessels**
C. **MR angiography of the intracranial vessels**
D. **Anti-Xa levels**
E. **Electroencephalogram (EEG)**

CASE 13

A 69-year-old woman attends a general elderly care clinic. She has recently been diagnosed with human immunodeficiency virus type 1 (HIV-1) infection, but has no other significant past medical history. She is concerned about her future health and asks what screening tests she would require.

Which of the following screening tests is most relevant in planning her future management?

A. **Abdominal ultrasound scan**
B. **Annual colonoscopy**
C. **Annual mammogram**
D. **Dual-energy X-ray absorptiometry (DEXA)**
E. **Three-yearly cervical screening**

CASE 14

An 82-year-old retired politician is reviewed at the movement disorder clinic. He has had idiopathic Parkinson's disease for almost 18 years. Dyskinesias have proven difficult to manage. Drooling and erectile dysfunction are the patient's primary complaints. At the last review, three months ago, rasagiline was added. His wife reports problems with nocturnal agitation. When he wakes at night, he dismantles the radio and television, and can reorganise the books in his library. All tasks are left incomplete. In recent weeks when shopping or in their local bowls club, he has been vocalising inappropriately and loudly, often with sexual profanity. He currently takes co-beneldopa 125 mg six times/day, co-beneldopa dispersible 62.5 mg at 0600 hours, co-beneldopa controlled release at 2200 hours, rivastigmine 1.5 mg BD and rasagiline 1 mg OD.

What would be an appropriate next step?

- A. **Withdraw rasagiline**
- B. **Add galantamine**
- C. **Increase rivastigmine dose**
- D. **Add donepezil**
- E. **Stop co-beneldopa controlled release**

CASE 15

A 42-year-old hospital porter is seen to fall to the ground on the hospital's closed-circuit television by the security team at 0000 hours. You see him as a stroke thrombolysis call within 32 minutes of onset of symptoms. The National Institutes of Health stroke score (NIHSS) is 24. CT scan of brain and history identified no contraindication to thrombolysis. He receives IV tissue plasminogen activator. At two hours, his NIHSS is 12. On the consultant ward round the next morning, he has deteriorated. The Glasgow Coma score is 12/15 and NIHSS is 25. Repeat CT brain is shown in Figure 5.3.

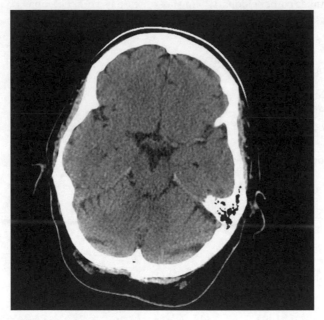

Figure 5.3

What is the diagnosis?

  A. Haemorrhagic transformation of acute ischaemic stroke
  B. Non-convulsive status epilepticus
  C. Malignant middle cerebral artery syndrome
  D. Further acute ischaemic stroke
  E. Aspiration pneumonitis

CASE 16

A 90-year-old man is found by his carers on the floor actively seizing. He is brought to hospital immediately by ambulance. A non-contrast CT brain scan does not reveal any acute abnormality. Delirium persists. He is noted to have a history of gradual cognitive decline in the preceding year. The MRI is shown in Figure 5.4.

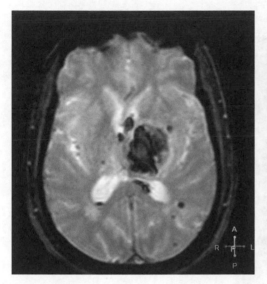 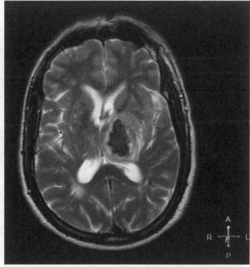

Figure 5.4

What is the most likely diagnosis?

    A. **Cerebral amyloid angiopathy**
    B. **Chronic small vessel disease**
    C. **Subarachnoid haemorrhage**
    D. **Corticobasal degeneration**
    E. **Acute cerebral infarct**

CASE 17

A 76-year-old man has been attending the movement disorder clinic for three years. He is now falling almost thrice weekly. He has significant postural instability and retropulsion. Orthostatic hypotension and flushing episodes are problematic. In the last year, he has suffered from 'sun-downing', rapid-eye-movement sleep behaviour disorder, marked cognitive decline and visual hallucinations. An MRI is undertaken and is shown in Figure 5.5.

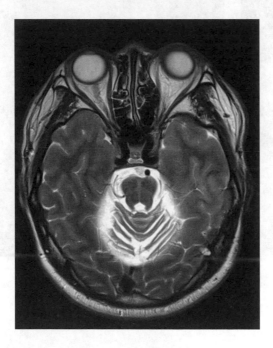

Figure 5.5

What is the most likely diagnosis?

    A. **Progressive supranuclear palsy (PSP)**

    B. **Dementia with Lewy bodies**

    C. **Vascular parkinsonism**

    D. **Idiopathic Parkinson's disease**

    E. **Multisystem atrophy**

CASE 18

You are the medical registrar on-call in a district general hospital. An elderly woman has suffered an intracranial haemorrhage and is presently unconscious. The admitting house officer has spoken with her next of kin and suggested that the likelihood of survival at one month is around 10%. This was on the basis of using a largely unvalidated prognostication tool. You are asked to see her by a nurse on the ward regarding stopping fluids. On examination her Glasgow Coma score is 4/15 (E1 V1 M2). You notice fluctuations in pupillary size and regular, non-volitional eye movements.

What is the most appropriate next step?

A. **Urgent CT scan of brain**
B. **IV benzodiazepines**
C. **Undertake an electroencephalogram**
D. **Erect a continuous subcutaneous infusion containing midazolam 30 mg**
E. **Stop IV fluids**

CASE 19

An otherwise fit and well 70-year-old woman with an overactive bladder and urinary incontinence has tried all conservative treatments for her problems and multiple drugs have proved ineffective. You review her at the multidisciplinary continence clinic and discuss surgical and non-surgical options. She is adamant she will not self-catheterise and really does not like the idea of botulinum toxin therapy, as a friend had a terrible experience when she had it injected as part of a cosmetic procedure.

What is the most appropriate next therapeutic step?

A. **Transcutaneous sacral nerve stimulation**
B. **Percutaneous sacral nerve stimulation**
C. **Cystic intramural botulinum toxin A injection**
D. **Percutaneous posterior tibial nerve stimulation**
E. **Urinary diversion procedure**

CASE 1

E: Commence on an intravenous insulin infusion and fluid replacement

This is a not uncommon presentation, ie a care-home-dependent person with late onset dementia who retains significant independence. If a person is unable to provide you with a history personally, it is vital that you gather information from other sources to complete the picture.

This woman has a hyperosmolar, hypernatraemic, hyperglycaemic syndrome resulting from her being incapable of taking her oral hypoglycaemic agents. This is an entirely reversible condition and the appropriate course of action would be to correct her hyperglycaemic and dehydrated state rapidly using an intravenous insulin infusion and fluid replacement. It is possible to calculate her total body water, water deficit and a safe sodium correction rate. It may be several days before delirium and oral intake improve let alone a precipitant be identified. A urinary tract infection is a possible precipitant here, and elderly patients often do not generate a marked response in their inflammatory markers. Inserting a urinary catheter with the explicit purpose of obtaining a urine sample is not good clinical practice.

It would be inappropriate to opt for an end-of-life approach to care in the absence of an explicit advance care directive, particularly given the presence of potentially an easily reversible state. Patients with dementia have a foreshortened life expectancy, shortening further the later in life the diagnosis is made.

CASE 2

C: Stop glimepiride and liraglutide, and give rapid-acting insulin

This man is probably in the last few months of his life and potentially the last few weeks of his life. It is less likely that death is imminent within days. The Diabetes UK End of Life Strategy document offers guidance on a systematic approach to the management of diabetes in the last year, the last few months, few weeks and few days of life. This includes: the management of hypoglycaemic and hyperglycaemic episodes, drug selection, ethical considerations and high-quality care in different settings at the end of life.

Learning point

Aggressive modification of this man's cardiovascular risk factors is not a therapeutic priority at this stage in his dementia process. For this patient, the most appropriate action would involve discontinuing hypoglycaemics and his injectable GLP-1 analogue (liraglutide). There is time to establish an insulin monotherapy regimen. If he had a pre-prandial capillary blood glucose of > 20 mmol/litre or 2+ glycosuria, administration of rapid-acting insulin with a glucose recheck at two hours would be appropriate. If he needs two doses of rapid-acting insulin in 24 hours, insulin glargine would be appropriate. If he had already been on an insulin regimen, simplification of this to a once-daily injection would be preferable.

CASE 3

B: Semantic (logopenic) dementia

The many types of dementia present in different ways, usually converging to a similar conglomeration of symptoms and involvement of cognitive domains, and even physical examination findings, eg parkinsonian facies.

> **Learning point**
>
> If there is predominance in language difficulties at the outset, the disease process may well represent a semantic variant of Alzheimer's disease. Other cognitive domains may not be involved until later.

Similarly, posterior cortical atrophy usually presents with predominantly visual symptoms ranging from visual agnosia to failure to recognise graphemes (letters, numbers and symbols).

There is no mention of any impulse control disorder or personality changes that one may expect with fronto-temporal lobe dementia. Vascular dementia could well account for his symptoms, although the MRI brain did not support this. Patients who have dementia with Lewy bodies often have marked fluctuations in their behaviour, visual or auditory hallucinations, and go on to develop prominent parkinsonian features within 12 months. Patients with Parkinson's disease dementia usually develop cognitive impairment after the first 12 months of the physical features of parkinsonism.

CASE 4

E: Refer to local interventional neuroradiologist for clot removal and give IV tPA

> ### Learning point
>
>
>
> This patient has presented within the treatment window for thrombolysis of hyperacute ischaemic stroke. She has also presented within the timeframe for clot removal (mechanical thrombectomy). It is generally considered safe to use tissue plasminogen activator (tPA) when the INR is < 1.7. Her age is outside the European licence for IV tPA; however, evidence from IST-3, a large, randomised, controlled trial, suggests that it is safe and effective to use IV tPA in selected patients over the age of 80 years.[1] A 'normal CT brain' scan is not a contraindication to thrombolysis, as changes of acute ischaemia are not always evident. Diabetes and having had a previous stroke carries a higher risk of haemorrhagic transformation with thrombolysis and this should be mentioned during the consent process.

There is no evidence to support use of rapid anticoagulation in hyperacute stroke.

The NIHSS (National Institute of Health Stroke Scale) is a rapid examination tool used to assess hyperacute stroke patients. This patient's stroke symptoms are certainly disabling enough to consider thrombolysis. Since February 2015, the recommendation from the European Stroke Organisation is to offer intra-arterial options as a first line option. IV tPA can be given as a 'bridging therapy'. The evidence base is emerging rapidly. In the UK, in the vast majority of hospitals, intravenous thrombolysis is the first line of treatment.

CHAPTER 5
ANSWERS

CASE 5

A: Arrange left carotid endarterectomy

This history is suggestive of anterior ischaemic optic neuropathy of retrobulbar origin, ie amaurosis fugax. The ultrasound Doppler examination of his carotids has identified symptomatic carotid stenosis on the left side. The right-sided stenosis is currently asymptomatic.

Learning point

In male patients, the benefits of carotid endarterectomy are seen at the lower threshold of 50% stenosis, in comparison to 60% in women. Surgery reduces the risk of having a disabling stroke by almost 50% in symptomatic stenoses. Ideally, carotid endarterectomy should be performed within 48 hours and certainly within two weeks as per Royal College of Physicians guidelines.[2] Asymptomatic stenoses may merit surgery at 70% narrowing, with a 30% reduction of stroke at three years.

It would be prudent to also manage his blood pressure aggressively; however, this is not the immediate priority. A once-off hypertensive blood pressure reading may not necessarily be clinically significant; to that end, confirmation of a true hypertensive state with ambulatory blood pressure monitoring would be reasonable.

CASE 6

A: Aggressively lower systolic blood pressure to a target of 130–150 mmHg

The prevailing paradigm until fairly recently was that blood pressure should not be lowered due to the theorised increased risk of ischaemia on the basis of reduced cerebral perfusion pressure.

> ### Learning point
>
> The INTERACT and INTERACT-2 trials demonstrated that reduction in haematoma expansion and perihaematomal oedema volume reduces mortality and post-stroke disability.[3, 4] The target systolic blood pressure should be 130–150 mmHg.

Extraventricular drains can be helpful primarily in posterior fossa strokes. No clear guidance on their use currently exists. The CLOTS-3 trial demonstrated a reduction of venous thromboembolic events in patients in whom intermittent pneumatic compression hosiery is used, for patients with both haemorrhagic and ischaemic strokes,[5] but blood pressure control takes priority.

Prothrombin complex concentrate should only be used in patients who are known to have vitamin K antagonism. The dose will be guided by the international normalised ratio and the patient's weight.

CASE 7

C: Carotid body hypersensitivity

The NICE guidance on transient loss of consciousness (TLoC) recommends carotid sinus massage for patients over 65 years old. In this octogenarian, you have identified carotid body hypersensitivity resulting in a pause and subsequent TLoC. It is often the case that cardiogenic syncope is misdiagnosed as epileptiform seizure activity due to the movements that are seen with cerebral hypoxia. His Barthel index indicates a good functional status despite cognitive impairment. 'Timed get up and go' and Berg balance score are indicative of a fairly sprightly man. It is likely that providing him with a permanent pacemaker will have a significant impact on his quality and quantity of life.

CASE 8

A: New fracture of lumbar vertebra

There is a trick here. There has been deterioration in hip T-scores but a simultaneous and counterintuitive improvement in the collective lumbar vertebral scores. Positioning of the patient in the scanner can account for variations in results obtained, but in this patient the improvement in the score is sizeable.

> ### Learning point
>
> The explanation in this case is a crush fracture of L4 being interpreted as an increase in bone mineral density by the computer algorithm. This highlights the importance of not being a slave to numbers and the need to review the accompanying image.

It is important to educate patients on how to take bisphosphonates correctly, ie upright, on an empty stomach, with plenty of water. Otherwise the drug effectiveness can be markedly reduced. Bisphosphonate 'holidays' (ie time off therapy) can be deployed in some patients in whom long-term therapy is anticipated. The trial data are emerging.

CASE 9

D: Refer for vertebroplasty

You may note the absence of lidocaine patch as an option for pain relief. The only licensed indication for these patches is post-herpetic neuralgia. Calcitonin is indicated for the prevention of acute bone loss due to sudden immobilisation, such as in patients with recent osteoporotic fractures; however, this therapy is not commonly used as it not infrequently causes nausea.

Non-invasive treatments in the form of back braces and immobilisation are poorly tolerated, but should be explored nonetheless.

Percutaneous vertebroplasty and balloon kyphoplasty are options for relieving pain, supporting the spine and reducing the risk of future fractures. The former procedure involves direct injection of bone cement into the vertebral body. The latter involves the insertion of a balloon into the vertebral body, slowly inflating it until vertebral height is restored (with the option for metal stenting) and then filling both with cement. NICE recommend that stents should not be used.[6]

> **Learning point**
>
> Vertebroplasty or kyphoplasty should be offered to any patient in whom there is inadequate pain control, failure of other conservative measures and pain confirmed to be where the fracture is.

CHAPTER 5 ANSWERS

CASE 10

B: 10–29%

Learning point

Risk factors for delirium include: age over 65 years, polypharmacy, premorbid functional dependence, premorbid cognitive impairment, metabolic/electrolyte disturbance, hip fracture, stroke and HIV infection.

Post-operative cognitive dysfunction is most probably under-recognised. Post-operatively, 15–53% of patients will have delirium and this figure increases to 70–87% of patients in intensive care settings. Some evidence would suggest 10–20% of medical patients have delirium at presentation and a further 10–30% develop it during hospitalisation. Patients with delirium have an increased length of stay, increased mortality and increased risk of institutional placement. Hospital mortality rate of patients with delirium range from 6 to 18% and are twice that of matched controls. There is a higher risk of hospital-acquired complications such as pressure sores and falls. The one-year mortality rate associated with cases of delirium is 35–40%. Delirium sufferers are three times more likely to develop dementia.

There are a multitude of instruments that can be used as screening tools for delirium, eg CAM-cog, 4AT.

CASE 11

D: Deep brain stimulator device

The direction of the leads confirms the nature of the device. Note that they are directed cranially. Implantable loop recorders do not have tunnelled leads. Spinal stimulators normally have a lead anchor point and stimulation areas can number 4–8 (quadripolar and octrode); multiple leads are required for bilateral spinal cord stimulation. Cardiac resynchronisation devices and pacemakers will be self-evident, with leads directed towards the myocardium.

Devices are likely to become increasingly common, more particularly with the wider use of implantable loop recorders, cardiac resynchronisation devices and deep brain stimulators.

CASE 12

B: CT angiography of the craniocervical vessels

> ### Learning point
>
> Patients with an acute ischaemic stroke can deteriorate because of intracranial haemorrhage, further ischaemic stroke, seizure activity, hypoglycaemia, cerebral oedema and sepsis.

This patient is fully anticoagulated yet continues to have ischaemic events, making atrial fibrillation less likely to be the cause. Anti-Xa levels are not a clinically reliable mechanism for testing the effectiveness of rivaroxaban.

EEG interictally is less useful than a trace recorded during a seizure. Although the post-seizure state can mimic stroke symptoms for several days, this man has radiologically confirmed stroke changes, making seizures alone an unlikely explanation for his developments. Stroke can of course act as a substrate for seizures.

The likely aetiology here is stenosis of the craniocervical vessels. This could be intracranial or extracranial, hence CT is to be preferred above Doppler ultrasound in this instance, and in preference to limited intracranial vessels with the MR option. Dependent upon the scanner in use and clinical question to be answered, CT is often superior to MR angiography and for this reason you should discuss the options with your radiology department.

CASE 13

D: Dual-energy X-ray absorptiometry (DEXA)

HIV screening is frequently neglected in the older age groups, with over half those living with HIV in the UK aged 30–49 years. The number of people living with HIV in the UK has trebled in the last decade. Given that the life expectancy of many of those carrying the virus is now nearing that of seronegative patients, geriatricians of the future can expect to encounter the condition more often than they do presently.

> ### Learning point
>
> Some antiretroviral regimens can result in a reduction of bone mineral density with a resultant increased risk of fragility fracture. Vigilance in that respect is prudent through the use of DEXA scanning.

There is evidence that seropositive women are at higher risk of cervical and vulval cancer, and that all seropositive individuals are at higher risk of anal neoplasia, non-Hodgkin's and Hodgkin's lymphoma, hepatocellular carcinoma and Kaposi's sarcoma. The risk is due to co-infection with other oncogenic viruses and the reduced immune response to development of neoplasia.

There is no known increased risk of breast, colorectal, prostate and many other cancers so screening programmes should follow the national strategies for the general population. Use of antiretroviral therapy can help reduce the risk of AIDS-defining malignancies.

CASE 14

A: Withdraw rasagiline

A convenient rule of thumb with regard to medications in parkinsonism is: 'last in, first out'. Punding is a behaviour seen with dopamine stimulation, taking the form of complex, prolonged, repetitive and purposeless actions. The attempts by others to intervene are often greeted with irritability and dysphoria, but the patient often acknowledges the futility and disruptive nature of the behaviour.

Punding differs somewhat from impulse control disorders, which form a spectrum of disorders ranging from pathological gambling, shopping and hypersexuality to skin-picking and impulsive eating. It may exist in up to 9% of patients with Parkinson's disease. Dopamine agonists are the most common precipitating drugs, so reducing or stopping these drugs as a priority is the preferred course of action.

If behaviours persist, rivastigmine could be increased or attempts made to reduce dopaminergic stimulation. The patient and their carers' therapeutic priorities should be negotiated.

CASE 15

C: Malignant middle cerebral artery syndrome

Learning point

Malignant middle cerebral artery (MCA) syndrome is a crucial diagnosis to make, as it is amenable to decompressive craniectomy. It should be considered in patients under 60 years old, with NIHSS over 15, a Glasgow Coma score drop of more than one point, and over 50% MCA territory involvement with sparing of anterior cerebral artery and posterior cerebral artery territories. Surgery must be undertaken within 48 hours from stroke onset.

The number needed to treat (NNT) is two to prevent one death, two to prevent a modified Rankin scale (mRS) less than or equal to four at one year, and four to achieve a mRS less than or equal to three at one year.

CASE 16

A: Cerebral amyloid angiopathy

This condition is often not seen on CT scans and requires the interpretation of T2 sequences on MRI scanning for a more definitive radiological diagnosis. Cerebral amyloid angiopathy (CAA) is characterised by amyloid beta peptide deposits in medium-sized blood vessels of the brain and leptomeninges. It can occur sporadically, in association with Alzheimer's disease, or as a familial syndrome. It becomes increasingly prevalent with each decade of life: 2.3% between 65 and 74 years and 12.1% over 85 years.

Some patients can present predominantly with seizures; others display cognitive deterioration as the predominant feature.

Learning point

The Boston criteria standardise the diagnosis.[7] Definite CAA is a post-mortem diagnosis revealing lobar, cortical or cortical/subcortical haemorrhage and pathological evidence of cerebral angiopathy. Probable CAA with supporting pathological evidence is when one has clinical data plus an evacuated haematoma or cortical biopsy specimen. Probable CAA is reserved for patients over 55 years who have MRI findings with multiple haemorrhages of varying sizes/ages without an alternative explanation and who give an appropriate clinical history. The criteria for diagnosing *possible CAA* are: age > 55years; AND an appropriate clinical history; AND MRI findings that show either a single lobar haemorrhage OR a haemorrhage with an atypical location OR cortical/subcortical haemorrhages without an alternate explanation.

CASE 17

E: Multisystem atrophy

> ### Learning point
>
> Multisystem atrophy (MSA) is a neurodegenerative synucleinopathy. It differs pathologically from other synucleinopathies (Parkinson's disease and dementia with Lewy bodies) as the intracellular deposits are not only found in neurones but also in oligodengroglia. MSA-C has predominance of cerebellar symptoms (also known as olivopontocerebellar atrophy) and MSA-P has predominance of parkinsonian signs and symptoms (striatonigral degneneration). Shy–Drager syndrome is a form of MSA in which autonomic features predominate.

Progressive supranuclear palsy (PSP) is a rare tauopathy. Parkinson's-plus or PSP-P, is a form of parkinsonism in which there are features of PSP such as faucalisation of the voice (when the voice takes on a raspy quality), dysexecutive features, nuchal dystonia and slowed vertical saccades. 'Sun-downing' is a phenomenon seen frequently in hospital settings with delirious and/or dementia patients in whom behavioural disturbances, such as wandering and vocalisations, occur 'as the sun goes down' in later afternoon and early evening.

Ultimately, the neurodegenerative processes outlined above converge to a similar end-point. Parkinson's disease patients will have autonomic features and psychological symptomatology at some stage of the disease process.

Dementia with Lewy bodies has a predominance of visual symptoms as the deposition usually occurs in the occipital lobes earlier in the process. This can be identified on positron emission tomography.

The trajectories of the parkinsonian variants follow different arcs, often facilitating diagnosis.

The 'hummingbird (or king penguin) sign' and the 'mickey mouse sign' are seen in progressive supranuclear palsy. These are absent in the MRI shown. They are due to atrophy of the midbrain.

CASE 18

B: IV benzodiazepines

One of the reasons why the Liverpool Care Pathway fell out of favour and out of common use was the risk of undertreating patients. This patient appears to be actively seizing (non-convulsive status epilepticus) and therefore an attempt to rapidly reverse this should be undertaken with IV benzodiazepines and potentially other IV anti-epileptics such as phenytoin or valproate.

If there is no response to anti-epileptic therapies, focus on a palliative approach would perhaps be more appropriate at that juncture. The use of midazolam via continuous subcutaneous infusion can serve the dual purpose of raising the seizure threshold and helping to manage dyspnoea/restlessness in the palliative setting.

Decisions regarding discontinuation of clinically assisted hydration should be taken on an individualised patient basis.

CASE 19

B: Percutaneous sacral nerve stimulation

Urinary incontinence is rarely life-threatening but can have a destructive impact upon the physical, psychological and social wellbeing of affected individuals. Absorbent products, urinals and toileting aids are only a coping strategy pending definitive treatment or an adjunct to ongoing therapy.

Percutaneous posterior tibial nerve stimulation for overactive bladder (OAB) should only be offered after multidisciplinary assessment, failure of drug treatment and when the patient has declined botulinum toxin A treatment or percutaneous sacral nerve stimulation. There is insufficient evidence to recommend the use of percutaneous posterior tibial nerve stimulation to routinely treat OAB.

Percutaneous sacral nerve stimulation is the preferred option in this patient. It does carry a long-term commitment with a potential requirement for surgical revision. The transcutaneous option should not be offered (this takes the form of surface electrode deployment).

The preferred option would normally be botulinum toxin; however, this patient has declined this option, albeit on a fairly irrational basis, and her wishes must be respected. A smaller dose of botulinum toxin A can be used if the patient wishes to have a lower likelihood of a requirement for intermittent self-catheterisation post procedure.

A urinary diversion procedure and augmentation cystoplasty are the last-line options.

References

1. The IST-3 collaborative group. 2012. The benefits and harms of intravenous thrombolysis with recombinant tissue plasminogen activator within 6 h of acute ischaemic stroke (the third international stroke trial [IST-3]): a randomised controlled trial. Lancet, 379, 2352–2363

2. National Collaborating Centre for Chronic Conditions. 2008. Stroke: national clinical guideline for diagnosis and initial management of acute stroke and transient ischaemic attack. London, Royal College of Physicians

3. Anderson C et al. 2010. Effects of early intensive blood pressure lowering treatment on the growth of hematoma and perihematomal edema in acute intracerebral hemorrhage: the Intensive Blood Pressure Reduction in Acute Cerebral Haemorrhage Trial (INTERACT). Stroke, 41, 307–312

4. Anderson C et al. 2013. Rapid blood-pressure lowering in patients with acute intracerebral hemorrhage. New England Journal of Medicine, 368, 2355–2365

5. CLOTS Trials Collaboration. 2013. Effectiveness of intermittent pneumatic compression in reduction of risk of deep vein thrombosis in patients who have had a stroke (CLOTS 3): a multicentre randomised controlled trial. Lancet, 382, 516–524

6. NICE. 2013. Percutaneous vertebroplasty and percutaneous balloon kyphoplasty for treating osteoporotic vertebral compression fractures. NICE technology appraisal guidance 279. www.nice.org.uk/guidance/ta279

7. Knudsen K et al. 2001. Clinical diagnosis of cerebral amyloid angiopathy: validation of the Boston criteria. Neurology, 56, 537–539

CASE 1

A 70-year-old woman presents with increasing confusion and tiredness.

Blood testing shows: Haemoglobin 88 g/litre, MCV 102 fl, White cells 13.4 × 10^9/litre, Platelets 90 × 10^9/litre, Creatinine 193 µmol/litre, Albumin 31 g/litre, Bilirubin 12 µmol/litre.

Immunoglobulin analysis with serum electrophoresis shows low levels of IgG, IgA and IgM with no paraprotein.

A bone marrow aspirate is shown in Figure 6.1.

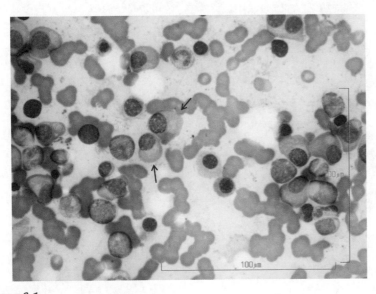

Figure 6.1

What is the most likely diagnosis?

A. **Acute myeloid leukaemia**
B. **Burkitt's lymphoma**
C. **Multiple myeloma**
D. **Basophilic leukaemia**
E. **Acute lymphoblastic leukaemia**

CASE 2

A 12-year-old boy visiting his ailing grandmother in Malawi presents with fatigue and tiredness. He appears to be jaundiced and has been passing dark-coloured urine.

His full blood count shows: Haemoglobin 53 g/litre, White cells 12×10^9/litre, Platelets 334×10^9/litre.

A blood film is shown in Figure 6.2.

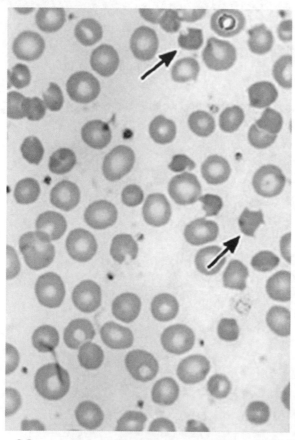

Figure 6.2

Which would be the best investigation to diagnose his underlying condition?

    A. **Osmotic fragility test**

    B. **Pyruvate kinase level**

    C. **Flow cytometry**

    D. **Glucose 6 phosphate dehydrogenase (G6PD) level**

    E. **Sickle solubility test**

CASE 3

A 69-year-old man is referred to the haematology clinic with an abnormal full blood count picked up on his annual 'well man clinic' screening.

The test shows: Haemoglobin 138 g/litre, White cells 24×10^9/litre, Platelets 257×10^9/litre.

He has no palpable lymphadenopathy or splenomegaly. A blood film is provided in Figure 6.3.

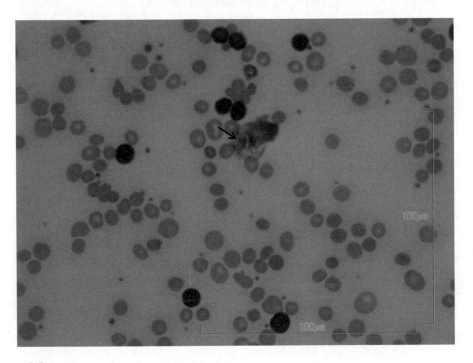

Figure 6.3

The best current management plan for him would be:

- A. **Watch and wait**
- B. **Prescribe antivirals**
- C. **Commence on chemotherapy with purine analogues**
- D. **Start imatinib**
- E. **Consider a broad spectrum antibiotic awaiting results of blood cultures**

CASE 4

A 33-year-old lady with two prior miscarriages is referred to the clinic with an abnormal clotting profile.

Her coagulation profile is as follows: PT–12 s, APTT–73 s, TT–13 s, Fibrinogen 3.7 g/litre.

A 50 : 50 mix on the prolonged activated partial thromboplastin time (APTT) does not correct the extended time. The most likely diagnosis is:

    A. **Heparin contamination**
    B. **Haemophilia A carrier**
    C. **Haemophilia B carrier**
    D. **Disseminated intravascular coagulation**
    E. **Antiphospholipid antibody syndrome**

CASE 5

A 33-year-old man presents after a major road traffic accident with multiple limb fractures and a trauma-related coagulopathy. He has been stabilised and his vital parameters are normalised by the resuscitation team. Fifteen minutes in to his fresh frozen plasma infusion he becomes unwell and short of breath. The oxygen saturation is 82% breathing room air, respiratory rate 38 breaths/min, pulse rate 118 bpm and a blood pressure of 100/80 mmHg. A chest radiograph on admission was normal. A repeat film is shown in Figure 6.4.

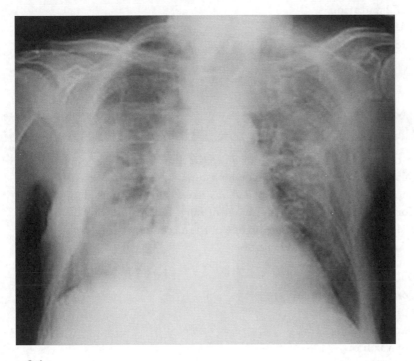

Figure 6.4

What is the most likely diagnosis?

    A. **Transfusion associated lung injury (TRALI)**
    B. **Transfusion associated cardiac overload (TACO)**
    C. **Transfusion transmitted bacterial infection**
    D. **Adult respiratory distress syndrome**
    E. **Post-transfusion purpura**

CASE 6

A 61-year-old lady is referred to the clinic with asymptomatic thrombocytosis.

Her full blood count shows: Haemoglobin 118 g/litre, White cells 9×10^9/litre, Platelets 810×10^9/litre.

Your investigations should include all of the following except:

A. **Serum ferritin**
B. **C-reactive protein**
C. *JAK2* **mutation**
D. *CAL-R* **mutation**
E. *C282Y* **mutation**

CASE 7

A 65-year-old man has self-referred himself to the clinic for a change of his anticoagulant treatment. He has been on long-term warfarin after an aortic valve replacement and for atrial fibrillation, and has recently been admitted for warfarin reversal for rectal bleeding caused by an out-of-range INR reading of 9.3 while on antibiotics. He is keen to be changed to one of the newer direct anticoagulants. The best choice for this patient would be

A. **Dabigatran**
B. **Continue on warfarin**
C. **Apixiban**
D. **Danaparoid**
E. **Rivaroxiban**

CASE 8

A 27-year-old man presents to the emergency department with fatigue and epistaxis.

His full blood count shows: Haemoglobin 77 g/litre, White cells 23×10^9/litre, Platelets 43×10^9/litre.

Examination reveals a mild splenomegaly with no lymphadenopathy. A blood film is shown in Figure 6.5.

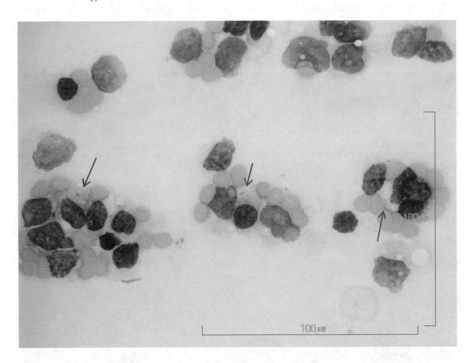

Figure 6.5

The most likely diagnosis is

    A. **Chronic myeloid leukaemia**

    B. **Acute myeloid leukaemia (AML)**

    C. **Acute lymphoblastic leukaemia (ALL)**

    D. **Hodgkin's lymphoma**

    E. **Acute promyelocytic leukaemia**

CASE 9

A 31-year-old primigravida presents at 24 weeks of gestation with the acute onset of hemiplegia. A CT scan of the head demonstrates a lacunar infarct in the internal capsule. She is a non-smoker with a body mass index of 27 kg/m² and has no family history of thrombophilia. She is normotensive with no proteinuria.

Investigations reveal the following: Haemoglobin 90 g/litre, White cells 4.5 × 10⁹/litre, Platelets 44 × 10⁹/litre, PT 12 s, APTT 31 s, Fibrinogen 4.7 g/litre, Creatinine 275 μmol/litre, Bilirubin 33 μmmol/litre, ALT 35 U/litre, Albumin 40 g/litre, lupus anticoagulant (LA) – undetectable.

A blood film has been provided in Figure 6.6.

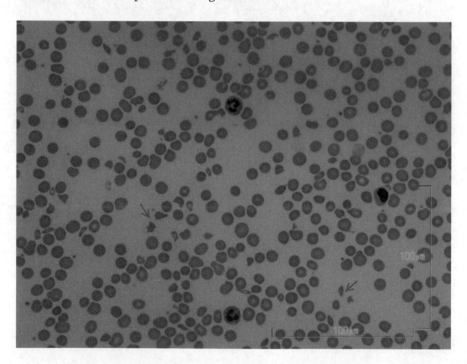

Figure 6.6

The most likely diagnosis is:

 A. **Thrombotic thrombocytopaenic purpura (TTP)**

 B. **Disseminated intravascular coagulation**

 C. **Haemolytic uraemic syndrome**

 D. **Heparin-induced thrombocytopaenia**

 E. **HELLP syndrome**

CASE 10

A 17-year-old boy known to have homozygous sickle cell anaemia presents with increasing back pain and lethargy. His oxygen saturations are 97% on room air and his chest X-ray is normal.

Investigations reveal: Haemoglobin 59 g/litre, White cells 16 × 10⁹/litre, Platelets 450 × 10⁹/litre, Reticulocytes 4 × 10⁹/litre, C-reactive protein 23 mg/dl, Creatinine 103 μmol/litre, Bilirubin 29 μmol/litre, Albumin 33 g/litre, Haemoglobin electrophoresis shows: HbA 5%, HbS 89%, HbF 6%.

Which of the following treatment plans would be most appropriate?

    A. **Exchange transfusion**
    B. **Top-up transfusion**
    C. **Broad spectrum IV antibiotics**
    D. **Rest, analgesia and supplemental oxygen**
    E. **Hydroxycarbamide**

CASE 11

A 50-year-old Indian man is referred with increasingly irritability, anorexia and constipation.

His investigations reveal: Haemoglobin 89 g/litre, MCV 88 fl, White cells 12×10^9/litre, Platelets 243×10^9/litre.

A blood film is provided in Figure 6.7.

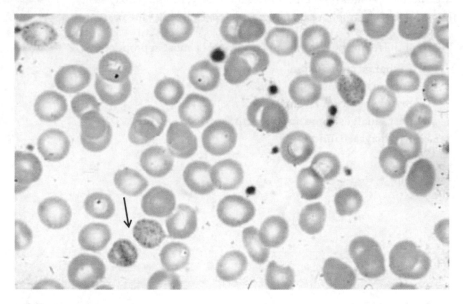

Figure 6.7

The most likely diagnosis is

    A. **Sideroblastic anaemia**
    B. **Thalassemia intermedia**
    C. **Malarial parasitemia**
    D. **Lead poisoning**
    E. **Leishmanaiasis**

CASE 12

A HIV positive individual presents with increasing fatigue and inguinal lymphadenopathy. He is well maintained on triple, highly active antiretroviral therapy, with low levels of viral load and a CD4 count > 200/mm^3.

A bone marrow smear has been provided in Figure 6.8.

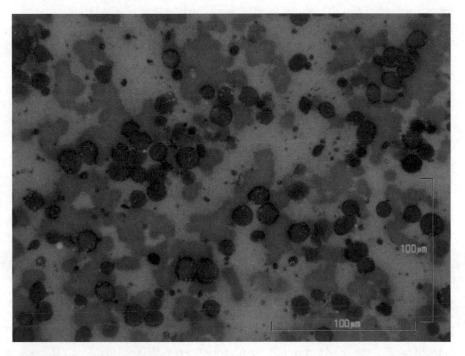

Figure 6.8

What is the most likely diagnosis?

A. **Burkitt's lymphoma/leukaemia**
B. **Hodgkin's lymphoma**
C. **Plasma cell leukaemia**
D. **Acute basophilic leukaemia**
E. **CMV infection**

CASE 13

A 77-year-old resident of a warden-controlled flat experiences intense lethargy and fatigue after coming back from her Christmas shopping on a snowy morning. She has no fever or previous cardiac issues but admits to passing dark-coloured urine.

An hour later she collapses and is brought to the emergency department, where investigations reveal the following: Haemoglobin 64 g/litre, MCV 110 fl, White cells 15.5 × 10⁹/litre, Platelets 333 × 10⁹/litre, Reticulocytes 285 × 10⁹/litre, Direct anti-globulin test: IgG negative, C3d 3+, Creatinine 122 µmol/litre, C-reactive protein 65 mg/dl, LDH 565 U/litre.

Which of the following is the most likely diagnosis?

A. **Cold agglutinin disease**
B. **Warm autoimmune haemolytic anaemia**
C. **Paroxysmal cold haemoglobinuria (PCH)**
D. **Cryoglobulinaemia**
E. **Paroxysmal nocturnal haemoglobinuria**

CASE 14

A three-year-old Indian child presents to the emergency department with increasing lethargy, irritability and cyanosis. He has accidentally swallowed his mother's medication that she is currently taking for tuberculoid leprosy. The child is tachycardic, cyanosed but not in respiratory distress. His pulse rate is 115 bpm, blood pressure is 112/76 mmHg and oxygen saturations are 99% breathing room air.

Which of the following would be the best investigation to confirm the diagnosis?

A. **Mass spectrometry**
B. **Glucose 6 phosphate dehydrogenase levels**
C. **Arterial blood gas analysis**
D. **Pyruvate kinase levels**
E. **P50 on an oxygen dissociation curve**

CASE 15

A 56-year-old woman underwent an elective hip replacement and required the transfusion of two units of blood. She developed spontaneous bruising and epistaxis six days after the surgery while in the orthopaedic ward.

Her full blood picture showed: Haemoglobin 96 g/litre, White cells 12×10^9/litre, Platelets 8×10^9/litre, having been completely normal pre-surgery. Her clotting screen is normal and she has been on no antibiotics likely to cause thrombocytopaenia. Which of the following represents the best next stage in her management?

A. **Platelet transfusion**
B. **Steroids**
C. **Rituximab**
D. **Intravenous immunoglobulin (IVIG)**
E. **Fondaparinux**

CASE 16

A 19-year-old girl presents to the clinic with drenching night sweats and cervical lymphadenopathy. She has recently returned back from an African safari. She has lost a stone in weight unintentionally over the last two weeks. Her lymph node biopsy appearances have been provided in Figure 6.9.

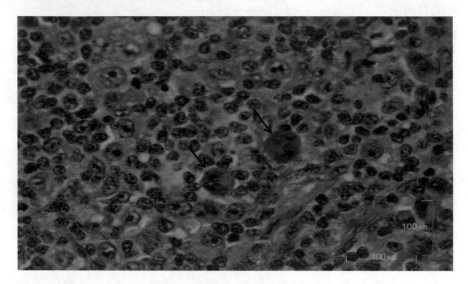

Figure 6.9

Which of the following is the most likely diagnosis?

- A. HIV sero-conversion illness
- B. Hodgkin's lymphoma
- C. Non-Hodgkin's lymphoma
- D. Tuberculosis
- E. Kaposi's sarcoma

CASE 17

A 31-year-old lady is diagnosed with an above-knee, deep vein thrombosis in the second trimester of pregnancy. She has no family history suggestive of thrombophilia and has not had any previous thrombotic episodes. Her risk factors are pre-eclampsia, cigarette smoking and obesity. What is the best way to monitor her anticoagulation with low-molecular-weight heparin?

A. **No monitoring required**
B. INR
C. APTT
D. **Anti-Xa levels**
E. **Thrombin time**

CASE 18

A 23-year-old man presents to the emergency department with persistent epistaxis and gum bleeding. He is otherwise fit and well. He has recovered from a diarrhoeal illness four weeks ago. He has no family history of increased bruising and is on no medications.

His investigations show the following: Haemoglobin 135 g/litre, White cells 10.3 × 10⁹/litre, Platelets 8 × 10⁹/litre.

A blood film confirms thrombocytopaenia with a few giant platelets and no blasts. The liver, renal and clotting function tests are within normal limits. The best first-line management would be:

A. **Observation only**
B. **Anti-D**
C. **Prednisolone**
D. **Intravenous immunoglobulin**
E. **Rituximab**

CASE 19

A 33-year-old man from India is being investigated for pyrexia of unknown origin with worsening cytopaenias and massive splenomegaly. The blood film has confirmed no blasts. His bone marrow aspirate is provided in Figure 6.10.

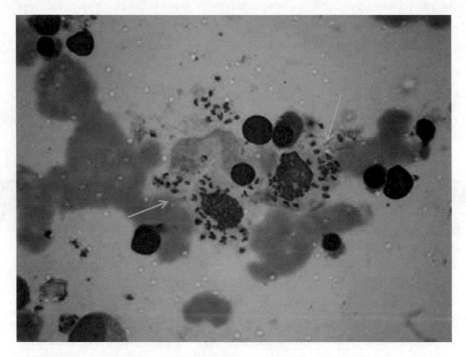

Figure 6.10

What is the most likely diagnosis?

    A. **Leishmaniasis**
    B. **Tuberculosis**
    C. **Myeloma**
    D. **Haemophagocytic syndrome**
    E. **Histoplasmosis**

CASE 20

A 14-year-old patient with severe haemophilia A presents with two episodes of haemarthosis despite being on thrice-weekly prophylaxis with a third-generation recombinant factor VIII concentrate. The factor VIII level is recorded as undetectable. The platelet function analyser-100 is normal. The most likely cause for this clinical profile is:

A. Tachyphylaxis to factor VIII infusions
B. Inhibitor to factor VIII
C. Ingestion of non-steroidal anti-inflammatory drugs (NSAIDs)
D. Accompanying von Willebrand's disease
E. Underdosing of factor VIII

CASE 1

C: Multiple myeloma

This question tests your ability to identify plasma cells in the bone marrow. The fact that there is no paraprotein on serum electrophoresis may be misleading, since a majority of myeloma patients (95%) present with a distinct IgG or IgA paraprotein. However, a few patients belong to the diagnostic category of light chain myeloma, which presents with reduced gamma globulins, no paraprotein and free light chains (Bence–Jones) in the urine only.

This patient has a diagnosis of light chain myeloma with abundant plasma cells (red arrows) in the bone marrow. Plasma cells are easy to diagnose on morphology since they have a distinctly basophilic cytoplasm, an eccentric nucleus and a perinuclear halo (expanded Golgi zone). Burkitt's lymphoma blasts are basophilic but are intensely vacuolated and lack the eccentric nucleus.

Learning point

Myeloma is a common theme in the MRCP exam. Patients typically present with the characteristic CRAB criteria:
 	
    C – high calcium
    R – renal impairment
    A – anaemia, often mildly macrocytic
    B – bone lytic lesions, with classical punched-out lesions in skull

This patient certainly has the 'A' and possibly the 'C', since hypercalcemia may be the cause of her confusion.

CASE 2

D: Glucose 6 phosphate dehydrogenase (G6PD) level

Learning point

The combination of anaemia, jaundice and dark urine should alert you towards a haemolytic anaemia with intravascular haemolysis (IVH). The blood film portrays changes of oxidative haemolysis with irregularly contracted cells (blue arrow) and bite cells (red arrow), which are characteristically seen in G6PD deficiency.

Hereditary spherocytosis, pyruvate kinase deficiency and sickle cell anaemia all are various subtypes of Coombs' negative haemolytic anaemias with pathologies in the red cell membrane, enzymes and haemoglobin, respectively. The seat of red cell destruction in hereditary spherocytosis and pyruvate kinase deficiency is commonly extravascular (in the liver and spleen), and patients seldom present with signs of intravascular haemolysis, eg dark urine.

Paroxysmal nocturnal haemoglobinuria presents with intravascular haemolysis but is a rare acquired condition with the clinical triad of aplasia, haemolytic anaemia and thrombosis (which this patient does not have). There are no sickle cells in the blood film to support a diagnosis of sickle cell anaemia.

Glucose 6 phosphate dehydrogenase deficiency is an X-linked disorder (this patient is a boy!) commonly seen in patients of Black and Mediterranean ethnicity (the patient visiting his grandmother in Malawi probably hints towards this). Patients present with intermittent IVH upon exposure to drugs and fava beans that cause oxidative haemolysis. This patient has presumably taken antimalarial prophylaxis with primaquine, which might have caused his current G6PD crisis.

CASE 3

A: Watch and wait

The blood film depicts a smear cell (black arrow) and classical chronic lymphocytic leukaemia (CLL) cells (green arrow), which are small uniform (monomorphic) lymphocytes with a condensed nucleus and basophilic scanty cytoplasm.

The commonest presentation of CLL is an asymptomatic patient found to have abnormal leukocytosis, predominantly lymphocytosis with a preserved haemoglobin and platelet count.

> ### Learning point
>
> The standard management is to watch and wait (meta-analysis proven). Indications of treatment would be B symptoms (weight loss, night sweats, fevers), bulky lymphadenoapthy, haemoglobin < 110 g/litre, platelets < 100 × 10⁹/litre or a lymphocyte doubling count < 6 months. This patient has none of the above to consider treatment with chemotherapy currently.

Imatinib, a tyrosine kinase inhibitor, is the drug of choice for chronic phase chronic myeloid leukaemia (CML). However, the blood film does not show any changes of CML such as basophilia, eosinophilia, myelocytes and metamyelocytes.

Viral infections such as infectious mononucleosis would show pleomorphic lymphocytes with plentiful cytoplasm and scalloping edges, and the patient would probably be symptomatic. Bacterial infections would cause abundant neutrophils with toxic granulation on the blood film.

CASE 4

E: Antiphospholipid antibody syndrome

An isolated prolongation of the APTT would indicate either a deficiency of the intrinsic factor pathway (factor VIII, IX, XI or XII) or the presence of an inhibitor to these factors – commonly a lupus anticoagulant. A complete correction of the extended APTT on a 50:50 mix would favour a factor deficiency (since the added 50% normal plasma to the patient's plasma in the test tube will correct the deficiency and hence normalise the APTT). An inhibitor-like lupus anticoagulant will show an uncorrected prolonged APTT on a 50:50 mix.

Heparin contamination would prolong both the APTT and the thrombin time. Disseminated intravascular coagulation would result in prolonged PT, APTT, and low fibrinogen and platelets with a few fragments on the blood film.

CASE 5

A: Transfusion associated lung injury (TRALI)

> ### Learning point
>
>
>
> Transfusion associated lung injury is defined as an acute lung injury that is temporally related to a blood transfusion. Specifically, it occurs within the first few minutes or up to six hours following a transfusion. It is typically associated with plasma components such as platelets and fresh frozen plasma, although cases have been reported with packed red blood cells since there is some residual plasma in the packed cells. Bilateral pulmonary infiltrates on a chest X-ray post transfusion are suggestive of TRALI. Unlike adult respiratory distress syndrome, TRALI is self-limiting, and there is usually clinical improvement within 48–96 hours provided prompt respiratory support (commonly with mechanical ventilation) is provided. A high index of clinical suspicion is required as TRALI is a diagnosis of exclusion.

It is hypothesised that TRALI may be precipitated by the infusion of donor antibodies directed against recipient leukocytes. The infusion of donor anti-HLA (human leukocyte antigens) or anti-HNA (human neutrophil antigens) antibodies is thought to directly cause complement activation, resulting in the influx of neutrophils into the lung, followed by neutrophil activation and release of cytotoxic agents, with subsequent endothelial damage and capillary leak. Donor-derived antibodies to HLA class I antigens and neutrophils have been demonstrated in up to 89% of TRALI cases examined in the literature.

Transfusion associated cardiac overload is commonly seen in elderly patients with compromised cardiac reserve who develop pulmonary oedema after hasty and overzealous transfusion, and is often associated with hypertension. The age and the blood pressure of this patient make the diagnosis of TACO unlikely.

CASE 6

E: *C282Y* mutation

Common causes of thrombocytosis include inflammatory/infective aetiologies, malignancy, iron deficiency anaemia and myeloproliferative neoplasms.

This platelet count of 810×10^9/litre is considerably high and should raise the possibility of a myeloproliferative neoplasm such as essential thrombocythaemia (ET), although the reactive causes mentioned above need to be ruled out with a serum ferritin and C-reactive protein.

Both *JAK2* and *CAL-R* mutations are associated with ET, and are mutually exclusive, accounting for 90% of cases of the condition (*JAK2* ~ 50% and *CAL-R* ~ 40%).

C282Y is the commonest mutation identified in patients with genetic haemochromatosis which does not affect the platelet count.

CASE 7

B: Continue on warfarin

Newer anticoagulants such as direct thrombin inhibitors (dabigatran) and anti-Xa inhibitors (rivaroxiban and apixiban) have created a splash in the anticoagulation domain since they have a safe pharmacokinetic profile with fewer drug interactions and no need for constant monitoring as compared to warfarin. The trials in non-valvular atrial fibrillation (AF) show that they are all non-inferior to warfarin with a lesser incidence of intracranial bleeds. They are licensed for this indication.

Learning point

However, this patient has valvular AF for which these agents do not currently have a license. A recent trial of dabigatran vs. warfarin was prematurely closed because of more haemorrhagic manifestations in the dabigatran arm. Hence, this patient will not be deemed suitable/eligible for the direct newer anticoagulants. Reversal of these agents is also a sticky issue since there is no antidote available currently.

The patient should be advised about potential warfarin interactions. Proactive steps to monitor dose changes with closer monitoring should be advocated in future when the patient is prescribed any interacting new drugs such as antibiotics.

CASE 8

B: Acute myeloid leukaemia (AML)

Learning point

The blood film shows plentiful blasts with a high nucleo-cytoplasmic ratio and an immature chromatin pattern in the nucleus with distinct nucleoli. The distinctive feature is that these blasts demonstrate Auer rods (arrows) which strongly favour a diagnosis of AML. Auer rods (clumps of azurophilic granular material that form elongated needles) can only be found in myeloblasts, and so help to differentiate AML from ALL. They are composed of fused lysosomes/primary neutrophilic granules and contain peroxidase, lysosomal enzymes and large crystalline inclusions. However, if Auer rods are not seen, that does not mean that the blast is not a myeloblast!

Acute promyelocytic leukaemia blasts may contain Auer rods too, but have a characteristic morphology with a very granular cytoplasm and a perinuclear lucency. This leukaemia often presents with disseminated intravascular coagulation, has the characteristic translocation t(15;17) and is responsive to all-trans retinoic acid. Hodgkin's lymphoma typically presents with lymphadenopathy, B symptoms and has no circulating blasts or Reed–Sternberg cells on a blood film. The diagnosis must be made on an excisional lymph node biopsy.

CASE 9

A: Thrombotic thrombocytopaenic purpura (TTP)

The blood film shows florid fragments (broken red cells, indicated by blue arrows), which favour a diagnosis of microangiopathic haemolytic anaemia (MAHA). Disseminated intravascular coagulation (DIC) can cause MAHA and lead to both haemorrhage and thrombosis, but a normal coagulation profile with a normal fibrinogen concentration goes against that diagnosis.

> ### Learning point
>
> TTP is the pentad of MAHA (plentiful fragments), thrombocytopaenia and neurological manifestations such as stroke, convulsions, confusion, renal impairment and low-grade pyrexia. It classically leads to thrombotic complications in the face of thrombocytopaenia.

Heparin-induced thrombocytopaenia would give rise to a similar phenotype (paradoxical clots in the face of the thrombocytopaenia), but is not associated with MAHA. This patient fits well with a diagnosis of TTP and will need urgent plasmapheresis and steroids.

Haemolytic uraemic syndrome is often associated with preceding diarrhoea, and predominantly manifests with severe renal impairment without significant neurology.

HELLP (haemolysis, elevated liver transaminases and low platelets) syndrome can give rise to MAHA, but this patient does not have elevated liver enzymes to support the diagnosis.

CASE 10

B: Top-up transfusion

Learning point

The clue is the profoundly low reticulocyte count of 4×10^9/litre. Sickle cell anaemia is a haemolytic anaemia and will have a constant state of reticulocytosis ($> 100 \times 10^9$/litre), which will escalate in the event of a sickle cell crisis. A low reticulocyte count signifies an aplastic crisis with parvovirus B19, which is generally self-resolving and can be managed by top-up transfusions.

Chronic parvovirus infection might need treatment with intravenous immunoglobulin. Exchange transfusion is the treatment of choice for chest cell crisis, stroke and priapism in the context of sickle cell crisis, with an aim to get the HbS < 30%. Do not be tempted to label this as an infection with the high white cell count, since most patients with sickle cell disease have an erroneously reported leukocytosis because of nucleated red cells in the peripheral blood being wrongly counted as white blood cells by most laboratory counters!

CASE 11

D: Lead poisoning

The most conspicuous abnormality on the blood film is basophilic stippling (red arrow). Basophilic stippling implies the presence of small basophilic inclusions dispersed throughout the erythrocyte cytoplasm which can be demonstrated to be RNA. The symptoms of irritability, anorexia, constipation and normocytic anaemia fit very well with the diagnosis of lead poisoning. This gentleman was consuming Indian ayurvedic medicines, some of which can contain lead.

Abundant numbers of cells with basophilic stippling can be seen in poisoning by heavy metals such as lead, arsenic and mercury, all of which inhibit the enzyme pyrimidine 5' nucleotidase which is pivotal for RNA degradation.

Thalassemia major and intermedia can show basophilic stippling, but the MCV will be strikingly low (microcytosis), with other predominant features on the blood film such as nucleated red cells, target cells and aniso-poikilocytosis. Sideroblastic anaemia will show predominant Pappenheimer bodies and a dimorphic blood film.

Malaria and leishmanaisis demonstrate parasite rings and Donovan bodies, respectively.

CASE 12

A: Burkitt's lymphoma/leukaemia

The classical morphology is basophilic blasts which are intensely vacuolated. These unique, vacuolated blasts raise strong suspicions for Burkitt's lymphoma/leukaemia, which is common in the HIV population. The most common variant is t(8;14)(q24;q32), which accounts for approximately 85% of cases. The endemic variant seen in Africa with huge jaw tumours (famously published in most medical textbooks) is now rare.

CASE 13

C: Paroxysmal cold haemoglobinuria (PCH)

This history of having intravascular haemolysis (as evidenced by dark-coloured urine) with temperature changes is very classical of PCH. This is an anti-P antibody (popularly known as Donath–Landsteiner in textbooks) condition with dual temperature specificity. The antibody attaches the complement at cold temperatures (when the woman was out shopping on a cold December day) without causing haemolysis. However, when warmed up to room temperature and beyond (as the lady returns back to her heated flat), the complement is activated, which then ensues the intravascular haemolysis.

Learning point

Paroxysmal nocturnal haemoglobinuria comprises the triad of intravascular haemolysis, aplasia and thrombosis. Warm autoimmune haemolytic anaemia would be significantly positive for IgG on the direct anti-globulin test.

CASE 14

A: Mass spectrometry

The paradoxical history of cyanosis with a normal pulse oximetry reading (pulse oximetry and blood gases overestimate the oxygen saturation) should make you think of methaemoglobinaemia. Excessive dapsone ingestion (used for tuberculoid leprosy in his mother) is notoriously known to induce oxidative haemolysis and methaemoglobin production. Methaemoglobin is formed by the oxidation of haem iron, ie by conversion from the ferrous (Fe^{2+}) to the ferric (Fe^{3+}) form. The best way to measure it is by mass spectrometry. Patients with severe symptoms can be considered for plasma exchange or methylene blue treatment.

CASE 15

D: Intravenous immunoglobulin (IVIG)

The history of severe isolated thrombocytopaenia post transfusion should raise the possibility of post-transfusion purpura (PTP).

> ### Learning point
>
> PTP is an adverse reaction to a blood transfusion or platelet transfusion that occurs when the body produces alloantibodies to the introduced platelets' antigens. These alloantibodies behave like autoantibodies and destroy the patient's platelets leading to thrombocytopaenia. PTP usually presents 5–12 days after transfusion, and is a potentially fatal condition. The mechanism of an alloantibody destroying self-platelets is not well understood. PTP is rare, but usually occurs in women who have had multiple pregnancies or in men who have undergone previous transfusions. It is usually self-limiting, but IVIG is effective in 85% of cases.

Heparin-induced thrombocytopaenia is another possibility (which can be treated with fondaparinux), but often presents with moderately low platelets (40–60 × 10⁹/litre), and thrombosis rather than bleeding. Immune thrombocytopaenia which can present with severe isolated thrombocytopaenia (responsive to steroids and IVIG) is a diagnosis of exclusion and the occurrence post transfusion is unlikely to be just a coincidence, especially in the exam setting!

CASE 16

B: Hodgkin's lymphoma

The classical cells strikingly prominent are the Reed–Sternberg cells (black arrows) which are a sine qua non for Hodgkin's lymphoma. Reed–Sternberg cells are large and are either multinucleated or have a bi-lobed nucleus (so resembling an 'owl's eye') with prominent eosinophilic inclusion-like nucleoli. Reed–Sternberg cells are CD30 and CD15 positive, but are usually negative for CD20 and CD45. The presence of these cells is necessary in the diagnosis of Hodgkin's lymphoma. The absence of Reed–Sternberg cells has very high negative predictive value. The African safari is a distracting red herring in this case!

CASE 17

D: Anti-Xa levels

Pregnancy is a prothrombotic physiologic state with a four- to five-fold increase in the incidence of venous thromboembolism. This risk is even higher in the post-partum period.

> ### Learning point
>
> Low-molecular-weight heparin therapy in general does not need monitoring. However, there are a few indications in pregnancy where monitoring with anti-Xa levels is recommended. The four main indications for monitoring during pregnancy with a four-hour post-dosing anti-Xa level are: extremes of weight (this patient is obese and hence would need monitoring), impaired renal function, mechanical heart valves and recurrent thrombosis with string thrombophilia traits.

INR is used to monitor warfarin and APTT is used to monitor unfractionated heparin.

CASE 18

C: Prednisolone

Severe isolated thrombocytopaenia in an otherwise young, fit patient should strongly raise the possibility of immune thrombocytopaenia (ITP). The diarrhoeal illness four weeks ago might indicate tweaking of the immune system (live vaccines, pregnancy, infections are often triggers for ITP). There is no confirmatory diagnostic test for ITP and one needs to have a high index of suspicion to intervene since it is largely a diagnosis of exclusion. Disseminated intravascular coagulation, drugs and leukaemia are ruled out in this case.

First-line management is with oral steroids. Intravenous immunoglobulin can be used in patients with imminent potentially serious bleeds (eg intracranial or retinal haemorrhage) for a quicker response. Rituximab, an anti-CD20 antibody, is effective as second-line management for ITP. The relatively newer thrombopoietin receptor agonists such as romiplastim and eltrombopag are being increasingly used as third-line agents for relapsed/refractory cases. Anti-D, once popular for the management of ITP, has fallen into disrepute in Europe because of the haemolysis that it induces.

CASE 19

A: Leishmaniasis

The bone marrow smear demonstrates the amastigotes of *Leishmania donovani* (LD bodies), indicated by the orange arrows in Figure 6.10. They classically have a double dot appearance with the nucleus and kinetoplast. Cytopaenias and splenomegaly would fit in well with the clinical profile of visceral leishmaniasis transmitted by the bite of infected female phlebotomines and flies. Haemophagocytic syndrome would fit clinically with the profile provided, but would demonstrate hungry macrophages and histiocytes phagocytosing haematopoietic precursors in the bone marrow. Histoplasmosis is not prevalent in India.

CASE 20

B: Inhibitor to factor VIII

Severe haemophilia A (factor VIII levels < 1 U/dl) are routinely treated with thrice-weekly prophylaxis of a third-generation recombinant factor VIII. This profile with undetectable factor VIII levels in the event of recurrent haemarthosis is indicative of inhibitor formation, which can happen in up to 25% of these patients on regular infusions.

Platelet function analyser-100 (PFA-100) is the standard test used instead of the archaic 'bleeding time' as a surrogate marker of the first phase of coagulation. Platelet dysfunction and von Willebrand's disease would cause prolongation of the closure times on PFA-100. Please note that haemophilia A, which is deficiency of factor VIII, disrupts the second phase of coagulation and hence patients with this condition will have a normal PFA-100. The normal PFA-100 rules out NSAID ingestion and von Willebrand's disease.

Haemophilia A inhibitors are treated with bypassing agents such as Novo-7® (recombinant factor VII) or FEIBA (factor eight inhibitor bypassing agent) in the short term and with immunosuppression in the long term.

CHAPTER 7

Infectious Diseases and Genito-urinary Medicine

Emilia Mamwa and Paul H. McGurnaghan

CASE 1

A 19-year-old boy presents three days after returning from a holiday abroad. He is admitted with headaches, fever, neck stiffness and reduced level of consciousness. He admits to having unprotected sexual intercourse while on holiday and recalls a vesicular rash on his genitals during his trip. His CT scan of brain is unremarkable and his cerebrospinal fluid (CSF) analysis shows no organisms on gram stain and has no growth after 48 hours culture. He was not given any antibiotics before having CSF sampled. The CSF has 150 leukocytes (95% lymphocytes and 5% polymophocytes).

What is the most appropriate next stage of management?

- A. **No further medical intervention required**
- B. **Commence antibiotics for bacterial meningitis**
- C. **Request CSF virology and PCR, and start IV aciclovir**
- D. **Request CSF PCR and await the result before starting any treatment**
- E. **Refer to the infectious diseases team**

CASE 2

A 79-year-old gentleman presents to the emergency department with fever, headaches, vomiting, drowsiness, dysarthria and left-sided weakness. He had a witnessed tonic-clonic seizure at the time of admission. He had recently completed a course of antibiotics prescribed by his GP for a facial throbbing pain that developed a few days after a chest infection. He has low-grade pyrexia.

Blood tests reveal: White cells 16×10^9/litre, C-reactive protein 340 mg/litre, Blood cultures – results awaited.

His brain MRI image is shown in Figure 7.1.

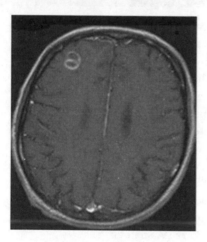

Figure 7.1

He is empirically started on IV ceftriaxone. Based on the likely diagnosis, what would be the most appropriate definitive management for this condition?

A. **Perform an urgent lumbar puncture and request CSF culture and PCR**

B. **Urgent referral to the stroke team**

C. **Combination antibiotics and urgent neurosurgical referral for drainage of pus**

D. **Continue with current antibiotics and await culture results**

E. **Refer for a brain biopsy**

CASE 3

A 35-year-old man presents with malaise and fever six months after an extended visit to rural India during which time he had been treated for amoebic dysentery. On examination he is tender in the right upper quadrant, but is not icteric.

Blood tests reveal: White cells 14×10^9/litre (neutrophils 11×10^9/litre), C-reactive protein 230 mg/litre, ESR 70 mm/1st hour, Liver enzymes: normal.

His temperature chart, abdominal CT and chest X-ray images are shown in Figures 7.2, 7.3 and 7.4.

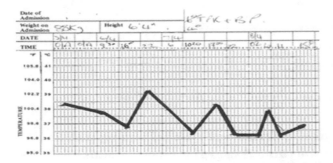

Figure 7.2

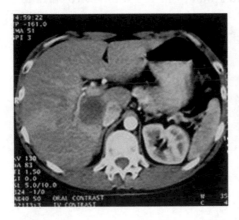

Figure 7.3   Figure 7.4

What would be the most appropriate next step in this patient's management?

    A. **Radiological intervention**

    B. **Combination IV antibiotics**

    C. **IV antihelmetics and radiological intervention**

    D. **Conservative management**

    E. **IV metronidazole**

CASE 4

A 32-year-old man presents with jaundice, malaise and right hypochondrial tenderness. He admits to pale stools and dark urine.

Blood tests reveal: Total bilirubin 360 μmol/litre, AST 1100 U/litre, ALP 370 U/litre.

A blood sample is sent to virology and the report reveals:

- ✦ Hepatitis A IgG   Negative
- ✦ Hepatitis B surface antigen   Positive
- ✦ Hepatitis B e antigen   Positive
- ✦ IgM core antibody   Positive
- ✦ IgG core antibody   Negative
- ✦ Hepatitis C total antibody   Negative

In untreated infection with hepatitis B, all of the following are true except:

A. **15–25% of those chronically infected will die from liver failure**
B. **2–10% of adults become chronically infected with hepatitis B**
C. **1 in 10 people with cirrhosis caused by chronic hepatitis B will go on to develop liver cancer**
D. **Fulminant hepatitis B occurs in around 1 in 100 adults with chronic hepatitis B**
E. **Up to 90% of infected adults become carriers**

CASE 5

A 75-year-old man with a background of type 2 diabetes and a left ureteric stent presents with recurrent urinary tract infections. He has had multiple antibiotic courses in the past few months. He now presents with rigors and severe flank pain. His temperature is 39 °C and blood pressure is 90/52 mmHg. A recent urine sample shows the presence of moderate quantities of pus cells and growth of *Candida albicans*. Ultrasound and CT imaging of the renal tracts scan show a collection in the left perinephric space.

Which of the following is true?

   A. **Percutaneous drainage is contraindicated in most patients**
   B. **Percutaneous drainage has the best outcome in fungal abscesses**
   C. **Follow-up urine cultures and imaging are recommended to rule out recurrent infection**
   D. **Systemic fluconazole therapy is not indicated in this case**
   E. **The mortality rate approaches 100% even with modern surgical therapy**

CASE 6

A 45-year-old man is seen four months after having unprotected sex while on holiday abroad. He presents with malaise and a scaly papular rash on the trunk and palms of his hands. He denies genital ulceration. Further examination reveals the presence of generalised non-tender lymphadenopathy. You are provided with the following serology results:

   ✦ VDRL   Negative
   ✦ TPPA   1/160
   ✦ Total antibody EIA   Reactive
   ✦ TP IgM   Negative

What is the most likely diagnosis?

   A. **Secondary syphilis**
   B. **Treated syphilis**
   C. **Primary syphilis**
   D. **False positive serology**
   E. **Latent syphilis**

CASE 7

You are asked to see an elderly lady who has become increasingly confused. Her temperature is 38 °C and blood pressure 100/60 mmHg. Chest examination is normal and urinalysis is negative. Her chest X-ray appears unremarkable. She is currently on oral flucloxacillin for cellulitis of her left wrist associated with a previously infected intravenous catheter site. You examine her wrist and notice it is markedly swollen with surrounding erythema and a reduced range of movement. An ultrasound scan of the wrist shows no collection or joint involvement.

A swab taken previously from the site has grown *Staphylococcus aureus* resistant to penicillin and flucloxacillin, but sensitive to doxycycline, vancomycin, gentamicin and fusidic acid.

What is your immediate management plan for this lady?

- A. **Send blood cultures, no change of antibiotics until culture results back**
- B. **Change antibiotics to oral doxycycline and isolate the patient**
- C. **Isolate the patient and change antibiotics to IV flucloxacillin**
- D. **Send cultures, isolate the patient and change antibiotics to IV vancomycin**
- E. **Isolate the patient, no antibiotic change**

CASE 8

A 67-year-old lady, who was previously fit and healthy, presents with a vague history of constitutional upset, sore throat, dry cough with pleuritic chest pain, myalgia and malaise for more than one week. The dry cough is persistent despite a course of amoxicillin from her GP. On examination she has a fine rash over her upper limbs and chest. Her chest X-ray shows diffuse infiltrates. Her respiratory rate is 22 breaths/min and blood pressure 110/78 mmHg.

Blood tests reveal: White cells 17×10^9/litre, C-reactive protein 89 mg/litre, Urea is 8.7 mmol/litre.

Sputum and throat swab cultures: negative at 48 hours.

Urine for legionella and pneumococcal antigens: negative.

Respiratory PCR test: positive for mycoplasma pneumonia.

What would be your treatment of choice?

A. **Start IV piperacillin-tazobactam**
B. **No antibiotics since this is probably a viral infection**
C. **Treat for mild community-acquired pneumonia with oral amoxicillin**
D. **Add a macrolide such as clarithromycin to her treatment**
E. **Treat for severe community-acquired pneumonia with IV co-amoxiclav**

CASE 9

A 23-year-old student presents with malaise, fever, sore throat and cervical lymphadenopathy. Serology results come back showing: Monospot positive (titre 240).

Which of the following viruses is most unlikely to cause a similar clinical presentation?

A. **HIV**
B. **Cytomegalovirus**
C. **Epstein–Barr virus**
D. **Herpes simplex virus**
E. **Adenovirus**

CASE 10

A 57-year-old lady presents with a history of weight loss and general malaise over several weeks following a dental procedure. On examination, she has low-grade pyrexia, pallor and left flank tenderness. CT scanning of the abdomen and pelvis shows hepatosplenomegaly with the spleen measuring 18 cm in long axis. Her urine shows microscopic haematuria. A bedside transthoracic echocardiography is performed and shows an ejection fraction of 54%, moderate aortic stenosis but no obvious evidence of regurgitation of, or vegetation on, the valves. Three sets of blood cultures are positive for the organism shown in Figure 7.5.

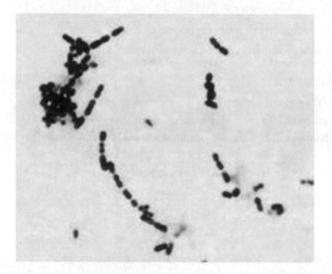

Figure 7.5

How should the patient be managed?

- A. **Treat for infective endocarditis with IV benzylpenicillin and gentamicin**
- B. **Withold antibiotics and arrange a trans-oesophageal echocardiography**
- C. **Send more blood cultures and only start antibiotics if positive with the same organism**
- D. **Investigate for haematological causes of her enlarged liver and spleen**
- E. **Refer to the surgical team for investigations of her splenomegaly**

CASE 11

You are asked to review a 33-year-old female patient commenced on gentamicin for a urinary tract infection two days ago. She has a documented penicillin allergy. Her temperature has settled and inflammatory markers are coming down. You notice that a trough level taken early that morning is 2.4 mg/litre. Her renal function tests are normal. What would be the most appropriate action in relation to this result?

    A. **Reduce the dose of gentamicin**

    B. **Check the time of the trough in relation to the last dose**

    C. **Skip one dose of gentamicin**

    D. **Stop gentamicin and prescribe an alternative**

    E. **Continue at current dose**

CASE 12

A 50-year-old man is diagnosed with viral hepatitis. His serology is reported as hepatitis C positive.

All of the following are true regarding the risk factors for hepatitis C except:

    A. **Like many other blood-borne viruses, sexual transmission is thought to be relatively common**

    B. **The risk of a mother infecting her newborn baby with hepatitis C is estimated to be less than 10%**

    C. **Intravenous drug use is the most common way to acquire hepatitis C virus infection in the UK**

    D. **In the UK, blood donations have been screened for hepatitis C since September 1991**

    E. **Infection is not acquired through normal social contact**

CASE 13

An 82-year-old male patient with a myelodysplastic syndrome requiring regular blood transfusions is admitted with pyrexia and malaise. He has been unwell with rigors at home during the previous five days. On examination, his temperature is 37.8 °C and his blood pressure is 144/83 mmHg. His chest is clear and the abdomen is soft and non-tender. He has an erythematous discharging wound from a cat bite, on the dorsum of his right hand. He has been given a tetanus booster in the emergency department. You receive a call from microbiology informing you of the presence of gram-negative bacilli in his blood cultures.

What organism should you be mostly concerned about?

A. *Pseudomonas auriginosa*
B. *Eschericia coli*
C. *Pasteurella maltocida*
D. *Clostridium tetani*
E. *Brucella arbotus*

CASE 14

An eastern European gentleman was treated for pulmonary tuberculosis (TB) a few years ago. He now presents with a productive cough and night sweats. On examination, he is cachexic, and a CT scan of his chest shows a cavitating lesion and hilar lymphadenopathy. Sputum samples sent to the laboratory come back with the following results:

+ Sputum sample: a few acid fast bacilli seen
+ Nucleic acid amplification test: *Mycobacterium tuberculosis* (MTB) complex
+ No resistance to rifampicin detected

Which of the following options is most accurate?

A. **This is unlikely to be multi-drug-resistant (MDR) TB**
B. **This history suggests he has MDR TB**
C. **Culture is no longer required in this instance**
D. **Typically two drugs will be used during the first eight weeks, then three or four drugs for the remaining duration**
E. **Visual acuity should be monitored during rifampicin use**

CASE 1

C: Request CSF virology and PCR, and start IV aciclovir

The likely diagnosis is encephalitis. The initial site of pathogen entry may have been the respiratory tract (eg measles, mumps and varicella zoster viruses), the genital tract (eg herpes simplex virus (HSV)), the gastrointestinal tract (eg enteroviruses) or subcutaneous tissues (eg arboviruses, ricketsiae, trypanosomes or rabies). A good travel history including exposure to insects and animals would be important. In a patient presenting with meningeal symptoms and a prior history of genital vesicular rash after unprotected intercourse, HSV infection would be a likely cause.

Learning point

Patients with HSV encephalitis present with fever, neck stiffness and reduced levels of consciousness. Some may have focal neurological signs, seizures and temporal lobe lesions on imaging. CSF analysis will usually show a lymphocytosis and bacteriology culture is negative – hence the importance of CSF virology tests including PCR. Empirical and prompt treatment with aciclovir reduces mortality to less than 20%. Referral to an infectious disease specialist would be required for further investigations, including HIV testing, but this would not be the first priority.

CHAPTER 7
ANSWERS

CASE 2

C: Combination antibiotics and urgent neurosurgical referral for drainage of pus

Meningeal signs and symptoms following an episode of sinusitis and the appearance of a space-occupying lesion on neuroimaging suggests the diagnosis of a brain abscess. Brain abscesses are caused by contiguous spread from para-meningeal infections, foreign bodies or haematogenous spread. Infection can be due to bacteria (often polymicrobial with staphylococci, *Streptococcus* species, *Enterobacteriaceae* and anaerobes), fungi (eg *Candida* species, *Aspergillus* species and mucormycosis) or protozoa/helminths (eg trypanosomes, *Toxoplasma gondii* or neurocysticercosis). Patients may present with headaches, fever, reduced consciousness level and focal neurology. Differential diagnoses include bacterial meningitis, brain neoplastic disease (primary or metastatic), cryptococcosis, cysticercosis, focal encephalitis, mycotic aneurysm, septic cerebral emboli causing infarction or septic dural sinus thrombosis.

Signs of raised intracranial pressure and seizures may be present. Radiological imaging, eg CT scanning, is often diagnostic. Lumbar puncture is contraindicated because of the high risk of cerebellar herniation. Drainage of pus for culture is recommended and treatment with a combination of antibiotics, which might include benzylpenicillin or cefotaxime/ ceftriaxone with metronidazole or chloramphenicol

CASE 3

E: IV metronidazole

This patient has an amoebic liver abscess close to the inferior vena cava. Attempting to drain this abscess may be risky. Amoebic liver abscesses are caused by *Entamoeba histolytica*, an intestinal protozoa endemic in developing countries.

Learning point

Onset of symptoms usually occurs within 8–12 weeks from the date of travel and patients present with abdominal pain, fever, weight loss and diarrhoea, which may or may not be bloody.

E. histolytica exists in two forms, the cyst stage which is the infective form, and the trophozoite stage which causes invasive disease. There is a 10% risk of developing symptomatic invasive amoebiasis after acquiring a pathogenic strain of the protozoa. It cannot be distinguished morphologically from similar amoeba such as *E. dispar*, which is thought to be non-pathogenic, and hence differentiation requires analysis of faecal antigens or PCR. Ultrasound, CT or MRI scanning are very sensitive in the diagnosis of liver abscesses. Treatment is usually with a course of metronidazole followed by eradication of the intraluminal cysts with an amoebocide such as paromomycin or diloxanide to prevent relapse. Follow-on stool cultures are recommended to establish clearance.

CHAPTER 7 ANSWERS

CASE 4

E: Up to 90% of infected adults become carriers

Viral hepatitis is an infection of the liver by the hepatitis viruses. Most commonly, hepatitis A virus (HAV), hepatitis B virus (HBV) and hepatitis C virus (HCV) are implicated. Other causative viruses include cytomegalovirus and Epstein–Barr virus.

Learning point

Transmission of hepatitis B virus mostly occurs through blood contact, sexual intercourse and perinatal transmission from mother to infant. The majority of those infected during adulthood make a full recovery and acquire immunity. Diagnosis is made by the presence of hepatitis B surface antigen (HBsAg) in blood. All patients with positive HBsAg should have other hepatitis B markers and hepatitis B DNA checked. Chronic hepatitis B is defined as persistence of HBsAg for six months or more after an acute infection, and affects 2–10% of adults, 50% of young children and almost 100% of infected neonates. Presence of the 'e' antigen is a marker of infectivity. See Figure 7.6.

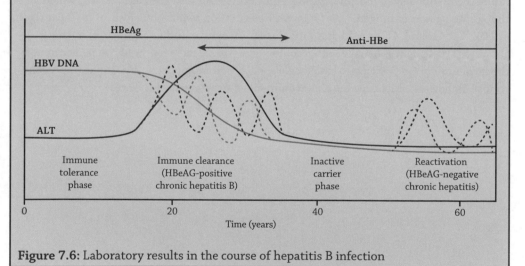

Figure 7.6: Laboratory results in the course of hepatitis B infection

Acute infection presents with general malaise, nausea and vomiting, abdominal pain and jaundice. Patients may present with mild flu-like symptoms. Chronic infection is asymptomatic in the majority of carriers, but a few may have persistent muscle aches, lethargy, nausea, lack of appetite, intolerance of alcohol, right upper quadrant abdominal pain, jaundice and depression. Complications include cirrhosis and hepatocellular cancer. Diagnosis may be aided by a blood liver enzyme profile, liver imaging, liver biopsy and virology results. Treatment options for chronic disease include lamivudine, adefovir, tenofovir and interferons. A vaccine is available to protect against hepatitis B and should be offered to those at increased risk of infection, eg sexual and household contacts of someone infected with hepatitis B. Pre- and post-exposure vaccination is available for healthcare workers. All pregnant women in the UK are offered a hepatitis B blood test. If a mother is infected, her baby is given hepatitis B antibodies and is also vaccinated.

CASE 5

C: Follow-up urine cultures and imaging are recommended to rule out recurrent infection

> **Learning point**
>
> Urinary tract infections (UTIs) in men are generally viewed as complicated in nature, because they result from an anatomic or functional anomaly, or occur after instrumentation of the genito-urinary tract. Conditions like prostatitis, chlamydial infection and epididymitis should be considered in the differential diagnosis of men with acute dysuria or frequency and appropriate diagnostic tests should be considered.

In all men with symptoms of UTI, a urine sample should be taken for culture. In all patients with a history of fever or back pain, the possibility of a complicated UTI should be considered. X-ray, ultrasound, CT and MRI imaging, as well as intravenous renography, may be used to confirm the presence of stones and retroperitoneal or perinephric collections. A perinephric abscess is an uncommon complication of a UTI, affecting patients with one or more anatomical or physiological abnormalities. The abscess may be confined to the perinephric space or extend into adjacent structures. Causative organisms are usually gram-negative bacilli but can also be staphylococci or *Candida* species. Mixed infections have also been reported.

Cultures are positive in up to 80% of cases. Even with modern surgical therapy, the mortality rate is 8–22% and significant morbidity occurs in 35% of patients. Empiric antibiotics that cover both gram-negative and positive organisms should be started before

continued

culture results are available. Treatment is often required for between one and three weeks after drainage of an abscess. Fluconazole is the treatment of choice for *Candida albicans* infections. See Table 7.1.

	Fluconazole	Itraconazole	Voriconazole	Ambisome	Caspofungin
Candida albicans	Yes	Yes	Yes	Yes	Yes
Non-albicans candida	Variable	Variable	Variable	Variable	Yes
Aspergillus spp.	No	Yes	Yes	Yes	Yes
Mucor	No	No	No	Yes	No
Fusarium	No	No	Yes	Yes	No
Cryptococcus	Yes	Yes	Yes	Yes	No

Table 7.1: Typical antimicrobial choices in fungal infections

CASE 6

A: Secondary syphilis

Syphilis is a complex systemic disease caused by *Treponema pallidum*, a spirorochete. Related treponemes cause non-venereal infections such as bejel, or endemic syphilis (*T. pallidum endemicum*), yaws (*T. pallidum pertenue*) and pinta (*T. carateu*). Syphilis can be acquired sexually or, rarely, through transfusion or congenitally. It can be classified into early (infectious) and late (non-infectious) stages. Early syphilis may be further divided into primary (painless chancre), secondary (papular rash) and early latent syphilis. Late syphilis includes late latent and the various forms of tertiary syphilis (eg neurosyphilis, cardiovascular or gummatous). Syphilis is most infectious during primary and secondary stages, but transmission can rarely occur during early latent syphilis. Mother to child transmission can occur throughout early syphilis (see Table 7.2).

Early infectious syphilis	
Stage	**Time post exposure**
Primary	9–90 days; usually 3 weeks
Secondary	6 weeks–6 months
Early latent	< 2 years
Late latent	> 2 years
Tertiary	3–20 years
Note: transmission to fetus can occur in late latent < 2 years since birth – early congenital syphilis stage > 2 years – late congenital syphilis	

Table 7.2: Stages of syphilis infection

Serology is the mainstay for the diagnosis of syphilis. Non-treponamal tests such as Venereal Disease Research Laboratory (VDRL) or Rapid Plasma Reagin (RPR) are useful as screening tests and to monitor response to treatment. Other screening tests include testing for antibodies to *T. pallidum* using enzyme immunoassays (EIA). Confirmatory tests include the *T. pallidum* particle agglutination assay (TPPA), dark ground microscopy or immuno-fluorescence tests of fluid from lesions. See Figure 7.7.

continued

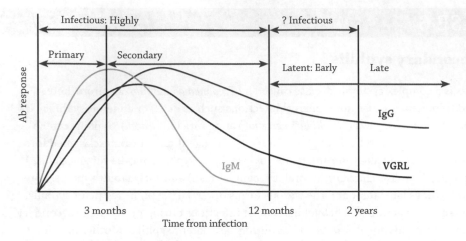

Figure 7.7: Laboratory results in the course of syphilis infection

All patients testing positive for syphilis should be offered tests for other sexually transmitted infections including HIV. Treatment is with penicillin.

Table 7.3 gives the differential diagnosis for genital ulcer disease.

	Syphilis	HSV	Chancroid	Lymphogranuloma venereum	Granuloma inguinale
Organism	Treponoma pallidum	Herpes simplex	Haemophilus ducreyi	Chlamydia trachomatis L1, L2, L3	Calymmatobacterium granulomatis
Geographical distribution	Worldwide	Worldwide	Africa, Asia, Latin America	Foci in tropics	All resource-poor countries
Incubation period	1–12 weeks	2–7 days	1–14 days	3 days–6 weeks	Up to 6 months
Primary lesion	Papule	Vesicle	Pustule	Papule	Papule
No. of lesions	Usually one	Multiple, may coalesce	Multiple, may coalesce	Usually one	Variable
Diameter (mm)	5–15	1–2	2–20	2–10	Variable
Edges	Elevated, round	Erythema	Ragged, undermined	Elevated, round	Elevated, irregular
Depth	Superficial or deep	Superficial	Excavated	Superficial or deep	Elevated
Induration	Firm	None	Soft	Variable	Firm
Pain	Unusual	Common	Common	Variable	Uncommon
Lymphadenopathy	Firm, non-tender	Firm, tender, bilateral	Soft, very tender, may suppurate	Tender, loculated, unilateral	Uncommon, firm, 'pseudobubo'

Table 7.3: Differential diagnosis for genital ulceration

CHAPTER 7 ANSWERS

CASE 7

D: Send cultures, isolate the patient and change antibiotics to IV vancomycin

Staphylococci are natural inhabitants of human skin. Patients and hospital personnel provide a reservoir of potential pathogens. Colonisation of intravascular devices often precedes infection, with central line-related bloodstream infection being the most common hospital-acquired infection. *S. aureus* is an obligate pathogen when isolated from blood and other sterile body fluids, and colonisation with methicillin-resistant *Staphylococcus aureus* (MRSA) is an important hospital infection control challenge. Cellulitis is a common condition, and common causative organisms include *Streptococcus pyogenes*, *Staphylococcus aureus*, and, rarely, gram-negative bacilli and anaerobes. Clinical features include erythema of the skin, warmth and swelling. Fever and pain may be present. In patients with cellulitis associated with intravascular devices, it is important to exclude deep-seated infections such as bacteraemia, septic arthritis, osteomyelitis, abscesses or phlebitis. The choice of antibiotic therapy depends on the following:

1. Site of infection: penetration of antimicrobials into tissues such as bone and joints.

2. Organism sensitivity: MRSA is resistant to flucloxacillin and hence to penicillin.

3. Allergies: range from mild gastrointestinal upset and skin rashes to severe anaphylactic reactions.

4. Age: use of clindamycin or cephalosporins may increase risk of super-infection, eg with *Clostridium difficile* in the elderly.

5. Route of administration: intravenous medication is suitable for severe life-threatening infections and oral treatment is ideal for community practice. Other routes include topical, intrathecal, vaginal and rectal.

6. Side-effect profile of the drug.

CASE 8

D: Add a macrolide such as clarithromycin to her treatment

Community-acquired pneumonia can be caused by viruses, eg influenza virus, or bacteria such as *Streptococcus pneumonia*, *Haemophilus influenzae*, *Mycoplasma pneumoniae*, *Chlamydophila* species, *Legionella* species or *Staphylococcus aureus*. The urea and electrolytes profile, C-reactive protein concentration, full blood count and liver function tests help to inform severity of infection. The severity can be assessed by using a scoring system such as the CURB65 score (see Table 7.4).

Confusion
Urea > 7 mmol/l
Respiratory rate ≥ 30/min
Low systolic (< 90 mmHg) or diastolic (≤ 60 mmHg) blood pressure
Age ≥ 65 years

Table 7.4: The CURB65 score for assessment of community-acquired pneumonia

Learning point

Mycoplasma pneumoniae can occur in otherwise healthy individuals. Patients often present with a history of a slow-onset decline over a few days or weeks with constitutional upset, fever, headaches, dry cough with pleuritic pain, myalgia, malaise and sore throat. The hacking, dry cough can be very persistent. Other features include rashes such as erythema multiforme, erythema nodosum and urticaria; neurological complications including Guillain–Barré syndrome, transverse myelitis, cerebellar ataxia and aseptic meningitis. Diagnosis is by serology and nucleic acid amplification testing on respiratory samples. Treatment is with macrolide antimicrobials such as clarithromycin.

CASE 9

D: Herpes simplex virus

This patient has infectious mononucleosis. This syndrome is most commonly caused by Epstein–Barr virus (EBV). In EBV infection, heterophile antibodies are present and these agglutinate non-human red blood cells resulting in the positive monospot or Paul–Bunnell test. The heterophile antibodies are detectable for up to six months after infection. False negative monospot testing can occur in children under 12 years of age, and false positive tests can be seen in lymphoproliferative disorders. Complications of the infection include splenic rupture, tracheal obstruction, chronic infectious mononucleosis, aplastic anaemia and thrombocytopaenia. Management is supportive.

CASE 10

A: Treat for infective endocarditis with IV benzylpenicillin and gentamicin

The patient has infective endocarditis. Patients commonly present with malaise and fever. Classical features such as arthralgia, variable heart murmurs, splinter haemorrhages, Osler's nodes and microhaematuria may or may not be present and are often seen with infections present for longer durations of time. Some patients may present with multiple septic emboli and stroke.

Infective endocarditis should be considered in the circumstances shown in Table 7.5.

A febrile illness and a murmur of new valvular regurgitation

A febrile illness and a pre-existing at-risk cardiac lesion and no clinically obvious site of infection

A febrile illness associated with any of:

✦ predisposition and recent intervention with associated bacteraemia

✦ evidence of congestive heart failure

✦ new cardiac conduction disturbance

✦ vascular or immunological phenomena: embolic event, Roth's spots, splinter haemorrhages, Janeway lesions, Osler's nodes

A new stroke or peripheral abscesses (renal, splenic, cerebral, vertebral) of unknown cause

A protracted history of sweats, weight loss, anorexia or malaise and an at-risk cardiac lesion

Any new unexplained embolic event (eg cerebral or limb ischaemia)

Unexplained, persistently positive blood cultures

Intravascular catheter-related bloodstream infection with persistently positive blood cultures 72 h after catheter removal

Table 7.5: When to consider infective endocarditis

Viridans streptococci form part of the resident flora of the oral cavity and are a common cause of endocarditis of native valves. The streptococci are a large group of gram-positive coccoid organisms appearing in chains or pairs. Differentiation can be made from the haemolytic appearance on blood agar. Alpha (partial) haemolysis is seen with viridans group streptococci, beta (complete) haemolysis with *Streptococcus pyogenes* for example, and non-haemolytic organisms include *S. pneumoniae*. Beta haemolytic streptococci can be further differentiated by means of a latex agglutination test (the Lancefield grouping test) into:

✦ Group A: *S. pyogenes* commonly causing pharyngitis, scarlet fever, skin and soft tissue infections

✦ Group B: *S. agalactiae* commonly colonises the female genital area and is an important cause of early neonatal sepsis and meningitis

✦ Groups C and G: *S. dysgalactiae* commonly cause skin and soft tissue infections

✦ Group D: *S. bovis* group associated with occult abscesses and enterococci species associated with biliary or urinary sepsis

✦ Group F: *S. anginosus* group (formerly milleri group) comprising *S. anginosus*, *S. constellatus* and *S. intermedius* associated with intra-abdominal pathology.

Streptococcus species are invariably susceptible to penicillin, which remains the treatment of choice for infections caused by these organisms.

CASE 11

B: Check the time of the trough in relation to the last dose

Gentamicin is an aminoglycoside antibiotic, as are amikacin and tobramycin. These agents act by preventing translation of mRNA into protein. They are usually given parenterally, are limited to the extracellular fluid and are excreted in the urine. Important side effects include toxicity to the kidneys and eighth cranial nerves, making careful monitoring of levels necessary. Trough levels should be taken immediately before the next dose. Checking the 'trough' too early may result in falsely high levels. Doses need to be adjusted based on changing renal function or volume status. A once daily dose of 5-7 mg/kg is usually given in adults with normal renal function with a target trough of < 1 mg/litre. For obese patients, a calculated ideal body weight (IBW) plus 40% of excess fat (actual body weight – IBW) should be used. For synergy with β-lactam-containing agents, in the treatment of gram-positive infections, a dose of 1 mg/kg 12 hourly is commonly used.

CASE 12

A: Like many other blood-borne viruses, sexual transmission is thought to be relatively common

Hepatitis C is a blood-borne viral infection with an estimated 170 million carriers worldwide. The prevalence of chronic hepatitis C infection in England is estimated to be around 0.4%.

Learning point

Intravenous drug use is the most common way to acquire hepatitis C virus infection. In the UK, blood donations have been screened for hepatitis C since September 1991, but it is possible to acquire the infection through blood transfusion in a country that does not screen its blood for the virus. Unlike many other blood-borne viruses, sexual transmission is thought to be relatively rare. Infection is not acquired through normal social contact, but it can occur in situations where blood can be transferred from one person to another, through sharing razors, toothbrushes or during body piercing if sterile needles are not used. The risk of a mother infecting her new born baby is estimated to be less than 10% and is highest in mothers who are also infected with HIV or have high viral loads.

CASE 13

C: *Pasteurella maltocida*

Pasteurella is a group of gram-negative bacteria that colonise the respiratory tract of animals and should be considered when there is a history of contact with pets which include bites, scratches or licking of wounds. Infection causes mild skin and soft tissue infections in healthy subjects, and severe systemic illnesses in immunocompromised hosts. The species *P. multocida* cause almost 70% of all cases, and *P. multocida bacteraemia* carries an overall mortality rate of 31%. Penicillins are the antibiotics of choice with ciprofloxacin and doxycycline as alternatives.

CASE 14

A: This is unlikely to be multi-drug-resistant (MDR) TB

TB is an infection caused by MTB complex (*M. tuberculosis*, *M. bovis*, *M. africanum*). It can either cause pulmonary or extra-pulmonary infections, with lymph nodes, meninges, pleura, pericardium, kidneys, joints, skin or intestines often being involved. *M. tuberculosis* and *M. africanum* are primarily from human hosts, with *M. bovis* from cattle. Most initial infections are asymptomatic, with up to 95% of affected individuals becoming latent carriers. Up to 10% of these latent carriers develop clinical disease in their lifetime and more than half do so in the first five years of infection.

continued

Learning point

Classical features include fatigue, weight loss, chronic cough or night sweats. Exposure to airborne droplet nuclei from people with pulmonary TB occurs during coughing or sneezing. The risk of acquisition is related to the degree of exposure. When inhaled, these bacilli can settle in the lungs causing a primary infection (ghon focus) and may remain viable for the lifetime of the host. The incubation period from exposure to primary infection is usually 4 to 12 weeks. Extra-pulmonary TB is usually not transmissible – a rare exception would include a procedure such as the draining of an abscess. TB may also be acquired through the ingestion of unpasteurised milk. Reactivation of latent TB occurs during periods of immunosuppression, alcoholism or debilitation, eg with diabetes mellitus, HIV, cancer, malnutrition or advanced age. The Mantoux skin test and the gamma interferon TB blood tests are useful to detect latent infection. Inspection of a chest X-ray is central to the diagnosis of pulmonary TB, as well as testing of sputum or early morning urine samples using Ziehl–Neelsen's stain and TB culture.

Gastric washing may be a suitable test for children unable to produce sputum. Other suitable samples for testing include lymph node and other organ biopsies, depending on the presentation. Nucleic acid amplification testing (NAAT) is now commonly used for TB diagnosis and detection of rifampicin sensitivity. The treatment for TB is lengthy and complex, and should therefore be supervised, since inadequate treatment or non-compliance can result in the emergence of drug-resistant organisms. Effective treatment with multiple antimicrobials usually eliminates infectivity within two weeks. First-line treatment usually consists of a combination of rifampicin, isoniazid, ethambutol and pyrazinamide. MDR TB is defined as TB resistant to two or more of the first-line antimicrobials, usually rifampicin and isoniazid with or without other drugs. MDR TB should be managed at facilities with expertise in its management, and patients should be isolated in negative pressure rooms.

CHAPTER 8

Neurology

Stella Hughes and Gavin McDonnell

A 14-year-old boy is brought to the emergency department by his parents at 0830 hours. He had been dressing for school that morning when his brother witnessed him collapse onto the bedroom floor. His mother attended and found him lying with his eyes closed, fists clenched and elbows flexed. She described his body 'shaking' for one or two minutes and he did not respond to her for another five to ten minutes. He has no past medical history. His parents were concerned that he had recently been staying up late and seemed slow and clumsy in the mornings. They did not think that he had been taking alcohol or illicit drugs. On assessment, his general observations were normal. He responded to voice and had no focal neurological signs on examination. He had bitten the side of his tongue.

Which of the following investigations is most likely to lead to a diagnosis in this case?

- A. **Blood alcohol level**
- B. **EEG**
- C. **CT scan of brain**
- D. **Serum prolactin concentration**
- E. **ECG**

CASE 2

A 56-year-old lady is admitted for the investigation of headache. The headache came on in the morning the day before and became 'excruciating' by that evening. It was worse on lying down. She describes nausea and intermittent visual disturbance. Past medical history includes ulcerative colitis, for which she was treated for a 'severe flare-up' one week ago. On initial assessment, blood pressure was 148/80 mmHg, and she was found to have mild right hemiparesis.

What is the most likely diagnosis in this case?

    A. **Subarachnoid haemorrhage**
    B. **Cerebral reversible vasoconstriction syndrome**
    C. **Cerebral venous sinus thrombosis**
    D. **Migraine**
    E. **Enterococcal meninigitis**

CASE 3

A 64-year-old man is brought to the emergency department by his wife. He had been well that morning on getting out of bed. One hour later he was standing shaving in the bathroom but seemed 'confused'. He repeatedly asked her 'Where am I?' and appeared agitated. Four hours later he was back to his usual self but had no memory of the events of the morning. He had no history of similar episodes in the past. Past medical history included osteoarthritis and paroxysmal atrial fibrillation. His general observations were normal, capillary blood glucose was 4.2 mmol/litre and ECG showed normal sinus rhythm. He had no focal neurological signs on examination.

What is the most likely diagnosis in this case?

    A. **Transient epileptic amnesia**
    B. **Complex partial seizure**
    C. **Transient ischaemic attack**
    D. **Cardio-embolic stroke**
    E. **Transient global amnesia**

CASE 4

A 22-year-old man is referred to the neurology outpatient clinic from the ophthalmology department. He had a recent diagnosis of optic neuritis in his right eye which has fully resolved. He describes an episode of vertigo and double vision 18 months ago which lasted for two weeks. Examination findings include visual acuity 6/6 in both eyes, right relative afferent pupillary defect, bilateral internuclear ophthalmoplegia and mild bilateral finger–nose ataxia.

His MRI scan of brain is shown in Figure 8.1.

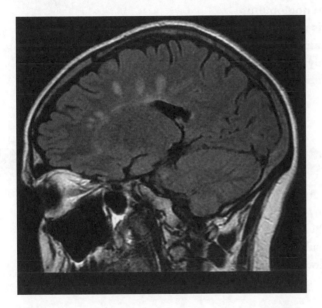

Figure 8.1

Which of the following treatments would you consider prescribing at this time?

    A. **Plasma exchange**
    B. **Rituximab**
    C. **Natalizumab**
    D. **Interferon beta**
    E. **Methylprednisolone**

CASE 5

A 48-year-old lady presents with generalised limb weakness which had worsened over the previous five days. She drinks a bottle of vodka (700 ml) each day and smokes 30 cigarettes per day. Examination reveals moderate weakness of the distal upper and lower limbs and neck flexion. Reflexes were reduced throughout the limbs. There was reduced pinprick sensation distally to the wrists and ankles. Cerebrospinal fluid protein was 0.77 g/litre.

Which treatment would you consider administering urgently in this case?

A. **Intravenous immunoglobulin**
B. **Intravenous fluids with potassium chloride**
C. **Intravenous thiamine**
D. **Intravenous methylprednisolone**
E. **Intramuscular hydroxocobalamin**

CASE 6

A 36-year-old lady suffers an out-of-hospital cardiac arrest. Cardiorespiratory resuscitation was started by a bystander within three minutes and was ongoing by paramedics on arrival at the emergency department. Cardiorespiratory function was restored and she was subsequently intubated and ventilated in the intensive care unit. Following withdrawal of sedation three days later, she is found to be comatose and further clinical assessment is undertaken to determine prognosis.

Which of the following markers will have the most prognostic value in indicating a poor outcome at this time?

A. **Presence of myoclonus status epilepticus**
B. **Longer duration of anoxia**
C. **Elevated body temperature**
D. **Absent or extensor motor responses**
E. **Type of cardiac arrhythmia leading to cardiac arrest**

CASE 7

A 66-year-old man has been given a recent diagnosis of motor neurone disease. His daughter has been researching the condition on the internet and they want to discuss management strategies for the disease. Which of the following interventions has been shown to improve survival in motor neurone disease?

    A. **Non-invasive ventilation**
    B. **Exercise programme**
    C. **Enteral feeding**
    D. **Diaphragmatic pacing**
    E. **Spinal stimulation**

CASE 8

A 44-year-old lady complains of increasing difficulty rising from a chair over three months. She has a history of hypothyroidism. She denied any excess alcohol intake. Liver transaminases were mildly elevated. Serum creatine kinase was over 6000 U/litre. On examination, there was proximal muscle weakness in the upper and lower limbs and weakness of neck flexion. Sensory examination was normal. There was mild tenderness on palpation of the quadriceps muscles. There was no skin rash.

Which of the following investigations is most likely to lead to a diagnosis?

    A. **Electromyography**
    B. **Muscle biopsy**
    C. **Tensilon® test**
    D. **Oral glucose tolerance test**
    E. **Thyroid-stimulating hormone level**

CASE 9

A previously well 52-year-old man is admitted with a 4-day history of headache and fever. He had been treated with oral antibiotics for suspected sinusitis for three days before admission. On the morning of admission, his wife had found him drowsy and confused and he had a witnessed generalised tonic-clonic seizure after arriving in the emergency department. On examination, he was drowsy and pyrexic (temperature 38.4 °C). He was not able to cooperate with a full neurological examination, but reflexes were brisk in the limbs and he had extensor plantar responses. He had no papilloedema. A CT scan of brain was normal. Lumbar puncture was performed and cerebrospinal fluid (CSF) analysis showed 48 leukocytes/mm^3 (60% lymphocytes), 4 erythrocytes/mm^3, protein 0.69 g/litre and glucose 3.5 mmol/litre (blood glucose 4.8 mmol/litre). Blood and CSF gram stain are awaited.

Which of the following treatments should be commenced immediately?

- A. **Intravenous amoxicillin**
- B. **Intravenous amphotericin**
- C. **Anti-tuberculous therapy**
- D. **Intravenous methylprednisolone**
- E. **Intravenous aciclovir**

CASE 10

A 72-year-old man attends the emergency department giving a 1-hour history of bilateral leg weakness. This had come on suddenly when he was working in the garden. He had back pain and urinary incontinence at onset. He has a history of hypercholesterolaemia, for which he takes a statin. On examination, he had a flaccid paraparesis with impaired temperature and pain sensation below the umbilicus.

Which of the following diagnoses is most likely?

- A. **Acute transverse myelopathy**
- B. **Spinal dural arteriovenous fistula**
- C. **Anterior spinal artery stroke**
- D. **Spinal haematoma**
- E. **Brown-Séquard syndrome**

CASE 11

A 38-year-old lady with a 10-year history of multiple sclerosis complains of bladder urgency, frequency and incontinence. She is able to walk at least 500 metres without a walking aid. She is currently taking detrusitol 4 mg daily. A post-void ultrasound scan of bladder is performed, and shows a residual volume of 32 ml.

Which additional management strategy may be useful for bladder management in this case?

    A. **Clean intermittent self-catheterisation**
    B. **An indwelling urethral catheter**
    C. **Botulinum toxin A injection into detrusor muscle**
    D. **Reduction in daily fluid intake**
    E. **Desmopressin twice daily**

CASE 12

A 15-year-old girl presents with involuntary movements. She had recently attended a child psychologist as she had struggled over the school year due to anxiety and low mood. Three months previously, she had presented to her GP with a sore throat and fatigue and was noted to have mild jaundice. Liver function tests at that time showed mild hepatitis. On examination, there was postural tremor and mild rigidity in the upper limbs. She had irregular, fleeting jerky movements of the trunk and limbs suggestive of chorea.

Which of the following blood tests is most likely to lead to the diagnosis in this case?

    A. **Huntington's disease genetic testing**
    B. **Serum caeruloplasmin**
    C. **Anti-double-stranded DNA antibody**
    D. **Anti-streptolysin titre**
    E. **Anti-basal ganglia antibody**

CASE 13

A 48-year-old man presents with a 3-hour history of left-sided weakness which had been present on wakening. He had been diagnosed with non-small cell lung cancer four months previously, for which he had radiotherapy. Adjuvant chemotherapy was under consideration by the treating oncologist. He is taking a statin as his last fasting serum cholesterol was 6.3 mmol/litre. On examination, he opens his eyes to voice and his speech is normal. He has a left hemiplegia with neglect and the left plantar response is extensor. Blood glucose is 5.4 mmol/litre and blood pressure 158/84 mmHg. An ECG shows normal sinus rhythm. His CT scan of brain is shown in Figure 8.2.

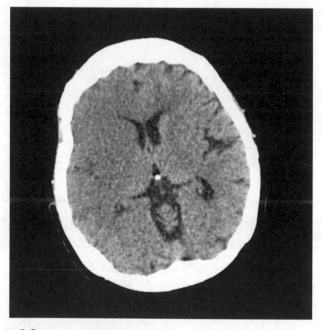

Figure 8.2

Which treatment should be initiated immediately in this case?

A. **Dexamethasone**

B. **Mannitol**

C. **Tissue plasminogen activator**

D. **Aspirin 300 mg**

E. **Enoxaparin**

CASE 14

A 58-year-old lady attends the clinic with a 1-year history of tremor and difficulty walking. She has had several falls in the last two months and complains of urinary frequency and incontinence. She was diagnosed with Parkinson's disease by her GP, who had gradually titrated co-beneldopa over the past nine months with no clinical improvement.

On examination, there was a jerky tremor and rigidity in the upper limbs. Reflexes were brisk throughout the limbs and the left plantar response was extensor. There was past-pointing in the upper limbs. Sensory examination was normal. There was mild dysarthria. The gait was slow and wide-based. Supine blood pressure was 122/76 mmHg and on standing was 104/70 mmHg.

Which of the following diagnoses is most likely in this case?

    A. **Multiple system atrophy**
    B. **Idiopathic Parkinson's disease**
    C. **Progressive supranuclear palsy**
    D. **Corticobasal degeneration**
    E. **Primary autonomic failure**

CASE 15

A 42-year-old smoker presents with generalised weakness in his muscles. His wife had recently noticed that his eyelids seemed to droop. He denied double vision or difficulty swallowing or talking. He had recently required over-the-counter laxatives for constipation. He had a history of hypertension for which he was prescribed amlodipine 5 mg daily, but this was stopped as he felt weaker and lightheaded with this treatment. On examination, there was bilateral partial ptosis which was non-fatigable on sustained upgaze. Eye movements were full. There was moderate weakness in the proximal upper and lower muscles. Tendon reflexes were reduced but were easier to obtain after exertion. He had a waddling gait.

Which of the following treatments is likely to result in an improvement in muscle strength in this patient?

    A. **Vitamin D**
    B. **Thyroxine**
    C. **Riluzole**
    D. **Guanidine**
    E. **3,4-diaminopyridine**

CASE 16

A 24-year-old pregnant lady of 14 weeks gestation is admitted to the maternity ward for management of hyperemesis gravidarum. On the day after admission she complains of double vision. On assessment, she is agitated and has poor attention and recall. Her cooperation with the neurological examination is limited, but a horizontal gaze palsy to the right is observed. Blood glucose was 4.1 mmol/litre. Which of the following treatments should be commenced immediately in this case?

A. Therapeutic dose enoxaparin
B. Intravenous immunoglobulin
C. Intravenous thiamine
D. Intravenous Hartmann's solution
E. Intravenous methylprednisolone

CASE 17

A 61-year-old man is referred to the neurology clinic with a 3-year history of dizziness. He describes brief attacks of a 'feeling of the room spinning around' which was associated with nausea. Attacks seemed to be triggered by suddenly turning his head and have sometimes occurred when he turned over in bed at night. He has a history of hypertension, ischaemic heart disease and paroxysmal atrial fibrillation. He is taking aspirin, ramipril, atorvastatin and had recently commenced betahistine. Neurological examination was normal. Which of the following management strategies should be initiated in this case?

A. Refer for carotid endarterectomy
B. Commence warfarin therapy
C. Commence dipyridamole and continue aspirin
D. Canalith repositioning manoeuvres
E. Neck physiotherapy

CASE 18

A 28-year-old right-handed nurse is admitted to hospital with a 1-week history of left-sided weakness and sensory loss. She has a history of eczema and irritable bowel syndrome and occasionally takes loperamide. On examination, she walks with one stick with her ankle held in eversion. There is moderate weakness globally in the left upper limb. In the left lower limb, there is severe weakness of hip flexion, knee extension and ankle plantar flexion, and moderate weakness of knee flexion and ankle dorsiflexion. There is full power throughout the right-sided limbs and Hoover's sign was present. Tendon reflexes are normal and symmetrical, and plantar responses are flexor. Cranial nerve examination is normal. Which is the most likely diagnosis in this case?

A. **Multiple sclerosis**
B. **Functional neurological symptoms**
C. **Right anterior cerebral artery stroke**
D. **Cervical myelopathy**
E. **Syringomyelia**

CASE 1

B: EEG

In this case, an adolescent presents with a first generalised tonic-clonic seizure (GTCS). There are features in the history to suggest a diagnosis of juvenile myoclonic epilepsy (JME). In JME, seizures tend to first occur around puberty and can be precipitated by sleep deprivation, often occurring soon after awakening in the morning. There may be a history of myoclonic jerks before the first GTCS. This may have been observed by others as 'clumsiness' in the mornings, earning the condition a nickname of 'cornflake epilepsy'.

Learning point

JME is an idiopathic generalised epilepsy, with a characteristic finding on interictal electroencephalogram (EEG) of polyspike-and-wave activity. EEG is therefore the most useful test.

The case history does not suggest alcohol-related seizures, therefore an alcohol level is unlikely to be helpful. Serum prolactin can be elevated after a seizure but is rarely measured. It is sometimes used to provide supportive evidence of an epileptic rather than non-epileptic attack (or 'pseudoseizure'). Brain imaging is not necessary in this case if the EEG is typical of JME. An ECG should be performed in all cases of collapse but the event in this case is suggestive of a seizure rather than syncope. See Figure 8.3.

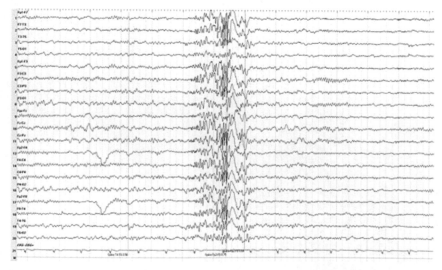

Figure 8.3 Typical EEG appearances in JME

CASE 2

C: Cerebral venous sinus thrombosis

This lady is at risk of cerebral venous sinus thrombosis given the pro-coagulant state produced by active inflammatory bowel disease. This diagnosis is supported by the associated visual disturbance and focal neurological signs. The history is not in keeping with thunderclap headache which would be the most common presenting complaint of subarachnoid haemorrhage and cerebral reversible vasoconstriction syndrome. Hemiplegic migraine is a possible diagnosis but it would be imperative to exclude a structural lesion in this case, especially in the absence of a previous history of this condition. There are no features in the history, such as pyrexia or meningism, to suggest bacterial meningitis.

CASE 3

E: Transient global amnesia

Learning point

The case history is typical of transient global amnesia (TGA) in which there is a sudden onset of anterograde amnesia and often repetitive questioning. Episodes last less than 24 hours and do not tend to recur. Precipitating factors include emotional stress, acute pain, physical exertion, sexual intercourse, immersion in cold water (bathing, swimming) or performance of a Valsalva manoeuvre.

A complex partial seizure due to temporal lobe epilepsy can produce amnesia alone (transient epileptic amnesia), but episodes tend to have a shorter duration (usually less than one hour) and are more likely to recur than TGA. Memory disturbances in isolation are uncommon presentations of stroke or transient ischaemic attack.

CHAPTER 8 ANSWERS

CASE 4

D: Interferon beta

The diagnosis is relapsing remitting multiple sclerosis (RRMS) as the patient has had two clinical attacks and there is objective evidence of optic nerve and brainstem lesions on examination. The MRI scan of brain (T2-weighted imaging) shows white matter lesions consistent with the diagnosis of multiple sclerosis (MS).

The current prescribing criterion for first-line treatment for RRMS in the UK is two clinically significant relapses in the previous two years.[1] The patient is therefore eligible for treatment with interferon beta or glatiramer acetate, which are injectable therapies. Oral agents such as fingolimod, teriflunomide and dimethyl fumarate have also recently become available for RRMS. Natalizumab, a monoclonal antibody, would be considered in those with rapidly evolving severe RRMS. The current UK prescribing criteria for natalizumab is two or more disabling relapses in one year with evidence of active disease on MR imaging.[2]

There is currently insufficient evidence to support the use of rituximab in MS. Methylprednisolone (and other corticosteroid preparations) may be used for significant relapses of MS, with the aim of hastening recovery. Plasma exchange is generally reserved for severe relapses in which there has been incomplete recovery following steroid therapy. The patient's recent episode of optic neuritis has resolved and therefore there is no current indication for steroids or plasma exchange.

CASE 5

A: Intravenous immunoglobulin

This lady has progressive muscle weakness, hyporeflexia and distal sensory loss, suggesting a diagnosis of Guillain–Barré syndrome (GBS). GBS is usually diagnosed based on clinical findings and should be considered and treated early since good supportive care reduces morbidity and mortality. Clinical trials have shown that intravenous immunoglobulin and plasmapheresis are equally efficacious. However, IV immunoglobulin is typically used initially as this is more readily available. There is no evidence to suggest that steroids improve outcomes in GBS. Respiratory function requires close monitoring with forced vital capacity (FVC) to allow for early referral to the high-dependency or intensive care unit.

IV potassium is not indicated as the predominantly distal weakness and sensory involvement would argue against a diagnosis of hypokalaemic periodic paralysis and no biochemical evidence of hypokalaemia is provided. The clinical examination lacks features to suggest Wernicke's encephalopathy, such as ataxia and ophthalmoplegia, although IV thiamine may be warranted given the history of alcohol misuse and possible low dietary intake of thiamine. There are also insufficient findings to suggest subacute combined degeneration of the spinal cord, and so the serum vitamin B12 level should be measured before considering hydroxocobalamin replacement therapy.

CASE 6

D: Absent or extensor motor responses

The American Academy of Neurology (AAN) has produced a *Summary of evidence-based guidelines for clinicians on prediction of outcome in comatose survivors after cardiopulmonary resuscitation.*[3]

Learning point

The clinical markers which have the strongest evidence for prognostic value are the Glasgow Coma Scale, motor responses to pain and brainstem reflexes (pupillary light reflexes, corneal reflexes and eye movements). Clinical features for which there is good evidence for prognostic value include seizures or myoclonus status epilepticus and circumstances of cardiopulmonary resuscitation (CPR) (anoxia time, duration of CPR and type of cardiac arrhythmia).

There is insufficient evidence to determine the utility of brain imaging (CT, MRI, PET) for prognostication. Regarding electrophysiological studies, in the AAN guidelines, somatosensory evoked potentials (N20 response) appear to have a superior prognostic value to that of EEG.

CASE 7

A: Non-invasive ventilation

Respiratory failure is the main cause of death in people with motor neurone disease (MND) and non-invasive ventilation (NIV) has been shown to improve survival. NIV is usually considered when orthopnoea first develops. Assessment for NIV includes nocturnal oximetry and pulmonary function testing including FVC, maximal inspiratory pressure and sniff nasal pressure measurement.

There is no convincing evidence for improved survival due to feeding via gastrostomy, although this is often used in people with MND who have bulbar weakness. There is no evidence for improved outcomes due to exercise or spinal stimulation. There are ongoing studies on diaphragm pacing in MND but no beneficial effect has been confirmed to date.

CASE 8

B: Muscle biopsy

The history is suggestive of polymyositis (PM) given the progressive proximal limb muscle and neck weakness with elevated muscle enzymes. There is no skin involvement to suggest that she has dermatomyositis (DM).

> ### Learning point
>
>
> Muscle biopsy is crucial to confirm the diagnosis of an inflammatory myositis and exclude mimics of the condition, such as metabolic myopathies or muscular dystrophies. Pathological findings specific to PM include the presence of cytotoxic CD8+ T cells and activated macrophages in the fascicles of non-necrotic muscle fibres. In DM, the hallmark histological feature is perifascicular atrophy. The lymphocytic infiltrate in DM is composed of B cells and CD4+ T cells, seen in the perivascular and perifascicular areas, consistent with a humorally mediated process.

Electromyography (EMG) is usually abnormal in inflammatory myopathies with neurogenic and myopathic changes. Classical findings include increased spontaneous activity (fibrillation potentials, positive sharp waves), early recruitment and small, polyphasic motor unit potentials (MUPs). However, these features are not specific for PM, and therefore muscle biopsy is required to distinguish between the inflammatory myopathies. EMG can be used to select the site for biopsy. However, a muscle which has recently undergone EMG study should not be biopsied as this may result in false positive inflammatory changes in the muscle sample.

There is no history of fatigability making myasthenia gravis a less likely diagnosis. A Tensilon® (edrophonium) test can be helpful in diagnosing myasthenia gravis when there is clinical uncertainty. It is mainly used for those presenting with ptosis rather than limb weakness, with an improvement in orbicularis oculi weakness sought by two examiners after administration of edrophonium. Given the history of thyroid disease, thyroid myopathy should be considered, but neck involvement is uncommon and serum CK would be expected to be normal or only mildly elevated. Diabetes mellitus can cause a proximal myopathy but there are no features in the history or examination (eg peripheral neuropathy) to suggest that this is the underlying cause.

CASE 9

E: Intravenous aciclovir

In this case, the history is in keeping with viral encephalitis, with clinical findings suggesting encephalomyelitis. The lymphocytic CSF with mildly elevated protein and normal glucose would be consistent with this condition. It would be prudent to commence IV aciclovir (10–15 mg/kg tds) immediately after lumbar puncture as poorer outcomes are associated with delays in receiving antiviral therapy.

Learning point

Virological tests performed on CSF and blood should include influenza, pertussis and measles, but the most likely pathogens in viral encephalitis are herpesviruses (usually herpes simplex virus type 1 but also simplex virus type 2, varicella zoster, Epstein–Barr, cytomegalovirus and human herpesviruses type 6 and 7). Other pathogens should be considered if there has been a history of travel.

EEG can provide supportive evidence of encephalitis and the commonest abnormality seen is diffuse slow waves. The Association of British Neurologists and British Infection Association have produced a guideline on *Management of suspected viral encephalitis in adults.*[4]

Other causes of CSF lymphocyte pleocytosis should also be considered and treated if felt likely. In this case, partially treated bacterial meningitis should be considered given that the patient has had antibiotics in the community. There is no suggestion that the patient is immunosuppressed and therefore treatment for listeria meningoencephalitis (with IV amoxicillin) would not be immediately necessary. IV amphotericin should be considered if cryptococcal meningitis is felt likely, eg in patients with HIV or other causes of immunosuppression, optic disc swelling, raised CSF opening pressure or low CSF glucose. CSF and blood should be sent for cryptococcal antigen and India ink staining should be performed on CSF to examine for cryptococci. Tuberculous meningitis can cause CSF lymphocytosis but CSF protein is often markedly elevated and CSF glucose is usually less than one third of the serum glucose. There is no indication for IV methylprednisolone in this case as there is no evidence to support use of corticosteroids in viral encephalitis.

CASE 10

C: Anterior spinal artery stroke

The diagnosis in this case is acute ischaemic spinal cord infarction in the anterior spinal artery territory. This artery supplies the corticospinal and spinothalamic tracts of the cord, with stroke resulting in paraparesis or quadriparesis, bladder dysfunction and impairment of pain and temperature below the level of infarction. Pain at the level of the infarct at onset is a common feature. There is sparing of the posterior columns. The anterior spinal artery is vulnerable to insult due to arterial hypotension but there are many other causes of ischaemia such as atherosclerosis, dissecting aortic aneurysm, trauma and vasculitis.

Acute transverse myelopathy is an acute cord syndrome with motor, sensory and autonomic dysfunction of the cord. In addition to the anterior cord syndrome in this case, transverse myelopathy will also have signs to suggest posterior (dorsal) column involvement (proprioception and vibration loss below the level of the lesion).

The onset is usually subacute and the main causes are infective (herpesviruses, HIV), demyelinating (multiple sclerosis, neuromyelitis optica) or other inflammatory disease (such as systemic lupus erythematosus or neurosarcoidosis).

Spinal dural arteriovenous (AV) fistulas are most commonly seen in elderly men presenting with a progressive paraparesis. They are usually found in the thoracolumbar cord and are suggested by cord oedema, dilated vessels and cord enhancement on MR imaging. Treatment options include endovascular embolisation or neurosurgical occlusion of the fistula.

A spinal haematoma is a possible diagnosis in this case as this can present with the abrupt onset of leg weakness, but there are no known risk factors for this, eg a preceding procedure such as lumbar puncture, coagulopathy or a known arterio venous malformation of the cord.

Brown-Séquard syndrome is a functional hemisection of the spinal cord with the following findings: contralateral spinothalamic tract signs (loss of pain and temperature), ipsilateral corticospinal tract signs (upper motor neurone weakness) and ipsilateral dorsal column signs (loss of proprioception and vibration). Brown-Séquard syndrome is more common with extramedullary spinal cord lesions but can be caused by any lesion which affects one half of the cord.

CASE 11

C: Botulinum toxin A injection into detrusor muscle

This lady with multiple sclerosis (MS) has bladder symptoms attributable to neurogenic detrusor activity, which have been refractory to anticholinergic therapy. She may benefit from botulinum toxin A injection into the detrusor muscle. There is evidence that this intervention improves urinary symptoms, urodynamic parameters and quality of life in people with MS who have failed first-line therapy. There is a need for intermittent self-catheterisation following this procedure.

In this case, intermittent self-catheterisation or indwelling urethral catheter placement is not required, as a post-void residual volume of less than 100 ml excludes significant urinary retention. Fluid intake should be maintained, with at least 1 to 2 litres per day recommended. Desmopressin is a vasopressin analogue which is generally reserved for night-time use to control nocturia. Caution is advised in relation to the fluid retention and hyponatraemia that can result from excessive use of desmopressin. See Figure 8.4.

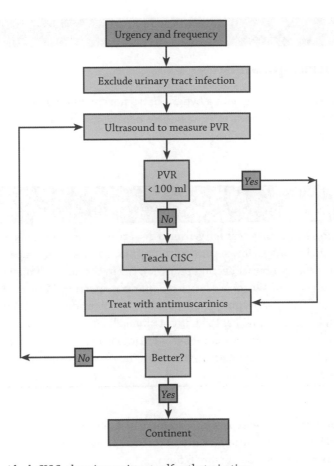

PVR, post-void residual; CISC, clean intermittent self-catheterisation.

Figure 8.4[(5)]: A UK consensus of the management of the bladder in multiple sclerosis.

CASE 12

B: Serum caeruloplasmin

This is an adolescent presenting with a hyperkinetic movement disorder. Given the extra-pyramidal signs, psychiatric features and possible hepatic involvement, the most likely diagnosis in this case is Wilson's disease.

Learning point

The most valuable laboratory test for Wilson's disease is serum caeruloplasmin. The typical biochemical profile is low serum caeruloplasmin, low serum copper and elevated urinary copper (on a 24-hour collection of urine). Given the large number of possible mutations in the gene for Wilson's disease (copper transporting ATPase – ATP7B, chromosome 13q14.3), genotyping is not usually helpful for diagnosis. A liver biopsy is sometimes required for diagnosis. The patient should have ophthalmological assessment with slit lamp examination for Kayser–Fleischer rings (granular deposition of copper in Descemet's membrane of the cornea), found in the vast majority of cases of Wilson's disease with neurological involvement.

The treatment of Wilson's disease is with a copper chelating agent, such as D-penicillamine or trientine, which should be initiated early to prevent progressive damage to the neurological system and liver. See Figure 8.5.

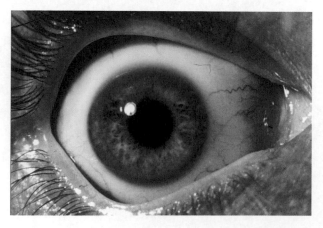

Figure 8.5: Kayser-Fleischer ring

The differential diagnosis for chorea is wide, including structural (commonly vascular), metabolic, drug-induced and genetic causes. Chorea can also occur in association with immune-mediated disorders such as systemic lupus erythematosus, antiphospholipid syndrome, Behçet's disease and polyarteritis nodosa. In children, Sydenham's chorea and PANDAS (paediatric autoimmune neuropsychiatric disorders associated with streptococcal infection) can present with chorea, tics and neuropsychiatric symptoms (obsessive compulsive disorder) in the weeks or months following group A streptococcal infection. Anti-basal ganglia antibodies have been detected in some children with PANDAS but the significance of the antibody in this condition is not fully understood. Post-streptococcal chorea is generally self-limiting but can recur with a subsequent streptococcal infection. Refractory cases may respond to immunotherapy.

Huntington's disease (HD) is the most common inherited cause of chorea. It is a CAG trinucleotide repeat disorder and inheritance is autosomal dominant. Like Wilson's disease, HD can also present as a hyperkinetic movement disorder with neuropsychiatric symptoms. However, the onset of HD is typically in the fourth or fifth decade, and cognitive impairment is a prominent feature. An earlier age of onset is observed in individuals with a larger number of CAG repeats. For instance, juvenile onset cases tend to have over 60 CAG repeats.

CASE 13

D: Aspirin 300 mg

The patient has presented with a large ischaemic stroke in the right middle cerebral artery (MCA) territory. The history given includes two vascular risk factors – hypercholesterolaemia and a potentially hypercoagulable state associated with malignancy. He is not eligible for consideration for intravenous thrombolysis which is licensed for administration within 4.5 hours of stroke onset, since the acute event could have taken place during his sleep. He should have a loading dose of aspirin immediately as there is no evidence of haemorrhage on the CT scan.

There is evidence of oedema and mild mass effect and therefore he is at risk of developing malignant MCA syndrome. He should have close monitoring of his Glasgow Coma Scale and have brain imaging repeated urgently if there is any clinical deterioration. He should be referred to the neurosurgical team within 24 hours of stroke onset as decompressive craniectomy may be considered. This should be performed within 48 hours of stroke onset as earlier intervention has been associated with better outcomes.

The criteria for decompressive craniectomy are shown in Table 8.1.[6]

✦ Aged 60 years or under

✦ Clinical deficits suggestive of infarction in the territory of the MCA with a score on the National Institute of Health Stroke Scale (NIHSS) of above 15

✦ Decrease in the level of consciousness to give a score of 1 or more on item 1a of the NIHSS

✦ Signs on CT scanning of an infarct of at least 50% of the MCA territory, with or without additional infarction in the territory of the anterior or posterior cerebral artery on the same side, or infarct volume greater than 145 cm³ as shown on diffusion-weighted MRI.

Table 8.1: Criteria for consideration for decompressive hemicraniectomy in MCA infarction (all criteria must be met)

CASE 14

A: Multiple system atrophy

This is a case of multiple system atrophy (MSA), a sporadic neurodegenerative disorder with parkinsonism, cerebellar features and autonomic dysfunction. Pyramidal signs may also be present. The typical age of onset is in the fifties. There are two subtypes: MSA-P (predominant parkinsonism, the more common subtype) and MSA-C (with prominent cerebellar features). Early in the disease course, it may be difficult to discriminate the 'atypical' parkinsonian syndromes, such as MSA and progressive supranuclear palsy (PSP), from 'typical' idiopathic Parkinson's disease (IPD). However, there are a number of clinical 'red flags' which can help to differentiate between the conditions.

A lack of (or a short-lived) response to levodopa suggests atypical parkinsonism. The tremor also differs in MSA, as it is an irregular jerky tremor (with posture and action), rather than the pill-rolling rest tremor typical of IPD. Early falls are more common in PSP and MSA than in IPD. Male erectile dysfunction is common and occurs early in MSA. In MSA, bladder symptoms include urinary incontinence and retention, in addition to the urinary frequency and urgency seen in IPD and PSP. Orthostatic hypotension can occur in both MSA and IPD, more commonly due to dopaminergic therapy in the latter disease. There is a distinctive abnormality of the speech in MSA with a croaky, strained quality to the voice. Speech in PSP tends to be low-pitched in comparison. Dysphagia is more common with MSA or PSP than in IPD, in which it occurs as a late complication. Emotional lability is more common in MSA or PSP than in IPD.

The hallmark features of corticobasal degeneration (CBD) are parkinsonism, cortical dysfunction and prominent early cognitive impairment. In some cases of CBD, there is an 'alien limb' phenomenon, due to apraxia and cortical sensory loss.

CASE 15

E: 3,4-diaminopyridine

> **Learning point**
>
> The diagnosis is Lambert–Eaton myasthenic syndrome (LEMS), with the classical features of proximal myopathy, ptosis (but usually normal eye movements) and improvement in reflexes after exercise. There was exacerbation of muscle weakness with a calcium channel antagonist, as has been described in LEMS. The history is also suggestive of orthostatic hypotension and he has been constipated, suggesting autonomic involvement. Other autonomic features, such as dry mouth, erectile dysfunction or urinary retention, should be enquired about if LEMS is suspected.

The patient is a smoker and requires thorough investigation for malignancy given that LEMS can complicate cancer (diagnosed in approximately 60% of cases), with the most common association being with small cell cancer of the lung. Careful surveillance is needed following diagnosis as LEMS can precede the discovery of the malignancy. Antibodies to the voltage-gated calcium channel are present in the majority of cases of LEMS and are more commonly found in those with small cell lung cancer.

Treatment of LEMS is directed towards managing any associated malignancy. In the UK, symptomatic treatment usually includes 3,4-diaminopyridine (a potassium channel blocker), which has been shown to improve muscle strength in several clinical trials in LEMS. Pyridostigmine (a cholinesterase inhibitor) also improves strength in some patients with LEMS. If there is no evidence of cancer, immunotherapy may be considered. There is limited evidence for intravenous immunoglobulin, plasmapheresis, steroids and steroid-sparing agents in LEMS.

CASE 16

C: Intravenous thiamine

This lady has Wernicke's encephalopathy (typical features include ophthalmoparesis, ataxia and confusion), which is caused by thiamine deficiency, in this case due to persistent vomiting. This is a medical emergency and IV thiamine replacement should be initiated urgently to prevent permanent neurological impairment.

CASE 17

D: Canalith repositioning manoeuvres

The symptoms are suggestive of benign paroxysmal positional vertigo but this should be confirmed with a Dix–Hallpike manoeuvre. Brain imaging is required if this test is negative or there are abnormal neurological signs or history of headache, vomiting or hearing loss. There is usually an excellent response to vestibular rehabilitation and canalith repositioning techniques such as the Epley manoeuvre.

CASE 18

B: Functional neurological symptoms

In this case, the pattern of muscle weakness is unusual and there is a greater degree of weakness on grading power than would be expected for a patient who is walking. This suggests functional weakness and the additional sign which supports this diagnosis is Hoover's sign (voluntary lack of effort of hip extension in the 'strong' leg when hip flexion is tested in the 'weak' leg).

CHAPTER 8
ANSWERS

References

1. Association of British Neurologists. 2009. Guidelines for Prescribing in Multiple Sclerosis. www.mstrust.org.uk/competencies/downloads/abn_ms_guidelines_2009_final.pdf

2. NICE. 2004. Natalizumab for the treatment of adults with highly active relapsing–remitting multiple sclerosis. NICE technology appraisal guidance 127. www.nice.org.uk/guidance/ta127

3. Wijdicks E et al. 2006, reaffirmed 2009. Practice Parameter: Prediction of outcome in comatose survivors after cardiopulmonary resuscitation (an evidence-based review). Neurology, 67, 203–210

4. Solomon T et al. 2012. Management of suspected viral encephalitis in adults. Association of British Neurologists and British Infection Association National Guidelines. Journal of Infection, 64, 347–373

5. Figure 8.4 adapted from Fowler C et al. 2009. A UK consensus on the management of the bladder in multiple sclerosis. Journal of Neurology, Neurosurgery and Psychiatry, 80, 470–477

6. National Collaborating Centre for Chronic Conditions. 2008. Stroke: national clinical guideline for diagnosis and initial management of acute stroke and transient ischaemic attack. London, Royal College of Physicians

CHAPTER 9

Nephrology

Gareth Lewis

CASE 1

A 36-year-old man is reviewed every two months in the renal transplant clinic. He received a kidney transplant from his sister 18 months previously and his primary disease was reflux nephropathy. Since transplantation, his clinical course has been unremarkable and graft function stable with a creatinine of 80–90 µmol/litre. He has no other past medical history. He presents with a 2-day history of tremor and perioral tingling, with watery diarrhoea up to five times per day for the last week, which began on return from a weekend break in Spain. He had been maintaining good oral intake of food and fluids and denies use of any medications or medicinal substances other than those listed below.

On examination he appears euvolaemic. The pulse rate is 66 bpm regular, blood pressure 170/105 mmHg with no postural drop. The abdomen is soft and non-tender with a transplanted kidney palpable in the right iliac fossa. A bladder is not palpable. There is a fine but prominent tremor on holding his hands outstretched. There is no goitre, reflexes are normal and cranial nerve examination unremarkable.

Medication list: prednisolone 7.5 mg once daily, mycophenolate mofetil 750 mg twice daily, tacrolimus 2 mg twice daily, ranitidine 150 mg twice daily, paracetamol 1 g PRN.

Urinalysis: Specific gravity 1.015, otherwise bland.

Blood tests: Haemoglobin 145 g/litre, White cells 7.4×10^9/litre, Platelets 280×10^9/litre, Sodium 136 mmol/litre, Potassium 5.9 mmol/litre, Bicarbonate 16 mmol/litre, Urea 12.6 mmol/litre, Creatinine 165 µmol/litre, Glucose 6.4 mmol/litre.

Measurement of which of the following in serum is likely to yield a unifying diagnosis?

- A. **Calcium**
- B. **Cortisol immediately before, and 30 minutes after, Synacthen® administration**
- C. **Mycophenolic acid levels**
- D. **Tacrolimus levels**
- E. **Thyroid function tests**

CASE 2

A 45-year-old lady is reviewed in the nephrology clinic. Her current eGFR is 22 ml/min per 1.73 m². She is a non-smoker and does not consume alcohol. She first presented with an eGFR of 34 ml/min per 1.73 m² and an albumin/creatinine ratio (ACR) of 245 that was discovered on a routine medical check five years previously. She is taking ramipril 10 mg and amlodipine 10 mg daily, and is concordant with her medication. She has previously declined renal biopsy. Apart from well-controlled hypertension she has no other past medical history other than having a body mass index (BMI) of between 45 and 60 kg/m² since adolescence. She is unable to recall any childhood or recent urinary tract infections, and her three sisters have normal renal function with no other family history of renal disease.

On examination, she has a BMI of 52 kg/m². Chest and cardiovascular examination is unremarkable. Distal pulses are strong and equal in both lower limbs; there are no vascular bruits detectable. There is no peripheral oedema and blood pressure is 145/85 mmHg. Fundoscopy is unremarkable.

Investigations reveal: Glucose 5.6 mmol/litre, HbA1c 32 mmol/mol, Albumin 38 g/dl, Urinary albumin/creatinine ratio 420, Urinalysis: protein ++++, normal otherwise.

What histological features would a renal biopsy be most likely to show?

A. **Discrete areas of scarring in portions of some, but not all, glomeruli**
B. **Florid interstitial infiltrate of inflammatory cells, predominantly neutrophils**
C. **Normal appearances on light microscopy but flattening of epithelial podocyte foot processes on electron microscopy**
D. **Onion skinning of arterioles with marked ischaemic wrinkling of glomeruli**
E. **Thickening of the glomerular basement membrane with nodular scarring and mesangial matrix expansion**

CASE 3

A 64-year-old lady is referred for a renal opinion from the urology ward. She was admitted two days ago with the sudden onset of left flank pain, frank haematuria and a temperature of 37.6 °C. A non-contrast CT scan of renal tracts was performed and her pain and other symptoms settled quickly with morphine and diclofenac. She is now felt to be surgically well for discharge on day four. She is a smoker of 25 cigarettes per day, is on no regular medications and denies any past medical history. Apart from an occasional dry cough, she does not volunteer the presence of any other symptoms. Results of observations and investigations are shown in Table 9.1.

	Admission	Day 1	Day 2	Day 4
Urea (mmol/litre)	8.5	12.3	18.6	17.6
Creatinine (μmol/litre)	105	135	250	249
Haemoglobin (g/litre)	142	138	134	133
White cells (× 10^9/litre)	7.5	16.8	11.3	7.9
Differential white cell count	Normal	Neutrophils 14.5	Neutrophils 8.4	Normal
C-reactive protein (mg/litre)	15	35	30	25
AST (U/litre)	95	–	950	55
LDH (U/litre)	–	–	2400	650

Table 9.1: Results of observations and investigations

Urinalysis: blood +++, leukocytes ++, nil else.

Urine culture: no growth after 48 hours.

Blood cultures: no growth after 48 hours.

Non-contrast CT scan report: the left kidney is 10.8 cm and the right kidney is 11.1 cm. There is no hydronephrosis, and no obstructing calculus or collection is seen. Incidental note is made of peri-aortic lymphadenopathy which does not reach significance by size criteria.

The patient's ECG and chest radiograph are shown below in Figures 9.1 and 9.2.

continued

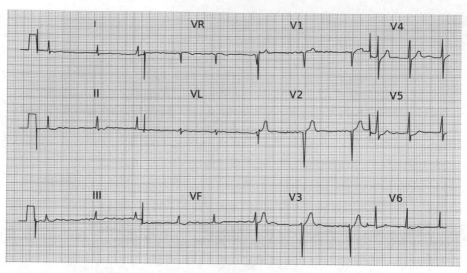

Figure 9.1

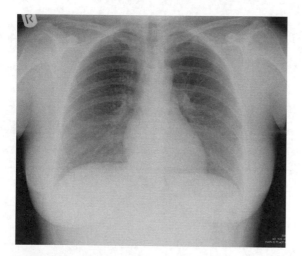

Figure 9.2

What now is the best course of action aimed at preventing further renal deterioration?

A. Start allopurinol, order a CT scan chest and abdomen, and begin intravenous fluid hydration at 150–200 ml/h

B. Commence therapeutic enoxaparin and request an echocardiogram

C. Document allergy to diclofenac, begin prednisolone 40 mg daily and schedule a renal biopsy

D. Advise fluid intake of 2.5–3 litres per day and a low-salt diet, organise dietetic review, and discharge when creatinine levels begin to fall

E. Take blood for complement levels, ANCA, anti-glomerular basement membrane and anti-nuclear antibody testing; commence intravenous steroids and oral cyclophosphamide

CASE 4

A 27-year-old man is referred by his GP for evaluation of intermittent frank haematuria. This has occurred six times in the past three years, most often noticed a couple of days after he develops a sore throat. The haematuria normally lasts for three to four days before clearing and on two occasions he had some lumbar discomfort which settled with paracetamol and non-steroidal anti-inflammatory drugs. He has no other medical history and is a non-smoker on no regular medications. He made an appointment on two occasions to see his GP one week after these episodes. Basic urine and blood investigations at that time were unremarkable.

On examination he is well with unremarkable cardiac, respiratory, abdominal and external genitalia examinations. Blood pressure is 116/74 mmHg.

Investigations reveal: Urinalysis: bland with no blood or protein, Creatinine 74 µmol/litre, Urinary albumin:creatinine ratio (ACR) < 3, Haemoglobin 170 g/litre, Platelets 310×10^9/litre.

ANCA, anti-glomerular basement membrane and anti-nuclear antibodies: all negative.

Complement C3 and C4: normal.

IgG 8.0 g/litre, IgA 7.4 g/litre, IgM 1.6 g/litre.

What is now the most appropriate advice to the GP?

- A. **Discharge from renal review; he requires psychological intervention for somatisation/malingering**
- B. **Discharge from renal review; he should attend his GP for annual blood pressure and ACR checks**
- C. **Discharge from renal review; he should commence lifelong penicillin V prophylaxis**
- D. **Discharge from renal review; the blood results permit a definitive diagnosis and so renal biopsy is not essential**
- E. **Keep under renal review; he requires a renal biopsy**

CASE 5

A 41-year-old man with a 34-year history of well-controlled type 1 diabetes is seen for the second time at a new GP practice. At his first attendance his blood pressure had been elevated and 24-hour monitoring revealed an average daytime blood pressure of 145/93 mmHg. Despite his good control of diabetes he does not like taking medications since he has had several family members who have had various side effects from antihypertensive and lipid-lowering treatment. He is reluctant to start medication having read about various antihypertensive side effects ahead of the most recent consultation. He speaks disparagingly of his previous GP whose prescription of allopurinol following two episodes of gout last year gave him a nasty rash. On review of his electronic record medication list he has intolerances to omeprazole, ibuprofen, ranitidine, allopurinol and fluoxetine documented. On examination he appears well. Cardiovascular, respiratory and abdominal examinations are unremarkable. He has very mild peripheral oedema. Fundoscopy reveals microaneurysms and a few scattered retinal haemorrhages.

His laboratory investigations are: Haemoglobin 160 g/litre, Sodium 138 mmol/litre, Potassium 5.6 mmol/litre, Urea 6.5 mmol/litre, Creatinine 115 μmol/litre, Glucose (fasting) 8.3 mmol/litre, HbA1c 46 mmol/mol, Uric acid 0.62 mmol/litre, Urinalysis: bland, Urinary albumin:creatinine ratio 28, Body mass index 26 kg/m^2.

What is the most appropriate course of action for this patient now?

A. **Commence amlodipine**
B. **Commence doxazosin**
C. **Commence losartan**
D. **Commence ramipril**
E. **Counsel on diet and lifestyle changes**

CASE 6

A 15-year-old girl is referred by her GP following a 2-week history of lethargy and vague bilateral flank discomfort. Because she looked pale, her GP requested blood and urine tests (shown below). She has an unremarkable past medical history except as a passenger in a road traffic collision six months earlier when she sustained a fractured wrist. Blood tests at that time were unremarkable. She was on no regular medications but took occasional analgesia for some residual stiffness in her wrist. She denied smoking cigarettes or taking alcohol. On examination, she was very pale. Blood pressure was 125/75 mmHg with no postural drop. Cardiovascular and respiratory examinations were unremarkable, and abdominal examination demonstrated mild, bilateral flank tenderness on deep palpation. There was no peripheral oedema and no rashes were visible.

Investigations reveal: Haemoglobin 70 g/litre, White cells 8.5×10^9/litre (normal differential), Platelets 280×10^9/litre, Sodium 137 mmol/litre, Potassium 3.1 mmol/litre, Bicarbonate 18 mmol/litre, Urea 11.5 mmol/litre, Creatinine 380 µmol/litre, C-reactive protein 8 mg/litre, Glucose 5.7 mmol/litre, Corrected calcium 1.95 mmol/litre, Magnesium 0.6 mmol/litre.

Anti-nuclear antibody: negative.

ANCA: negative.

Complement C3 and C4: unremarkable.

Anti-streptolysin O titre < 20 units/ml.

Rheumatoid factor: negative.

Urinalysis: protein +, specific gravity 1.010, glucose +++.

Urinary albumin:creatinine ratio 45.

In which of the following renal structures is the most likely primary site of pathology?

    A. **Glomerular endothelium**
    B. **Glomerular epithelium**
    C. **Tubulo-interstitium**
    D. **Urinary collecting system**
    E. **Vascular**

CASE 7

A 24-year-old lady who is 18 months post renal transplant for reflux nephropathy is inquiring about the possibility of pregnancy. She has normal renal function and her blood pressure is well controlled with no detectable proteinuria. She had been on maintenance haemodialysis for four years before a suitable donor was found. Otherwise, apart from ankle and wrist fractures following two trips on the pavement, her past medical history has been essentially unremarkable. She has had no prior pregnancies and her body mass index is 31 kg/m². Her immunosuppressive medications are as follows: tacrolimus 1 mg BD and mycophenolate mofetil 750 mg BD.

What is the best course of action?

- A. Counsel her that pregnancy is inadvisable at this stage
- B. Switch mycophenolate to azathioprine
- C. Switch mycophenolate to prednisolone
- D. Switch tacrolimus to ciclosporin
- E. Switch tacrolimus to prednisolone

CASE 8

A 55-year-old woman on long-term haemodialysis has her monthly blood tests reviewed by the dialysis unit team. She is taking aspirin, bisoprolol, calcitriol 250 ng on alternate days, esomeprazole, venofer® 100 mg IV fortnightly on dialysis and darbepoetin alfa 40 µg IV weekly.

Investigations reveal: Haemoglobin 137 g/litre, White cells 5.3 × 10⁹/litre, Platelets 385 × 10⁹/litre, Ferritin 450 ng/ml, Transferrin saturation 32%, Corrected calcium 2.42 mmol/litre, Phosphate 1.75 mmol/litre, Parathyroid hormone 155 pg/ml, C-reactive protein 6 mg/litre.

What change should be made to her treatment?

- A. Add a phosphate binder
- B. Decrease venofer® dose
- C. Decrease darbepoietin dose
- D. Increase calcitriol dose
- E. No change at this time

CASE 9

A 68-year-old gentleman is brought to the emergency department at 11pm after collapsing. He has a history of atrial fibrillation, hypertension, chronic kidney disease stage 3 and type 2 diabetes. He is taking warfarin, digoxin, ramipril and metformin. He, along with several family members, had had seven days of diarrhoea and vomiting following a bout of gastroenteritis. On arrival he is bradycardic at a rate of 30 bpm. Blood pressure is 80/45 mmHg, and oxygen saturation is 99% on high-flow oxygen. The Glasgow Coma Scale (GCS) is 14/15 and respiratory rate is 24 breaths/min. Results of a portable chest X-ray, ECG and point-of-care blood sampling are detailed below.

Sodium 128 mmol/litre, Potassium 8.4 mmol/litre, Bicarbonate 8 mmol/litre, Urea 55 mmol/litre, Creatinine 1150 μmol/litre, Digoxin level 6 ng/ml, INR 6.5, Glucose 14.5 mmol/litre, Lactate 6.5 mmol/litre.

See Figures 9.3 and 9.4.

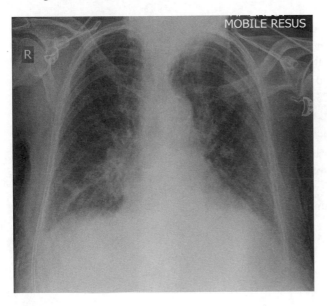

Figure 9.3

continued

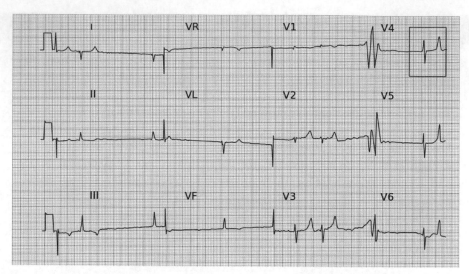

Figure 9.4

He is given a 2 litre bolus of 0.9% saline, 10 ml of 10% calcium gluconate, insulin, dextrose, DigiBind® antibody fragments, along with vitamin K and prothrombin complex concentrate for INR reversal. After this treatment, his pulse is 68 bpm in atrial fibrillation, blood pressure 130/60 mmHg, and oxygen saturation is 94% on high-flow oxygen; GCS is 15/15. He is catheterised and there is 15 ml residual urine. It is 90 minutes after arrival and the patient's observations remain stable. To where should the patient be transferred for further treatment?

A. **Acute medical unit**
B. **Coronary care unit**
C. **High-dependency/intensive care unit (HDU/ICU)**
D. **Remain in the emergency department**
E. **Renal ward**

CASE 10

A 58-year-old gentleman has been on haemodialysis for 11 years secondary to Henoch–Schönlein purpura. He presents with a new, exquisitely painful rash on both upper thighs (see Figures 9.5 and 9.6) which developed over five days and which is biopsied (see histological image of an affected blood vessel, Figure 9.7). His current medications include weekly erythropoietin, IV Venofer® fortnightly, calcitriol, calcium carbonate, cinacalcet, omeprazole, aspirin, amlodipine, doxazosin and rosuvastatin. He is a smoker of 15 cigarettes per day and does not consume alcohol.

His blood results are shown below: Haemoglobin 105 g/litre, White cells 6.8 × 10⁹/litre (normal differential), Ferritin 360 ng/ml, Parathyroid hormone 1850 pg/ml, Corrected calcium 2.55 mmol/litre, Phosphate 2.5 mmol/litre.

His blood results are shown below: Haemoglobin 105 g/litre, White cells 6.8×10^9/litre (normal differential), Ferritin 360 ng/ml, Parathyroid hormone 1850 pg/ml, Corrected calcium 2.55 mmol/litre, Phosphate 2.5 mmol/litre.

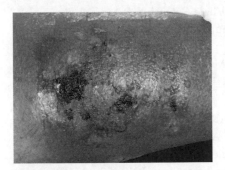

Figure 9.5

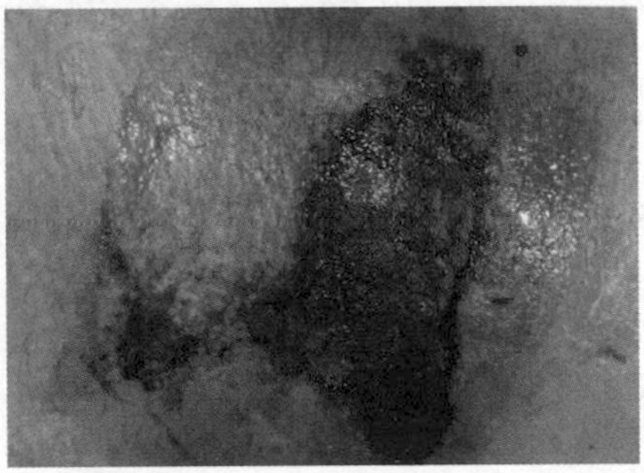

Figure 9.6

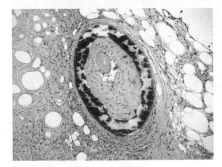

Figure 9.7

What is the most likely cause of these appearances?

- A. **Calciphylaxis**
- B. **Cholesterol emboli**
- C. **Henoch–Schönlein cutaneous vasculitis**
- D. **Porphyria cutanea tarda**
- E. **Pyoderma gangrenosum**

CASE 11

A 64-year-old woman is referred to renal outpatients with worsening renal function and ankle swelling. She gives a 3-month history of lethargy, and worsening lower limb swelling. She had been prescribed furosemide 40 mg daily, which has been increased to 80 mg, which aided the swelling somewhat. This was stopped two weeks ago after her GP found that her creatinine had doubled since last review. At the renal clinic, she denies taking any medication other than the prescribed furosemide. Her chest is clear, and cardiac auscultation is normal. There is mild to moderate pitting oedema in the legs. Her blood pressure is 115/75 mmHg lying, and 110/70 mmHg standing.

The following investigations are obtained:

Haemoglobin 98 g/litre, MCV 92 fl, White cells 9.1×10^9/litre (normal differential), Platelets 349×10^9/litre, Sodium 134 mmol/litre, Potassium 3.1 mmol/litre, Chloride 111 mmol/litre, Bicarbonate 17 mmol/litre, Urea 10.5 mmol/litre, Creatinine 170 µmol/litre, C-reactive protein 8 mg/litre, Corrected calcium: 2.4 mmol/litre, Phosphate 1.6 mmol/litre, Magnesium 0.55 mmol/litre, Bilirubin 11 µmol/litre, ALP 40 U/litre, AST 15 U/litre, GGT 50 U/litre, Albumin 39 g/litre.

Anti-nuclear antibody: negative, ANCA: P-ANCA 20, C-ANCA < 20, MPO < 0.2, PR3 < 0.2, Complement C3 and C4: normal, Anti-streptolysin O titre < 20, HBsAb: positive, HBsAg: negative, HBcAb: negative, Hepatitis C: non-reactive, HIV-1 and 2 antibody: negative, TSH 3.6 mU/litre, Nt-proBNP< 50 pg/ml.

Urinary sodium 55 mmol/litre, Urinary potassium 45 mmol/litre, Urinary chloride 20 mmol/litre, Urinary albumin/creatinine ratio 2, 24-hour urinary protein 4.6 g, Urinalysis: bland.

Chest X-ray: unremarkable, ECG: rate 84, sinus rhythm.

What is the likely cause of her renal impairment?

    A. **ANCA-associated vasculitis**
    B. **Hepatitis B-associated polyarteritis nodosa**
    C. **Interstitial nephritis secondary to furosemide**
    D. **Plasma cell dyscrasia**
    E. **Renal tubular acidosis**

CASE 12

A 57-year-old gentleman with an unremarkable past medical history except for smoking ten cigarettes per day is referred to a medical unit by his GP on account of fatigue, hypertension, arthralgia and shortness of breath on exertion. He last felt totally well three weeks previously, but then began gradually to deteriorate. His blood pressure was 210/120 mmHg, but there was no evidence of papilloedema or chronic hypertensive changes on fundoscopy.

Blood tests revealed the following: Haemoglobin 94 g/litre, White cells 11×10^9/litre, Platelets 234×10^9/litre, C-reactive protein 155 mg/litre, Sodium 144 mmol/litre, Potassium 6.2 mmol/litre, Bicarbonate 15 mmol/litre, Urea 45 mmol/litre, Creatinine 665 µmol/litre.

In the assessment unit, the patient complains of some mild chest discomfort. Two heart sounds are heard easily. Chest examination reveals slightly decreased air entry bilaterally. The abdominal examination is unremarkable. Blood pressure is 200/110 mmHg, pulse rate 85 bpm regular, oxygen saturation on room air 96% and temperature 37.2 °C. A chest X-ray shows diffuse patchy changes throughout both lung fields.

Repeat blood tests show the following:, Haemoglobin 88 g/litre, White cells 10.6×10^9/litre, Platelets 214×10^9/litre, C-reactive protein 160 mg/litre, Sodium 143 mmol/litre, Potassium 5.8 mmol/litre, Bicarbonate 15 mmol/litre, Urea 46.5 mmol/litre, Creatinine 690 µmol/litre, ANCA: C-ANCA < 20, P-ANCA < 20, MPO < 0.2, PR3 < 0.2, Anti-glomerular basement membrane antibody > 8, FEV_1: 95% predicted, FVC: 105% predicted, DLCO: 160% predicted.

Ultrasound renal tracts: left kidney 11.5 cm, right kidney 10.9 cm. No hydronephrosis.

Urinalysis: Blood +++, Protein +++.

What is now the best option for treatment?

- A. **Cyclophosphamide**
- B. **Haemodialysis**
- C. **Methylprednisolone**
- D. **Plasma exchange**
- E. **Rituximab**

CASE 13

A 44-year-old man, who has been commenced on peritoneal dialysis (PD) four months prior for end-stage renal disease due to hypertensive nephropathy, complains of abdominal discomfort. His discomfort began three days ago and has been worsening since then. He attends the PD unit where a sample of fluid is taken via his PD catheter and sent to the microbiology laboratory. On examination he appears well. The pulse rate is 75 bpm, blood pressure 145/82 mmHg, temperature 36.4 °C, oxygen saturation 99% on room air. His abdomen is mildly tender on palpation, and the fluid draining from the effluent bag is somewhat cloudy.

Peritoneal dialysis fluid white cells: $190 \times 10^6/mm^3$.

What is now the next best step in management?

A. **Admit for removal of PD catheter**
B. **Amoxicillin, metronidazole, fluconazole**
C. **Metronidazole and gentamicin**
D. **Tazocin and clarithromycin**
E. **Vancomycin and ciprofloxacin**

CASE 14

A 71-year-old gentleman with a history of type 2 diabetes, diabetic nephropathy, hypertension and ischaemic heart disease, with one previous non-ST elevation myocardial infarction with coronary artery stenting, is being considered for renal replacement therapy. He smokes ten cigarettes per day and has an exercise tolerance of half a mile on flat ground. His current eGFR is 17 ml/min per 1.73 m².

Which of the following statements is most accurate?

A. **Transplant graft survival is better with a 2-2-2 mismatched live donor kidney rather than a 0-0-0 mismatched deceased donor kidney**
B. **If he starts haemodialysis his survival rate is 60% at five years**
C. **Peritoneal dialysis, typically, could continue for up to eight years**
D. **Renal transplantation is unlikely to substantially prolong survival in this man**
E. **Transplantation should normally only be considered after starting peritoneal dialysis or haemodialysis**

CASE 15

A 65-year-old man with polycystic renal disease is approaching end-stage renal failure with an eGFR of 18 ml/min per 1.73 m². His father died on dialysis aged 73 and the patient has one son, aged 25. He is discussing options for renal replacement and would be keen for a transplant. His son is keen to donate a kidney to him. The son is very active. His blood pressure is 120/70 mmHg. He does not smoke and his urinalysis demonstrates no blood or protein. He understands there is a possibility that he may have polycystic renal disease himself and wants to know whether he is suitable to be a donor.

What should now be done to assess whether the son has polycystic kidney disease?

A. **Molecular genetic testing**
B. **MRI scan of kidneys**
C. **Renal biopsy**
D. **Ultrasound scan of renal tracts**
E. **Wait five years before further investigation**

CASE 16

A 34-year-old man is admitted to the ward with right-sided severe flank pain. A non-contrast CT scan demonstrates a 3 mm calculus in the right upper ureter. He is treated with non-steroidal analgesia, IV fluids and oral tamsulosin, and the stone passes. Fortunately the patient is able to retrieve this using a sieve and subsequent analysis shows it to be composed of calcium oxalate. This is the first presentation of stone disease in this patient and he denies any known family history. He has no other past medical history and works as an engineer. The blood pressure is 120/70 mmHg and body mass index is 23 kg/m². He is a non-smoker. Blood tests on admission show normal renal function and white cells.

What is the best intervention at this stage to reduce the risk of a recurrence of this presentation?

A. **Bendroflumethiazide**
B. **Low-calcium diet**
C. **Low-citrate diet**
D. **Low-sodium diet**
E. **Prophylactic antibiotics**

CASE 17

A 76-year-old gentleman is admitted to the medical ward with lethargy and fatigue. His GP performed blood testing which revealed a creatinine of 1450 μmol/litre. This was surprising as the man had had blood tests performed as part of a work-up for a respiratory illness three months ago and creatinine at that stage was 91 μmol/litre. On examination the most marked finding is a distended bladder on abdominal palpation. A urinary catheter is passed and 1.5 litres of residual urine drained. On questioning the man gives a long history of various lower urinary tract symptoms, which he had been too embarrassed to raise with his GP. Over the next eight hours his urine output from the catheter increases from 80 ml per hour to 700 ml per hour.

Repeat blood tests reveal the following: Sodium 139 mmol/litre, Potassium 6.0 mmol/litre, Bicarbonate 20 mmol/litre, Urea 45 mmol/litre, Creatinine 1490 μmol/litre.

Which of the following options is most appropriate regarding the management of his diuresis?

A. **Clamp the catheter for two to four hours after every litre of urinary output**

B. **Replace three quarters of the urine output volume using 5% dextrose**

C. **If blood pressure falls then give boluses of 2.7% saline until there is no postural drop**

D. **IV potassium supplementation will probably be required**

E. **The patient should be fluid-restricted to avoid prolonging the diuresis**

CASE 18

A 55-year-old man is being reviewed in the renal clinic; he has a long history of type 1 diabetes and diabetic renal disease. His blood pressure and urinary albumin/creatinine ratio (ACR) have been rising despite up-titration of his medications. His blood pressure is now 160/95 mmHg and ACR is 120. Current antihypertensive therapy is amlodipine 10 mg and ramipril 5 mg daily. Other medications include insulin given as insulin aspart three times daily and evening insulin glargine. He has had some recent episodes when his wife noticed he was a little confused and found his capillary blood glucose concentration to be 1.5 mmol/litre. The patient denies that he felt any different from usual during these times. On examination, he has mild ankle oedema, the chest is clear. Two heart sounds and no murmurs are heard.

Blood tests reveal: Sodium 141 mmol/litre, Potassium 6.0 mmol/litre (5.4 three months earlier), Chloride 114 mmol/litre, Bicarbonate 17 mmol/litre, Urea 7 mmol/litre, Creatinine 125 μmol/litre (105 three months previously pre Ramipril).

Urinary albumin:creatinine ratio 120 (was 180 three months earlier).

What is the best approach at this stage?

A. **Add bendroflumethiazide**
B. **Add bisoprolol**
C. **Add doxazosin**
D. **Add furosemide**
E. **Reduce ramipril dose**

CASE 19

A 73-year-old woman with difficult-to-control hypertension presents to her GP with muscle cramps and weakness two weeks after her dose of diuretic was increased. Her blood tests reveal a sodium level of 136 mmol/litre and a potassium level of 3.0 mmol/litre with normal calcium and magnesium values. Her GP considers the addition of amiloride to her therapy given these recent blood results.

Which of the following best describes the mode of action of amiloride?

A. **Blockade of an epithelial sodium channel**
B. **Competition for intracellular aldosterone receptors**
C. **Inhibition of a cytosolic enzyme**
D. **Inhibition of a symporter for sodium and chloride**
E. **Inhibition of a symporter for sodium, potassium and chloride**

CASE 20

A 66-year-old man with stage 4 chronic kidney disease with an eGFR of 22 ml/min per 1.73 m^2, congestive cardiac failure and severe restless legs is receiving inpatient treatment for endocarditis. He complains of tinnitus after the first week of treatment. Which of the following medications could be safely continued at this stage?

A. **Furosemide**
B. **Gentamicin**
C. **Quinine**
D. **Ramipril**
E. **Vancomycin**

CASE 21

A 45-year-old man with previously normal renal function, essential hypertension on ramipril 2.5 mg daily and chronic daily headache for which he takes a number of analgesics, is referred by his GP with a rash (as shown) and bilateral flank pain. On examination, there is a rash covering the flexor surfaces of both legs, the blood pressure is 145/85 mmHg and there is mild bilateral flank discomfort on abdominal palpation. There is nil else of note.

Investigations show: Haemoglobin 105 g/litre, White cells 10.5 × 10⁹/litre (neutrophils 5.5, lymphocytes 1.0, eosinophils 4.0), Platelets 189 × 10⁹/litre, Urea 15 mmol/litre, Creatinine 257 µmol/litre.

Urinary albumin:creatinine ratio: 8. Urinalysis: blood – trace; protein – trace; leukocytes and nitrites – negative. Ultrasound scan of renal tracts – 12.5 cm kidneys which are a little echobright; no hydronephrosis. See Figure 9.8.

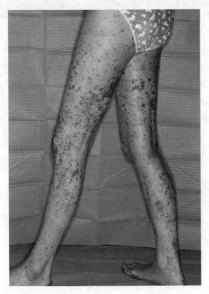

Figure 9.8

What findings would be expected on renal biopsy?

    A. **Amorphous nodular deposits with apple-green birefringence on Congo Red staining**

    B. **An infiltrate of inflammatory cells in the supporting tissues around tubules**

    C. **Destruction of Bowman's space with proliferative changes developing circumferentially**

    D. **Needle-shaped crystalline artefacts seen in tubular lumens**

    E. **Onion skinning of arterioles and diffuse scarring and tubular atrophy**

CASE 1

D: Tacrolimus levels

This case illustrates the clinical features of tacrolimus toxicity. Tacrolimus and ciclosporin are calcineurin inhibitors that are widely used in solid organ transplantation. Their metabolism and handling is based on a number of factors including metabolism by CYP450 enzyme isoforms. Therefore drugs that induce (eg barbiturates, phenytoin, rifampicin, carbamazepine) or inhibit (eg isoniazid, cimetidine, ketoconazole, some macrolide antibiotics, grapefruit juice) CYP450 enzymes can cause wide variability in tacrolimus and ciclosporin levels.

Learning point

Tacrolimus is unusual in that increased gut transit due to diarrhoea paradoxically causes increased blood levels. This is because tacrolimus is both absorbed from the intestinal lumen as well as excreted into the lumen by enterocytes. Transporter proteins, such as P-glycoprotein and other multi-drug resistance proteins actively pump absorbed tacrolimus drug back out into the lumen. These transporters can be downregulated or obliterated in the presence of inflammatory diarrhoea and also are less effective with increased gut transit.

Accumulation of tacrolimus acutely leads to several effects as seen in this case – neurotoxicity with tremor and perioral tingling, hypertension and creatinine rise due to vasoconstriction, as well as hyperkalaemia and metabolic acidosis. Chronic effects of tacrolimus include renal fibrosis and predisposition to developing diabetes mellitus. In this case, tacrolimus toxicity explains all the clinical features.

Low calcium levels can cause perioral paraesthesia, but this gentleman is not on regular calcium or vitamin D replacement and has maintained good oral intake. It would not explain the acute kidney injury or acidosis. Hyperkalaemia and metabolic acidosis can be found with hypoadrenalism but the elevated blood pressure and normal blood glucose in the context of the other clinical features make this diagnosis most unlikely. Mycophenolic acid levels can be measured. This drug commonly causes gastrointestinal side effects such as diarrhoea. In this case one might expect to see bone marrow suppression with pancytopaenia rather than the features described. Although diarrhoea is a common side effect of mycophenolate, this has only started recently in this patient and would not explain the other features.

Hyperthyroidism could explain his tremor and hypertension, but his normal pulse, normal reflexes and other features would not be explained by this diagnosis. See Figure 9.9.

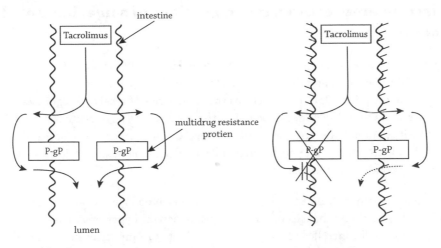

A: Normal
Tacrolimus absorbed across intestinal lumen.
P-glycoprotein pumps a proportion back
into the lumen where it is excreted.

B: Diarrhoea
Absorbtion of tacrolimus across an inflamed
gut wall or in the presence of increased transit
speed due to diarrhoea will both reduce
expression of P-glycoprotein as well as reduce
the effect of P-glycoprotein in pumping
tacrolimus back into the gut lumen.

Figure 9.9: Tacrolimus absorption in the normal state and with diarrhoea

CASE 2

A: Discrete areas of scarring in portions of some, but not all, glomeruli

This question requires a couple of steps in thinking. First of all, the most likely diagnosis needs to be decided upon and then that needs to be matched with the corresponding histological description. Option A describes the appearance of focal and segmental glomerulosclerosis (FSGS); option B would be the appearances in an acute bacterial pyelonephritis; option C describes the entity known as minimal change disease (MCD); option D is due to malignant hypertension and vascular changes; and option E is the classic description of diabetic nephropathy.

Diabetic nephropathy is unlikely here; she has a normal blood glucose and haemoglobin A_{1c} level with no diabetic changes on fundoscopy. Malignant hypertension is also less likely given her well-controlled blood pressure and lack of retinopathy either acutely or chronically. Minimal change disease could explain her significant levels of proteinuria; however, this often presents with nephrotic syndrome (including peripheral oedema and hypoalbuminaemia, which are not seen here). For such advanced renal impairment one would not expect to see normal light microscopic appearances. Chronic pyelonephritis could cause this presentation but evidence of scarring would undoubtedly be seen, the time course is too long and there is also no given history of recurrent urinary tract infections.

The most likely diagnosis is therefore FSGS. This is a condition that can be either primary (due to circulating immune factors) or secondary to a wide variety of conditions (see Table 9.2). Its hallmark is that not all glomeruli are scarred (focal sclerosis) and that only portions of those that are affected show scarring (segmental). The most likely aetiology in this case is her obesity with adaptive structural changes in her glomeruli that start to hyperfilter. Over time nephrons 'burn-out', are lost and scarring develops. This sets up a cycle of worsening pressure on remaining nephrons with further scarring. The end result is proteinuria, which often is in the nephrotic range, and declining renal function. The mainstay of treatment is the use of inhibitors of the renin–angiotensin system (ACE inhibitors or angiotensin receptor antagonists) to reduce blood pressure as well as reduce proteinuria. There is some evidence for the use of corticosteroids in those not improving with conservative management, and immunosuppressive strategies have been attempted with variable success.

Adaptive structural responses		
	Obesity	
	Reduced renal mass (low birth weight, renal malformations, nephrectomy, reflux nephropathy, chronic renal disease with nephron loss)	
Drug associated		
	Heroin Pamidronate Lithium	
Virus associated		
	HIV, parvovirus B19	
Genetic		
	Mutations in podocyte proteins – nephrin, podocin etc	

Table 9.2: Conditions associated with secondary FSGS

CASE 3

B: Commence therapeutic enoxaparin and request an echocardiogram

This lady has experienced a sudden episode of unilateral flank pain with acute kidney injury. Causes of such a presentation include stone disease, acute obstruction from blood clot or an abscess, acute interstitial nephritis (eg from drugs), acute vasculitis, or vascular or thrombo/atheroembolic events. Option A would be appropriate in the setting of tumour lysis syndrome (hinted at by the incidental but minor lymphadenopathy on CT scan and high LDH). However, LDH is a marker of cell turnover and will be raised in a number of conditions, not just lymphoma. With regard to option C, diclofenac could certainly have caused an acute interstitial nephritis with creatinine rise but this would not explain the prior pain, haematuria or the high LDH. Option D would be an appropriate management strategy if the patient had known stone disease with a transient rise in creatinine from obstruction. However, the CT did not demonstrate a stone or obstruction and again the LDH rise and fall is unaccounted for. Option E would be the correct course of action if vasculitis was the suspected cause (hinted at by acute kidney injury, haematuria and white blood cell count rise). However, this is not the most likely diagnosis and does not explain

continued

the LDH rise. Her dry cough could well be on the basis of her previous smoking history and there is nothing on the X-ray to suggest pulmonary haemorrhage, for example.

Therefore, taken as a whole, the most likely diagnosis is that this lady's previously undetected and untreated atrial fibrillation (her ECG shows atrial fibrillation) has resulted in thromboembolism to her left kidney with renal infarction.

Learning point

Renal infarction is an underdiagnosed condition, frequently mistaken for other causes, and is bilateral in approximately 10% of cases. In the setting of untreated atrial fibrillation, there is an up to four-fold higher rate of renal artery embolism than in the general population and many emboli found at autopsy were not detected clinically. Common signs and symptoms include flank pain, haematuria, leukocytosis and elevation of cell turnover markers such as LDH, transaminases and CK. Patients undergoing invasive vascular procedures may develop cholesterol emboli which can lodge not only in the renal vascular bed, but also in the lower limbs, leading to a livedo reticularis-type rash, peripheral blood eosinophilia and, if large enough, cause ischaemic toes/feet. Investigation is with angiography, often utilising CT with contrast or MRI with gadolinium. These investigations are complicated in the presence of severe renal impairment and the risk/benefit ratio needs to be decided.

Treatment, if embolism is suspected and demonstrated early, may be emergent vascular intervention. In this case however, four days afterwards, the damage has been done and there will almost certainly be a permanent loss of glomerular filtration. Therefore, anticoagulation and an echocardiogram to visualise any thrombus (which may now be obstructing the renal artery) is mandated.

CASE 4

B: Discharge from renal review; he should attend his GP for annual blood pressure and ACR checks

This young man presents with recurrent frank haematuria a couple of days after sore throat. His inter-morbid investigations are all totally normal with the exception of an elevated IgA level. In this case the most likely diagnosis is IgA nephropathy, which classically presents with flares in the setting of a sore throat.

Learning point

IgA levels can be normal or elevated at any time in this condition and are not diagnostic; the only definitive test is a renal biopsy which is required for diagnosis. Although biopsy is required for diagnosis, only the minority of people with suspected IgA nephropathy require a biopsy.

IgA nephropathy is the most common glomerulonephritis found on renal biopsy specimens. The cause is not totally clear but it is probably a combination of environmental, immune and infective factors. Demonstration of IgA deposition on biopsy is the hallmark of this disease. While most individuals who have IgA nephropathy have an essentially benign course, the condition can present with rapidly progressive renal failure.

This gentleman, however, has chronic kidney disease stage 1 – eGFR> 90 with haematuria but no proteinuria and normal blood pressure. In fact, there is not even demonstrated ongoing microscopic haematuria on urinalysis. His risk of progressive renal dysfunction is low and is equivalent to an otherwise healthy person of his age and gender. Therefore, he can be safely discharged from specialist renal review but annual checks with his GP should be required in case he does begin to develop proteinuria, hypertension or renal impairment. Option A makes an unwarranted and unevidenced assumption about the cause of his haematuria and is not an appropriate course of action. There is no benefit to penicillin prophylaxis for sore throat as suggested by option C, and tonsillectomy itself is not an evidence-based procedure in this disease. However, in some cases where recurrent tonsillitis is treated with tonsillectomy, those with IgA nephropathy have fewer flares. Regarding option D, an elevated IgA level is not diagnostic of this condition, and a normal level does not rule it out; biopsy is required. Regarding option E, he does not require a renal biopsy unless his ACR is over 70 (ie > 1 g/litre), his renal function starts to decline or the patient is very insistent on it to know the diagnosis. There are risks of bleeding associated with renal biopsy and, although modern practice is safe, there have been episodes of fatalities.

CASE 5

C: Commence losartan

This man has evidence of diabetic retinopathy as well as nephropathy (hypertension, microalbuminuria, elevated creatinine).

Learning point

In retarding the progression of diabetic nephropathy, renin–angiotensin system (RAS) blockade is the most effective strategy owing to both the antihypertensive and the specific anti-proteinuric effects of agents such as ACE inhibitors or angiotensin receptor blockers (ARBs). His target blood pressure should be < 125/75 mmHg, and therefore an ACE inhibitor or ARB is the logical choice.

His BMI is not overly elevated, so diet and lifestyle changes alone (answer E) are unlikely to reduce his proteinuria. He has had previous episodes of gout and uric acid is elevated. Losartan and ramipril are both options. In type 1 diabetes the evidence is mainly for the use of ACE inhibitors compared with type 2 diabetes where ARBs have been studied more. Clinically, however, their efficacy is judged to be equivalent and there is little to choose between them. Given the patient's stated concerns with side effects and reluctance to take extra medication it seems prudent to choose the agent which is likely to have fewer side effects. ACE inhibitors can cause a troublesome cough specific to their class and often necessitating switch to an ARB. Given that the patient has a long-term condition it is important, especially early in the patient's contact with a new healthcare professional, to maintain confidence in the therapeutic strategy and pre-empt possible issues with concordance due to foreseeable issues. An additional advantage of losartan is that it acts as a uricosuric and so may reduce the chance of further episodes of gout.

Given the patient's elevated potassium this would need to be rechecked at baseline (to ensure the sample has not been haemolysed from standing too long before transfer to the laboratory) and also one week after starting losartan to ensure it has not risen to > 6 mmol/litre. Further, a creatinine rise of 25% from baseline can be tolerated (in this case, that would equate to a rise of up to just over 140 μmol/litre). The patient may well require input from a dietician if his diet is high in potassium to maximise the benefit that he will gain from RAS inhibition. The aim in treating this patient would be to titrate up to the maximum tolerated dosage of the ARB. Note the strategy of combining ACE inhibitors and ARBs has fallen out of favour due to evidence of potential harm from dangerous hyperkalaemia.

Answers A and B are not the best options here as they have inferior proteinuric properties compared to ACE inhibitors and ARBs.

CASE 6

C: Tubulo-interstitium

Without a renal biopsy it can be difficult to ascertain the exact diagnostic process in a case of acute kidney injury. In this young girl's presentation, however, there are a number of clues to suggest that she has a condition affecting the tubulo-interstitium. Interstitial nephritis is the name given to the histological appearance of large numbers of inflammatory leukocytes invading the supporting, interstitial tissues on renal biopsy. There are many acute causes such as exposure to penicillin and non-steroidal anti-inflammatory drugs (hinted at in the question stem), as well as infectious agents such as viruses. Other conditions such as sarcoidosis, inflammatory bowel disease and autoimmune diseases can also cause a chronic interstitial nephritis. Chronic hypokalaeamia (eg from eating disorders) can also cause interstitial nephritis, as can exposure to lead and aristolochic acid found in some traditional herbal remedies. The time of onset after exposure to a causative drug can vary from days to months, and repeated exposure may be required. The treatment is withdrawal of the causative agent and consideration should be given to the use of steroids, eg prednisolone in a dose of 1 mg/kg per day. Steroids have a limited evidence base for hastening recovery.

Learning point

Hallmarks of interstitial nephritis include the presence of a rash and eosinophilia (not mentioned in the stem) and reduced glomerular filtration rate. The urinary sediment tends to be inactive (ie not heavily proteinuric or haematuric), and proteinuria tends to be less than 1 g/day (equivalent to an ACR < 70 as in this case). Anaemia occurs early and is often out of proportion to that expected, as seen here. Dysfunction of tubular mechanisms can lead to salt and electrolyte wasting as well as the development of Fanconi syndrome due to proximal tubular dysfunction. In this case, despite the normal serum glucose there is substantial glycosuria on urinalysis due to a reduced ability to reabsorb glucose from the renal tubules. Finally, the urine tends to be isothenuric, ie the specific gravity (a measure of urinary concentration) tends to stay stable at around that of protein-free plasma (approximately 1.01) as the urine can be neither concentrated nor diluted.

Option A is not correct as pathology affecting the glomerular endothelium (eg immune complex deposition from lupus or other vasculitic processes) would lead to dipstick positives, if not frank, haematuria. It would also be less likely to cause the tubular abnormalities seen here. Option B is not the best answer as pathology of the glomerular epithelium often leads to severe proteinuria and nephrotic syndrome (with ACR > 300)

continued

due to conditions such as minimal change disease, focal and segmental glomerulosclerosis, or membranous nephropathy. In those cases, flattening of the podocyte epithelial foot processes is seen on electron microscopy and this disrupts the molecular barriers to passage of albumin, resulting in large urinary losses.

Option D, obstruction to urinary flow, can be caused by a variety of stone types and cholesterol emboli can lodge here causing acute kidney injury, eosinophilia and rash (similar to interstitial nephritis). On renal biopsy it may be possible to see needles of cholesterol crystals in tubules. In this case, however, there is nothing to suggest cholesterol emboli from her examination and there would be no clear cause for this condition, which often occurs in older patients with atherosclerotic vascular disease or following interventional angiographic procedures.

Regarding option E, some types of glomerulonephritis as well as thrombotic microangiopathy can affect small- and medium-sized vessels but there is no suggestion from her clinical presentation, inflammatory markers, vasculitic screen or platelet count that this is the cause here. Blood pressure is normal, making scleroderma renal crisis or accelerated hypertension very unlikely, and there is nothing on her examination to suggest early disseminated cardiovascular disease.

CASE 7

B: Switch mycophenolate to azathioprine

Pregnancy in patients with renal disease can be associated with risks to both mother and fetus. The risk of pre-eclampsia, premature delivery and delivery of a small for gestational age baby are all increased when the mother has reduced glomerular filtration or uncontrolled blood pressure, hypertension or diabetes. With regards to immunosuppressive medications and risk of fetopathy, there is definite evidence that mycophenolate mofetil is teratogenic. Tacrolimus, ciclosporin and prednisolone are all considered safe, or at least there is no evidence of harm. In this case, mycophenolate should be stopped and switched to either azathioprine or prednisolone. In view of her elevated body mass index, previous fractures following minor falls (with the suggestion of prior renal bone disease given her time on dialysis), and the fact that tacrolimus and prednisolone are both diabetogenic, it seems prudent to use azathioprine rather than steroids. Answer A is incorrect as pregnancy can be advised 12 months post transplantation, provided blood pressure, creatinine and proteinuria are all favourable.

CASE 8

C: Decrease darbepoetin dose

Haemodialysis patients have a number of issues that need to be monitored regularly. These include fluid balance, blood pressure, uraemic symptoms, control of electrolyte disorders, minimising cardiovascular risk factors, control of renal anaemia and bone mineral disorder. Additionally, the presence of infection in lines or fistulas, or technical issues with dialysis may only become apparent when sought for either by clinical examination or on laboratory testing. The blood results given for the above patient demonstrate a phosphate level above the normal range and a parathyroid hormone level (PTH) three times above the normal range. This may suggest a problem with bone mineral disorder that could require adjustments in dosing. In this case, however, the calcium and phosphate are within acceptable limits for a patient on haemodialysis, and although the PTH is elevated, current guidelines stipulate that the PTH should be kept within the range of 2–9 times above the upper limit of normal (in this case between 100 and 450 pg/ml). PTH rises in advancing renal dysfunction due to several mechanisms and, left unchecked, can lead to worsening bone mineral disorder with risk of fractures, vascular calcification and worsening mortality. Uncontrolled hyperparathyroidism can not only result in severe symptoms such as lethargy, and itchy and red eyes, but can worsen renal anaemia. Medications such as vitamin D analogues (calcitriol) and phosphate binders (calcium carbonate, calcium acetate, sevelamer, lanthanum) are used to control bone mineral disorder. In this case there is no need to change current treatment as targets are met, therefore options A and D are incorrect.

The most significant issue with the blood result is the relatively high haemoglobin concentration. Current guidelines based on trial evidence suggest that the haemoglobin in dialysis patients should be maintained in the range 100–120 g/litre. Higher levels have been associated with increased cardiovascular mortality and thrombotic stroke risk. Iron indices are also acceptable here – ferritin should be between 200 and 500 ng/ml and transferrin saturations > 20%. Therefore the best strategy is to reduce, or temporarily stop, erythropoietin supplementation currently given in the form darbepoetin alfa. This will allow the haemoglobin to trend downwards safely. If haemoglobin becomes very high (> 14 g/litre) then one straightforward way to address this is to 'lose' a circuit of blood in the extracorporeal circuit of the dialysis machine when completing a dialysis session.

CASE 9

C: High-dependency/intensive care unit (HDU/ICU)

Decisions on patient transfer, especially out of hours, can be very difficult. This patient has a severe acute kidney injury with metabolic acidosis, is uraemic and has toxic digoxin levels with bradycardia and hypotension on a background of life-threatening hyperkalaemia. He responds well to therapy and remains stable. The next step in treatment, which will address many of his issues (hyperkalaemia, acidosis, uraemia, evolving fluid overload) is haemodialysis. Therefore, the renal ward is certainly an option. However, this gentleman is still potentially very unwell. He requires high-flow oxygen, being hyperkalaemic, digoxin toxic and acidotic means that his myocardium is 'irritable' and he is prone to further arrhythmias. This will be exacerbated if neck veins are accessed for a dialysis line and a guidewire is inserted. This can lead to atrial irritation and could potentiate a fatal episode of ventricular tachycardia/fibrillation. The patient may well require a temporary pacing wire additionally. Femoral access would probably be best in this patient; however, the possible need for a temporary pacing wire and the fact that reversal of digoxin toxicity with DigiBind® may precipitate pulmonary oedema or acute heart failure mean that this gentleman may require specialist coronary care unit support as well.

In view of this, the best answer is to transfer him to an HDU or ICU bed for close monitoring and where facilities exist for both dialysis and temporary pacing should it be required. Answer A is clearly inappropriate as this man requires dialysis for life-threatening hyperkalaemia. Remaining in the emergency department is also not appropriate as the patient requires definitive therapy in the form of dialysis. Note, digoxin is not cleared well by either haemodialysis or continuous veno-venous haemofiltration – DigiBind® or DigiFab® antibody fragments should be administered.

CASE 10

A: Calciphylaxis

This gentleman has a long vintage on haemodialysis with substantially deranged bone mineral biochemistry. The calcium level is toward the upper limit of normal, phosphate is elevated and PTH is grossly elevated. The rash has evolved quickly into a necrotic black eschar and is very painful. The histological image (Figure 9.7) shows a blood vessel with a fibrous intimal response causing almost complete occlusion. Surrounding the blood vessel is an infiltrate of neutrophils. The highly suggestive features of purple calcific deposits in the wall of the artery, in the context of the patient vignette, are typical of calciphylaxis.

CHAPTER 9 ANSWERS

Learning point +

Calciphylaxis, or calcific uraemic arteriopathy, is an extremely painful condition, typically associated with increasing time on dialysis, bone mineral disorder, obesity, hypoalbuminaemia and vitamin K antagonist treatment. It carries a 1-year mortality of 45%, often due to infection. Treatment is difficult but incorporates increased frequency of haemodialysis sessions, control of bone mineral disorder, consideration for emergency parathyroidectomy, hyperbaric oxygen, vitamin K supplementation and IV sodium thiosulfate (which acts as a calcium chelator) given during dialysis. Meticulous wound care and analgesia with combination opiate analgesia is also mandated.

Cholesterol emboli (option B) cause a livedo reticularis-type rash, often associated with an eosinophilia, and typically lodge in the peripheral circulation causing violaceous discoloration or gangrene of digits or toes. The histology may show cholesterol crystals in small blood vessels. Option C (Henoch–Schönlein cutaneous vasculitis) could present in this way although the rash tends to be more vasculitic in nature, rather than confluent as is the case here. A black eschar would not be typical and a skin biopsy may show positive immunofluorescence for IgA deposits. Answer D (porphyria cutanea tarda) tends to occur on sun-exposed areas (presumably not on the upper thighs, which would tend to have less sun exposure) in the context of liver disease or alcohol abuse. It tends to cause a blistering type rash, and calcific deposits in blood vessels would not be seen.

Answer E (pyoderma gangrenosum) could very well look like this and would explain the severe pain. However, the histology would comprise giant cells, granulomata and necrotic areas, which are not seen in the histological picture.

CASE 11

D: Plasma cell dyscrasia

This lady presents with a normocytic anaemia, renal dysfunction, a normal gap acidosis with a positive urinary anion gap (Na + K – Cl > 0) suggesting a renal tubular acidosis, and substantial proteinuria on a 24-hour timed collection, which is not detected using an ACR or urinalysis.

Learning point

The key here is to understand the discrepancy between the various urine tests. ACR measures the albumin/creatinine ratio and conventional urine dipsticks detect albumin mainly. In this case there is an excess of protein other than albumin, and given her renal impairment and nephrotic range proteinuria, the most likely diagnosis is a plasma cell dyscrasia with an excess of immunoglobulin light chains being produced, which are then filtered in the kidney and appear in the urine.

Light chains can injure the kidneys in various ways including obstruction, by inducing inflammatory damage and through direct tubular toxicity.

Option A, ANCA vasculitis, is unlikely given her normal inflammatory markers and lack of blood or protein on urinalysis (proliferative glomerulonephritides such as ANCA vasculitis will tend to cause non-selective loss of proteins including albumin which can be detected). Furthermore, this answer would not explain the excess of a protein other than albumin in the urine. The P-ANCA is mildly positive at a titre of 20 (the lowest limit of detection). This can be a false positive finding or be seen in other disorders such as inflammatory bowel disease. The negative MPO and PR3 staining is also reassuring.

Answer B is most unlikely – this lady has evidence of immunity to hepatitis B, most likely on the basis of a previous vaccination as her surface antibody is positive and all other markers are negative. Further, there is no other evidence of an inflammatory vasculitis. Polyarteritis nodosa tends to be associated with renal dysfunction and often weight loss and abdominal pain. Regarding option C, it is likely that the furosemide treatment has exacerbated the renal injury due to relative dehydration and precipitation of myeloma casts or light chains in the kidney. There is limited evidence of an interstitial nephritic process. Proteinuria in interstitial nephritis also tends to be non-selective and less than 1 g/day. Additionally, this would not fully explain the pre-treatment symptoms of fatigue and ankle swelling. With regard to option E, this lady does indeed have a renal tubular acidosis but this is secondary to an underlying cause – in this case a plasma cell dyscrasia. The renal tubular acidosis is not the cause of her creatinine rise per se.

See Table 9.3 for interpretation and comparison of different methods to detect proteinuria in clinical practice.

	Urine dipstick	ACR mg/mmol	PCR mg/mmol	24-h collection
Normal	Nil	< 3	< 5	< 0.15 g
Microalbuminuria	Nil or 'trace'	3–30	5–50	< 0.5 g
Proteinuria	+ or ++ 0.3–1 g/litre	70	100	1 g
	++ or +++ 1–3 g/litre	70–200	100–350	1–1.35 g
Nephrotic range proteinuria	+++ or ++++ 3–20 g/litre	> 200	> 350	> 3.5 g
Comments	Qualitative; easy to use, can detect blood, glucose, nitrites. Cannot detect microalbuminuria.	Quantitative; measures albumin excretion. Total proteinuria underestimated if proteins other than albumin present.	Quantitative; measures all urinary proteins. Divide PCR by 100 to derive proteinuria in grams.	Gold standard, but cumbersome and relies on appropriate collection techniques.

ACR, albumin/creatinine ratio; PCR, protein/creatinne ratio.

Table 9.3: Methods for detecting proteinuria

CASE 12

D: Plasma exchange

This gentleman presents with a 3-week history of symptoms suggestive of a systemic disorder. He has a significantly elevated creatinine, is acidotic and has a high titre of anti-glomerular basement membrane (GBM) antibody. This man has anti-GBM disease (Goodpasture's disease). In addition, he is moderately anaemic with patchy chest X-ray changes and a substantially increased transfer factor, which are all very suggestive of latent pulmonary haemorrhage. Given the fact that his creatinine is > 500 µmol/litre and he has anti-GBM disease, this is a compelling, evidenced-based indication for plasma exchange. Plasma exchange would also be indicated for pulmonary haemorrhage associated with anti-GBM or ANCA vasculitis at any creatinine level. The aim of plasma exchange is to rapidly remove pathogenic antibodies from the circulation to arrest further renal and lung damage. These antibodies are directed against the basement membranes of both renal and lung tissue and this is the explanation for the signs and symptoms seen. Goodpasture's disease is associated with smoking and petrochemical exposure, but these are by no means the only environmental modifiers. It tends to be a 'one-hit' disease and rarely recurs; however, it can cause substantial morbidity and mortality (if untreated). Many patients are rendered dialysis-dependent.

Alongside plasma exchange, IV methylprednisolone and oral or IV cyclophosphamide should be given, although here the priority is plasma exchange. Rituximab has been used with success as induction therapy in ANCA-associated vasculitis but not in anti-GBM disease. Haemodialysis may well be indicated soon but there is no compelling indication given the information in the vignette and despite there not being a baseline creatinine available, one would have to assume that this man's renal dysfunction was all very acute, especially given his normally sized kidneys on ultrasound.

CASE 13

E: Vancomycin and ciprofloxacin

This gentleman has a clinical diagnosis of PD peritonitis. The presence of the cloudy effluent and a PD white cell count of $> 100 \times 10^6/mm^3$ are diagnostic. The main organisms causing PD peritonitis are *Staphylococcus aureus*, coagulase negative staphylococci, *Escherichia coli*, *Pseudomonas* species and fungal organisms. Most cases are caused by bacteria and so appropriate gram-positive and gram-negative cover needs to be given. Pending microbiological testing and the fact that the patient is clinically well, it would be premature for the PD catheter to be removed. Indications for removal include fungal peritonitis, peritonitis not responding to antibiotics, or severe sepsis and recurrent infections.
The best answer of the ones given here is option E – vancomycin (conveniently given intraperitoneally) and ciprofloxacin (usually given orally). Gentamicin (intraperitoneally or IV) is an alternative, along with vancomycin. The others do not give broad enough or intensive enough coverage of the common organisms. Metronidazole may well be added at a later date if anaerobic infection is suspected or confirmed, and fluconazole added if fungi are present.

CASE 14

A: Transplant graft survival is better with a 2-2-2 mismatched live donor kidney rather than a 0-0-0 mismatched deceased donor kidney

The preferred form of renal replacement therapy is transplantation. It offers in almost all eligible cases substantial survival benefits over haemodialysis or peritoneal dialysis. Diabetes is the leading cause of end-stage renal disease and, of those with diabetes who require dialysis, only 30% will be alive at five years (not 60% as per answer B). Peritoneal dialysis (PD) usually has a lifespan of five years or fewer owing to the effects of the PD solutions on the function of the peritoneal membrane. Although there is an early increase in mortality in those with diabetes who undergo renal transplantation, there is substantial gain in survival odds after six months. Transplantation can take place 'pre-emptively', before a patient needs to start dialysis. This avoids exposure to a range of metabolic, nutritional, psychosocial and vascular problems associated with maintenance haemodialysis.

A poorly matched live donor transplant (2-2-2 is the least well-matched kidney one could receive – where the three major histocompatibility locus antigens tested on each chromosome are different at each location between donor and recipient) will have a greater likelihood of working compared to a well-matched deceased donor graft. This is due to both the circumstances of death, retrieval of the organ and the time taken for transportation and transplantation into a donor. With modern immunosuppressive regimens, the effects of poor matching on chances of subsequent rejection can be substantially minimised.

CASE 15

B: MRI scan of kidneys

Polycystic kidney disease in adults tends to be due to either mutations in the *PKD1* gene (chromosome 16; 85% individuals, mean age at end-stage renal disease = 54 years) or the *PKD2* gene (chromosome 4; 15% individuals, mean age at end-stage renal disease = 74 years). It is by no means certain which mutation this patient possesses.

Learning point

There are diagnostic criteria in the presence of a positive family history, but no documented mutation to assess whether patients have polycystic disease. Criteria are based on the number of cysts in each kidney with age-defined cut-offs. Usually over the age of 30, if there are fewer than two cysts on ultrasound in each kidney then the person is unlikely to have polycystic disease. Conversely, between the ages of 15 and 30 years, it can be difficult to tell how many cysts a patient has or whether they will go on to develop cysts. Therefore in the assessment of younger patients, especially those wanting to donate to a relative, MRI is the more sensitive diagnostic tool and will yield enough information to permit a diagnosis to be made or excluded in this setting.

A molecular genetic test that can be applied in all cases is not yet available. There are over 1000 different mutations in these genes and they are large. Therefore sequencing and analysing them for causative mutations is prohibitively expensive and time consuming at this present time; it does not normally occur outside a research programme. Renal biopsy is not performed in the evaluation of polycystic kidney disease as the chance of sampling a cyst is far too small (if not visible on ultrasound) and renal biopsy carries with it risks of bleeding. An ultrasound scan of renal tracts at this stage is too insensitive to the presence of smaller cysts that may be developing. Finally, waiting five years would be of no advantage – MRI can make a diagnosis or otherwise, and given the patient's renal function he will need to start dialysis soon.

CASE 16

D: Low-sodium diet

This gentleman has a first presentation with stone disease.

Learning point

Calcium oxalate stones are the most common type (50–60%) followed by calcium phosphate (15–20%), magnesium ammonium phosphate – associated with urease-splitting organisms such as *Proteus* species (5%), and uric acid (5%). Rare genetic syndromes or drug crystallisation comprise the remainder.

Stone formation is complex and there are physical and chemical promoters and inhibitors. Chemical factors promoting formation are high urinary calcium, oxalate and uric acid, and low urinary volume, citrate and magnesium. Additionally some stones form in alkaline urine (eg calcium phosphate, magnesium ammonium phosphate ('infection stones'), many drug-induced crystals such as HIV protease inhibitors and ciprofloxacin), whereas others tend to form in acidic urine (eg uric acid, cystine).

The acute treatment of renal colic due to stones is as described in the question. Tamsulosin is useful in relaxing ureteric smooth muscle and so promoting passage. Stones < 4 mm usually pass spontaneously. Long-term measures include maintaining adequate oral hydration (advise patients to drink 2–3 litres of fluid per day), replacement of citrate in the diet (especially if low urinary citrate) by consumption of citrus fruits or using potassium citrate, and avoidance of foods high in oxalate (eg strawberries, chocolate, nuts, tea, coffee). Dietary protein restriction is of value in those producing uric acid stones.

A low-calcium diet may appear intuitively correct but is the wrong thing to advise. People should maintain good intake of calcium and vitamin D. The reason is that calcium in the gut binds oxalate. If there is less calcium ingested, then more oxalate is reabsorbed and the risk of calcium oxalate formation in the urine is increased. Prophylactic antibiotics may be an option to consider if there are demonstrated recurrent urinary tract infections with stone-forming organisms. This is not relevant in this case.

Bendroflumethiazide, in common with other thiazide diuretics, has the effect of reducing urinary calcium excretion and so the risk of calcium stone formation. At this stage, however, it is not indicated, especially since the blood pressure is normal.

Excessive sodium in the diet, especially in combination with a low-potassium diet, leads to decreased calcium reabsorption from the tubular lumen and so increases the chance of stone formation in urine. Conversely, a low-sodium diet will permit calcium reabsorption.

CASE 17

D: IV potassium supplementation will probably be required

This gentleman has a post-obstructive diuresis that will require careful management to avoid large fluid and electrolyte shifts. The likely aetiology is bladder outlet obstruction from benign prostatic hypertrophy.

Learning point

To manage this it is helpful to understand that there are several factors driving his diuresis. These include:

+ Pre-existing sodium and fluid retention following the decline in glomerular filtration rate (GFR) with compensatory hormonal adaptation in the setting of bilateral obstruction.

+ High levels of osmotically active urea.

+ Circulating natriuretic factors that were not being excreted by the obstructed kidneys now able to have an effect in promoting sodium loss.

+ Insensitivity to the effects of antidiuretic hormone (ADH) on the renal tubules due to the obstructive damage and fall in GFR. Aquaporin channels are downregulated and there is less transport of water from the collecting tubules back into the interstitium.

+ Iatrogenic fluid resuscitation.

+ Damage to, and reduction in number of, active sodium transporters that create the needed electrochemical gradients which permit tubular fine-tuning of urinary concentration.

+ 'Wash-out' of the medullary concentration gradient. This is the gradient formed by active transport of small molecules into and out of the loop of Henle, which allows the production of both very dilute as well as very concentrated urine depending on fluid and electrolyte balance. The rapid flow of fluid in post-obstructive diuresis does not allow time for this to re-establish. The interstitial compartment remains with low concentration of solutes and so the gradient driving reabsorption of water out of the tubules to make a concentrated urine is reduced.

It is also helpful to realise that the composition of urine in a post-obstructive diuresis tends to mirror that of 0.45% saline. Measuring urinary electrolytes can confirm this. Additionally, potassium wasting is likely to occur due to the massive natriuresis with increased sodium delivery to the distal tubule which drives potassium excretion. This can be particularly welcome in those who are hyperkalaemic, but dramatic falls in serum potassium can ensue.

continued

Patients should have a regular fluid balance assessment, including pulse, blood pressure and postural blood pressure measurement. Weight should be recorded once or twice daily. If a patient is euvolaemic then the best strategy is to replace the previous volume urine lost per hour with alternating 5% dextrose and 0.9% saline, or Hartman's solution. If the patient is dehydrated, then the output plus 40 ml could be prescribed. This is best written in the fluid balance as 'Input = Output', or 'Input = Output + 40 ml'. Alternating bags of 1 litre of 0.9% saline and 5% dextrose should be written up.

The other options are much less satisfactory. Clamping the catheter will just lead to his bladder becoming distended again and will not stop his diuresis. The fluid being drained has already left the physiological compartments of the body so there is no advantage to keeping it in the ureter and bladder! Replacing three quarters of the volume lost with dextrose will probably lead to hyponatraemia and intravascular volume collapse due to the ongoing sodium losses. Additionally, if dextrose in water is given at too high a rate then it can lead to an osmotic diuresis due to the amount of dextrose given. Measuring blood pressure is important, but giving hypertonic saline as boluses can potentially lead to large swings in serum sodium. Additionally, sourcing this in adequate amounts can be quite difficult and will be unfamiliar to most staff. It is best to replace losses on an ongoing and predictable basis. The patient at this very early stage should not be fluid-restricted as it could take some days for the diuresis to settle as concentration gradients are re-established and various sodium pumps and hormonal systems re-establish. It may be a suitable strategy to keep the patient in a slightly negative fluid balance if a substantial diuresis persists after 24–48 hours, but not at this stage.

Potassium should be carefully monitored and fluid with added potassium should be used, so long as potassium is not infused at greater than 10 mmol/litre per hour on the medical wards. A separate IV line may be required to give this at a safe rate.

CASE 18

A: Add bendroflumethiazide

In deciding a treatment strategy for this gentleman there is a balance between ensuring patient safety and ensuring optimum treatment of pre-existing conditions. He has type 1 diabetes and has chronic kidney disease (CKD) stage 3 with substantial proteinuria and hypertension. His risk of progressive CKD is high. He has had a rise in creatinine following introduction of ramipril therapy, although this is within the accepted 25% rise allowed from baseline. His ACR has fallen but potassium is 6 mmol/litre. He runs a baseline high potassium and has a mild acidosis, and this is most likely due not to the severity of his renal dysfunction but to the effects of diabetes on the kidney causing a type 4 renal tubular acidosis. Further he appears to be developing hypoglycaemic unawareness.

There are therefore some issues that need to be addressed here: (a) the risk of progressive CKD is high; (b) he has uncontrolled proteinuria and hypertension; (c) his potassium is high and further up-titration of his ramipril may lead to dangerous hyperkalaemia.

Of the options given, adding bendroflumethiazide is best. It will not only assist blood pressure management but will also cause some potassium wasting and may permit further up-titration of his ramipril (helping to reduce ACR further). Its diuretic effect may help his ankle oedema which is presumably secondary to his amlodipine rather than proteinuria. Bisoprolol is also a useful antihypertensive agent but can worsen hyperkalaemia and, significantly, blunt hypoglycaemic symptoms leading to fatal hypoglycaemic coma. Doxazosin will not have as helpful an effect on hyperkalaemia. Furosemide will assist with ankle swelling but will not be as useful in the control of hypertension as bendroflumethiazide. This is because furosemide's effect occurs at the ascending loop of Henle. Inhibition of sodium reabsorption there means that it can potentially be reabsorbed later in the distal collecting tubule. Thiazide diuretics act at the distal tubule, and prevention of sodium reabsorption there means there is less chance for other downstream mechanisms to counteract the diuretic effect.

Stopping ramipril is not the best thing to do here – it is giving up too easily! A potassium level stably maintained at 6 mmol/litre is within the limits of current CKD guidelines and there is a chance his proteinuria might worsen on stopping ACE inhibition. In combination with the prescription of a thiazide diuretic, the patient should receive renal dietetic input for a low-potassium diet. It would also be sensible to commence him on oral sodium bicarbonate, eg 1 g BD PO. This will assist his acidosis with an expected improvement in serum potassium. It is also doubly important that he adhere to a no-added-salt diet to ensure the effects of these medication changes are not negated.

CASE 19

A: Blockade of an epithelial sodium channel

Not all diuretics are equal! A knowledge of where diuretics act can give clues to their best use in clinical practice. Amiloride is a potassium-sparing diuretic as its effects, unlike other diuretics such as loop and thiazides, do not lead to potassium wasting. Amiloride acts in the distal convoluted tubule on epithelial sodium channels (ENaC) in principal cells. These channels act to reabsorb sodium from the tubular lumen and to excrete potassium. Therefore **p**rincipal **c**ells **p**ee out **p**otassium. Inhibition of this process by amiloride prevents sodium reabsorption, leading to the diuretic effect, and also reduces potassium secretion, leading to its 'potassium-sparing' effects. Of note, ENaC also will reabsorb lithium ions. Lithium can easily enter principal cells, but it cannot leave as easily. Lithium can therefore accumulate, leading to some of the chronic damage seen in those on long-term lithium treatment. Amiloride blocks lithium uptake via ENaC and is one strategy to mitigate lithium-induced renal disease.

Competition for intracellular aldosterone receptors describes the effects of spironolactone. Carbonic anhydrase inhibitors such as acetazolamide inhibit the cytosolic version of this enzyme in proximal tubular cells. Thiazides inhibit the Na2Cl symporter in the distal convoluted tubule whereas loop diuretics inhibit the NaK2Cl symporter in the ascending loop of Henle.

CASE 20

D: Ramipril

Assuming of course the patient does not have roaring sepsis or hypotension, ramipril could be safely continued – it is not known to cause tinnitus. All the other options listed cause tinnitus. Vancomycin, gentamicin and furosemide are directly ototoxic. Quinine toxicity can cause cinchonism – flushed skin, tinnitus, blurred vision, confusion, abdominal pain, gastrointestinal symptoms and a skin rash. Of note, the combination of gentamicin and furosemide can be synergistic in their ototoxic effects. An audiological assessment should be conducted urgently and any ototoxic medications discontinued if possible.

CASE 21

B: An infiltrate of inflammatory cells in the supporting tissues around tubules

The clinical scenario, findings and rash are all suggestive of interstitial nephritis, possibly secondary to the non-steroidal anti-inflammatory drugs used. He has anaemia, renal dysfunction, eosinophilia and microalbuminuria. Cholesterol emboli can also cause the above signs; however, the rash is more typically a livedo reticularis-type rash and the patient would be quite young for this complication, which tends to occur in older vasculopaths. On renal biopsy the hallmark sign is an interstitial infiltrate of inflammatory cells that can also affect the tubules. Treatment is with oral corticosteroids and withdrawal of the offending agent.

Answer A details the findings seen in amyloidosis. Answer C describes a proliferative, crescentic glomerulonephritis that would be seen in eg ANCA vasculitis or Goodpasture's disease. Answer D details the appearance of cholesterol emboli syndrome, and answer E relates to the appearances of hypertensive nephrosclerosis, with onion skinning being a particular feature of malignant hypertension.

CHAPTER 10

Oncology and Palliative Medicine

Anna Ryan

CASE 1

A 59-year-old otherwise fit and healthy woman presents with a 3-month history of bloating. Her bowel habit and appetite are normal and she has had no postmenopausal bleeding or vaginal discharge. Abdominal ultrasound identifies a 5 cm complex cystic lesion arising from the left ovary and extending to involve the fallopian tube. There is also mild ascites. Blood tests demonstrate a CA125 level of 735 U/ml. A full staging CT scan shows no evidence of lesions elsewhere.

What is the most appropriate management?

- A. **Biopsy/FNA of the ovarian mass to obtain a tissue diagnosis**
- B. **Neoadjuvant chemotherapy**
- C. **Optimal cytoreductive surgery**
- D. **Local radiotherapy followed by surgical excision**
- E. **Monitor and repeat imaging and CA125 in six months**

CASE 2

A 47-year-old man presents with a mole on his shoulder which has been itching and bleeding for the last three weeks. Examination reveals a 0.8 cm irregularly pigmented asymmetrical lesion with a small 2 mm satellite nodule nearby. Enlarged lymph nodes are palpable in the ipsilateral axilla and cervical region. A CT scan of the chest and abdomen identifies three liver metastases.

Core biopsy of one of the affected nodes is performed and the pathology report is as follows:

+ Lymph node is replaced by atypical melanocytes. Poorly differentiated cells with a high mitotic index (> 50 mitoses/10 high-power fields).

+ Diagnosis: metastatic malignant melanoma

+ Mutational analysis performed: *BRAF* V600E mutation identified

Select the most appropriate systemic treatment for this patient:

A. **Dacarbazine (DTIC) chemotherapy**
B. **Ipilimumab**
C. **Interleukin-2**
D. **Vemurafenib**
E. **High-dose interferon**

CASE 3

A 79-year-old woman with metastatic breast cancer involving the liver, bones and brain is in the terminal stages of her illness. She has been admitted for symptom control and a hospice transfer is planned, but on the ward she is deteriorating and her family state they would prefer her not to be moved. Her tolerance of oral medications is diminished and you wish to convert her current analgesics to a subcutaneous syringe driver.

She is currently taking morphine sulfate tablets 60 mg BD and for breakthrough pain uses oramorph liquid 20 mg three times per day.

Which of the following prescriptions is most appropriate for her syringe driver?

A. **40 mg diamorphine s/c over 24 hours**
B. **60 mg diamorphine s/c over 24 hours**
C. **80 mg diamorphine s/c over 24 hours**
D. **100 mg diamorphine s/c over 24 hours**
E. **120 mg diamorphine s/c over 24 hours**

CASE 4

A 17-year-old boy with a stage IV testicular germ cell tumour and bulky, large-volume disease is started on his first cycle of combination chemotherapy as an inpatient. Thirty-six hours after initiating chemotherapy he complains of feeling generally unwell, nausea and of having palpitations. An ECG demonstrates a supraventricular tachycardia with a rate of 120 bpm. You note that his urine output has fallen and his biochemistry results from blood tests earlier that day are abnormal, leading you to suspect he has tumour lysis syndrome. Which of the following sets of blood results (see Table 10.1) are most suggestive of this diagnosis?

Answer	A	B	C	D	E
Sodium (mmol/litre)	140	140	156	125	140
Potassium (mmol/litre)	3.5	2.5	5.8	3.5	5.8
Urea (mmol/litre)	10	3.5	20	2.0	7.5
Creatinine (µmol/litre)	50	80	330	55	125
Corrected calcium (mmol/litre)	2.2	2.2	2.5	2.1	2.0
Phosphate (mmol/litre)	1.2	1.0	1.4	0.9	1.6
Urate (mmol/litre)	0.3	0.2	0.4	0.15	2.5

Table 10.1

CASE 5

Cytotoxic chemotherapy agents have been used for the treatment of cancer since the first experiments using nitrogen mustards in 1940s. Many different mechanisms of action are utilised by these agents. Three commonly used chemotherapy agents are listed. Identify the correctly matched list of their respective class from the list below:

    5-Fluorouracil; cyclophosphamide; doxorubicin

    A. **Antimetabolite; alkylating agent; camptothecin**
    B. **Antimetabolite; anthracycline; alkylating agent**
    C. **Alkylating agent; alkylating agent; anthracycline**
    D. **Antimetabolite; topoisomerase II inhibitor; taxane**
    E. **Antimetabolite; alkylating agent; anthracycline**

CASE 6

A 56-year-old man presents with a history of cough and wheeze of eight months duration. He is otherwise systemically well. He has a ten pack/year smoking history. A chest X-ray shows a right lower lobe opacity and CT scanning confirms the presence of a 2.5 cm lesion but no evidence of metastatic spread. A fine needle aspirate is obtained and demonstrates malignancy. A decision is made to perform a lobectomy. The histopathology report is as follows:

Malignant cells with well-differentiated neuroendocrine features. Mitotic count is < 1/10 high-power fields. There is no evidence of necrosis.

What is the most likely diagnosis?

A. **Typical bronchial carcinoid tumour**
B. **Atypical bronchial carcinoid tumour**
C. **Large cell neuroendocrine carcinoma**
D. **Small cell lung cancer**
E. **Squamous cell lung cancer**

CASE 7

You are reviewing a referral letter from a GP to the colorectal cancer clinic. In the text the patient is described as being of 'performance status 3'. Which of the following options most accurately describes the patients's current level of activity?

A. **Bedbound and unable to perform any self-care**
B. **Resting in a bed or chair more than 50% of the time**
C. **Fully fit and active**
D. **Generally active but unable to carry out heavy physical work**
E. **Active more than 50% of the time but tires easily and is unable to continue work**

CASE 8

Current estimates suggest that one in three people in the UK will be affected by cancer at some point, meaning that doctors in every medical speciality will deal with oncology patients on a regular basis. Having a broad idea of the prognosis of different cancers is important when reviewing these patients in the context of other medical problems. In Table 10.2 are listed some tumour types and expected median survival times. Pair the tumour types with their expected survival.

Tumour type	Approximate median overall survival
A: Metastatic breast cancer	1: 6–12 months
B: Stage I seminoma	2: Five years
C: Extensive stage small cell lung cancer	3: Two years
D: Metastatic small intestinal neuroendocrine tumour	4: No impact on survival
E: Metastatic prostate cancer	5: Ten years

Table 10.2: Match the tumour types in column one to the expected median survival times in column two

    A. **A5, B2, C1, D4, E3**
    B. **A2, B4, C1, D3, E5**
    C. **A3, B4, C1, D5, E2**
    D. **A3, B4, C1, D2, E5**
    E. **A2, B5, C3, D1, E5**

CASE 9

You have been referred a 41-year-old woman who has recently been diagnosed with renal cell carcinoma. She tells you that cancer 'runs in the family'. Examine the family pedigree shown in Figure 10.1 and select the most likely diagnosis from the listed conditions.

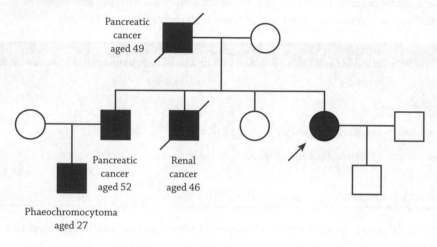

Figure 10.1

  A. **Multiple endocrine neoplasia type I**
  B. **Multiple endocrine neoplasia type II**
  C. *BRCA2* **mutation**
  D. **von Hippel–Lindau syndrome**
  E. **Neurofibromatosis**

CASE 10

A 59-year-old man presents to the emergency department complaining of headaches and difficulty breathing. He has had a cough for several months but over the last three weeks his symptoms have deteriorated and he now feels very unwell, is short of breath at rest and cannot lie flat. He tells you he has been a heavy smoker in the past but quit six months ago. On examination he looks distressed, respiratory rate is 35 breaths/min, heart rate 110 bpm, blood pressure 140/90 mmHg, oxygen saturation 86%. You notice facial oedema, venous distension around his neck and upper thorax, and on auscultation of his chest there is reduced air entry in the right upper zone. ECG shows sinus tachycardia. Examine his chest X-ray in Figure 10.2 and select the most appropriate initial management plan.

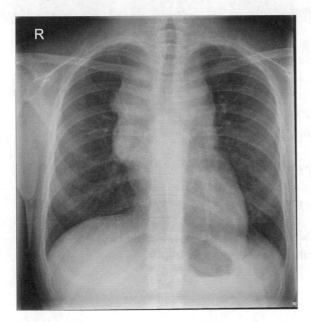

Figure 10.2

    A. **Nurse sitting up, oxygen, steroids (dexamethasone 16 mg per day with proton pump inhibitor), IV furosemide and bisoprolol**

    B. **Nurse sitting up, oxygen, steroids (dexamethasone 16 mg per day with proton pump inhibitor), discuss with an oncologist**

    C. **Nurse sitting up, oxygen, steroids (dexamethasone 4 mg per day), discuss with an oncologist**

    D. **Refer the patient for bronchoscopy**

    E. **Arrange emergency intubation and transfer to the intensive care unit**

CASE 11

Which of the following is the most significant cause of cancer-related mortality in the UK?

A. Breast cancer
B. Colorectal cancer
C. Lung cancer
D. Prostate cancer
E. Pancreatic cancer

CASE 12

A 77-year-old man is diagnosed with localised prostate cancer. Digital rectal examination and MRI scanning demonstrate T2a, N0 disease. His prostatic-specific antigen is 6.2 ng/ml, and template biopsy identifies a Gleason score of 3 + 3. He has no evidence of metastatic disease and is not symptomatic. What is the most appropriate management plan for this patient?

A. Radical prostatectomy plus adjuvant hormonal therapy for three years
B. Radical radiotherapy with no adjuvant treatment
C. Active surveillance
D. Cytotoxic chemotherapy with docetaxel every three weeks for six cycles
E. Hormonal therapy with a gonadotrophin-releasing hormone analogue and an oral anti-androgen

CASE 13

A 43-year-old man complains of weight loss, anorexia, nausea and fatigue. Past medical history is unremarkable and there is no relevant family history. Examination reveals cachexia, mild icterus and a palpable left supraclavicular lymph node.

His GP performs blood tests which reveal the following: Haemoglobin 97 g/litre, MCV 89 fl, White cells 6.1 × 10⁹/litre, Platelets 237 × 10⁹/litre, Sodium 139 mmol/litre, Potassium 4.2 mmol/litre, Urea 9.6 mmol/litre, Creatinine 50 μmol/litre, Bilirubin 42 μmol/litre, ALT 50 U/litre, AST 76 U/litre, ALP 130 U/litre, CA19-9 4398 U/ml, αFP 109 ng/ml, CEA 32 ng/ml.

A CT scan is performed (see Figure 10.3).

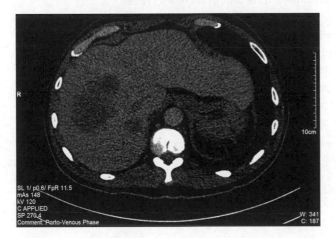

Figure 10.3

What is the most appropriate next investigation?

A. **Ultrasound guided liver biopsy**

B. **Colonoscopy**

C. **Upper gastrointestinal tract endoscopy**

D. **MRI scan of liver**

E. **PET scan**

CASE 14

A 42-year-old woman who is receiving adjuvant FEC-T chemotherapy following surgery for breast cancer presents to the emergency department. She last received chemotherapy eight days ago, and is now complaining of headache, fevers and rigors but denies any cough, dysuria or abdominal pains. She looks unwell. The temperature is 38.6 °C, blood pressure 108/60 mmHg, heart rate 112 bpm and oxygen saturation 98%. Blood results are awaited. Urinalysis testing shows the presence of white cells and nitrites. What is the most appropriate next step in management?

A. Give oral paracetamol and fluids. Await blood results to determine if patient is neutropaenic
B. Give bolus intravenous fluids and oral co-amoxiclav 625 mg three times daily to treat a presumed urinary tract infection
C. Give immediate intravenous broad spectrum antibiotics, rehydrate and monitor fluid balance
D. Give a subcutaneous injection of granulocyte colony-stimulating factor to treat presumed neutropaenic sepsis
E. Perform a lumbar puncture, send a cerebrospinal fluid sample for gram stain and culture, and treat for presumed meningitis

CASE 15

A 74-year-old man with known metastatic prostate cancer attends the emergency department. He describes three days of progressively worsening back pain which is preventing him from doing gardening. Examination demonstrates a mild weakness of hip flexion on the left side but is otherwise unremarkable and he is able to walk. Plain X-rays are difficult to interpret but appear to show vertebral collapse and an urgent MRI scan of spine is requested. Review the MRI scan (Figure 10.4) and identify the most appropriate management plan.

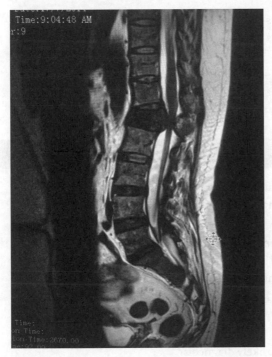

Figure 10.4

    A. Administer analgesia and steroids, arrange an urgent oncology outpatient appointment the next day for the patient, and advise him to return home until this time

    B. Refer the patient to the oncology day unit for urgent high-dose chemotherapy

    C. Discuss with the oncology and neurosurgery teams, admit the patient, give analgesia and high-dose steroids, and follow any further guidance from specialist teams

    D. Arrange immediate radiotherapy

    E. Prescribe analgesia and steroids, explain to the patient that his prognosis is poor and refer directly to the palliative care team

CASE 16

A 51-year-old woman was referred because of a change in bowel habit. She has not had any symptoms of gastrointestinal bleeding or weight loss. There is no relevant family history. Abdominal examination and digital rectal examination were unremarkable. Flexible sigmoidoscopy revealed a 5 mm polyp in the upper rectum, which was removed with forceps. Histology revealed a tubular adenoma.

What is the most appropriate next step in management?

A. **Barium enema now**

B. **Colonoscopy in two years**

C. **Colonoscopy in five years**

D. **Colonoscopy now**

E. **CT scan of the abdomen and pelvis**

CASE 17

A 69-year-old man complains of fatigue, shortness of breath and weight loss. He is a heavy smoker. Examination demonstrates stony dullness and reduced air entry at the left thoracic base.

Blood results are as follows: Haemoglobin 10.1 g/dl, White cells 4.6×10^9/litre, Platelets 200×10^9/litre, Sodium 138 mmol/litre, Potassium 3.6 mmol/litre, Urea 4.6 mmol/litre, Creatinine 110 μmol/litre, Corrected calcium 3.3 mmol/litre.

A CT scan demonstrates a 3 cm mass in the left lung and a pleural effusion.

An isotope bone scan is normal.

Which of the following is the most likely diagnosis?

A. **Typical bronchial carcinoid tumour**

B. **Mesothelioma**

C. **Small cell lung cancer**

D. **Bronchial adenocarcinoma**

E. **Bronchial squamous cell carcinoma**

CASE 18

After presenting with hip pain, an 89-year-old woman from a care home has been diagnosed with metastatic pancreatic adenocarcinoma affecting her liver and bones. She is admitted to hospital but deteriorates significantly. She is drowsy and in pain. A chest X-ray demonstrates right basal consolidation and pneumonia is diagnosed. What is the most appropriate management plan?

A. **Transfer to high-dependency unit for intravenous antibiotics, non-invasive ventilation and hydration**

B. **Intravenous antibiotics and oral analgesia**

C. **Intravenous antibiotics and subcutaneous diamorphine as required**

D. **Palliative care referral and a continuous subcutaneous diarmorphine infusion, with documentation of a 'do not attempt resuscitation' (DNAR) order in her notes**

E. **Intravenous steroids and antibiotics, and salbutamol nebulisers**

CASE 19

A 67-year-old woman with metastatic breast cancer attends the emergency department complaining of malaise, nausea and constipation. On examination her chest is clear, jugular venous pressure is not raised, heart rate is 70 bpm and blood pressure is 120/80 mmHg. She has some generalised abdominal tenderness and bony tenderness of the spine.

Her blood results are: Sodium 137 mmol/litre, Potassium 5.2 mmol/litre, Creatinine 130 μmol/litre, Corrected calcium 3.7 mmol/litre.

You note a recent re-staging scan has demonstrated multiple bony metastases. What is the most appropriate first-line treatment?

A. **IV fluids and intravenous bisphosphonates**

B. **IV fluids and furosemide**

C. **Haemodialysis**

D. **IV fluids and hydrocortisone**

E. **Oral fluids and oral bisphosphonates**

CASE 20

A 56-year-old woman, who is receiving adjuvant chemotherapy after surgery to resect ovarian cancer, presents with a painful swelling of the left calf. Examination demonstrates no evidence of infection and Doppler ultrasound confirms deep venous thrombosis. She has never had any previous episodes of venous thrombo-embolism. She is ambulatory and has normal renal function. What is the most appropriate management of her thrombosis?

A. Subcutaneous low-molecular-weight heparin (LMWH) until completion of chemotherapy, then convert to warfarin (target INR 2–3), total duration of therapy six months

B. Thrombolysis and no further anticoagulant therapy

C. Warfarin with target INR 2–3, subcutaneous LMWH for five days or until target INR is achieved

D. Subcutaneous LMWH for six months

E. Subcutaneous LMWH until completion of chemotherapy, then convert to warfarin (target INR 3–4), total duration of therapy six months.

CASE 21

A 29-year-old asymptomatic woman undergoes routine cervical screening. Liquid-based cytology (LBC) demonstrates moderate dyskaryosis. She has been sexually active since the age of 21 with two different partners. She states that she uses barrier contraception. She does not smoke, and a pregnancy test is negative. What is the next appropriate step in her management?

A. Human papilloma virus screening and, if positive, repeat LBC in six months

B. Repeat LBC in six months

C. Colposcopy now

D. Repeat LBC now, and if remaining positive, refer for colposcopy

E. Human papilloma virus screening and, if negative, repeat LBC in three years

CASE 22

A 62-year-old man has been diagnosed with malignant mesothelioma. Which of the following is **least** useful as a prognostic marker?

A. Total white cells
B. Haemoglobin
C. Performance status
D. Smoking history
E. Gender

CASE 23

A 15-year-old girl presents with knee pain of three weeks' duration. She denies any history of trauma and the symptoms are not related to exercise. She has no other symptoms. On examination her height is 1.65 m, weight is 50 kg, and a hard swelling is palpable at the distal end of the femur. Examination is otherwise unremarkable. What is the most likely diagnosis?

A. Chordoma
B. Osteosarcoma
C. Metastatic melanoma
D. Osteomyelitis
E. Malignant schwannoma

CASE 24

A 39-year-old woman presents with an itchy enlarging mole on her calf (see Figure 10.5).

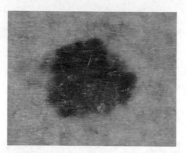

Figure 10.5

Which of the following would **not** be a poor prognostic marker in this case?

A. Diameter > 2 cm

B. Breslow thickness > 0.75 cm

C. Female gender

D. Amelanotic subtype

E. Ulceration

CASE 25

A male smoker presented with a cough of six weeks' duration. He was found to have a 2 cm lesion in his left lower lobe. Biopsy sampling confirmed a bronchial adenocarcinoma. Staging CT and PET scans demonstrated no evidence of disseminated disease. He is planned for curative surgical resection. Which of the following factors would be a contraindication to surgery in this case?

A. Age over 75 years

B. Myocardial infarction two months ago

C. $FEV_1 < 75\%$ of predicted

D. $FEV_1 < 50\%$ of predicted

E. Hypercalcaemia

CASE 26

A 15-year-old girl had been treated with 'mantle' field radiotherapy for Hodgkin's lymphoma in the 1980s. What long-term toxicity is she at greatest risk of developing now?

A. **Emphysema**
B. **Malignant melanoma**
C. **Left ventricular hypertrophy**
D. **Breast cancer**
E. **Hyperthyroidism**

CASE 27

A 63-year-old woman attends her GP complaining of a breast lump. He informs her that he will arrange for her to attend the rapid access breast clinic for 'triple assessment'. What would triple assessment involve for this patient?

A. **Mammography, breast MRI scanning, fine needle aspiration (FNA)/ biopsy**
B. **Mammography, breast ultrasound, FNA/biopsy**
C. **Clinical examination, breast ultrasound, FNA/biopsy**
D. **Clinical examination, breast ultrasound, mammography**
E. **Clinical examination, mammography, FNA/biopsy**

CASE 28

A 48-year-old woman attends her GP practice with multiple complaints: she feels tired all the time, and complains of low mood. She thinks that she is undergoing the menopause due to hot flushes. On systematic enquiry, she reports episodes of diarrhoea up to 4–5 times per day. She also has episodes of feeling 'tight chested'. She has lost almost 10 kg in recent months, which she says was intentional. Examination demonstrates mild bilateral wheeze and a mid-diastolic murmur. Abdominal examination is unremarkable. You note that she has had several attendances with similar symptoms over the last couple of years. Which investigation is most likely to establish the diagnosis?

A. Psychiatric evaluation
B. Flexible sigmoidoscopy
C. FDG PET scan
D. Measurement of carcinoembryonic antigen concentration
E. Measurement of urinary 5-hydroxyindoleacetic acid

CASE 29

A 45-year-old man is receiving adjuvant chemotherapy with 5-fluorouracil and oxaliplatin following resection of an early stage colon cancer. He attends the emergency department complaining of central crushing chest pain and shortness of breath. An ECG demonstrates widespread ST segment depression. You note he has a pump containing chemotherapy attached to an indwelling PICC line, which is approximately half-way through its dosage administration. In addition to standard measures for coronary ischaemia, what is the next step in his management?

A. Urgent Doppler ultrasound of his arm in case of line-associated DVT
B. Immediately remove the line in case of misplacement
C. Stop and disconnect the pump, aspirate the line
D. Rapidly administer the remaining chemotherapy in the pump before removing the line
E. Immediate thrombolysis

CASE 30

A 54-year-old man is brought into the emergency department by ambulance in status epilepticus. His seizures are controlled with a combination of benzodiazepines and phenytoin. His wife tells you that the patient has been complaining of headaches upon waking recently but otherwise seemed well. An urgent CT brain scan is performed and is shown in Figure 10.6. What is the next appropriate step in his management?

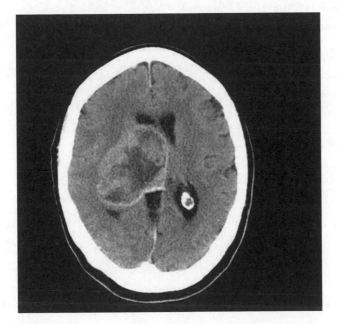

Figure 10.6

    A. Immediate intravenous broad spectrum antibiotics
    B. Immediate intravenous steroids
    C. Immediate palliative radiotherapy
    D. Immediate lumbar puncture
    E. Immediate CT chest/abdomen/pelvis

CASE 31

A 62-year-old man is diagnosed with oropharyngeal cancer. He is planned for radical resection and adjuvant radiotherapy. What is the most appropriate plan to manage his nutrition during this period?

    A. Total parenteral nutrition (TPN) until able to tolerate oral diet
    B. Soft diet and artificial saliva
    C. Percutaneous endoscopic gastrostomy tube feeding
    D. Nasogastric tube feeding
    E. Intravenous fluids for five days post-operatively then oral diet

CASE 1

C: Optimal cytoreductive surgery

This patient has ovarian cancer, the fourth commonest cancer in women. Epithelial ovarian cancer is the commonest subtype accounting for 70% of cases and median age at presentation is 55–59 years.

Characteristic features of ovarian malignancy on ultrasound are: multilocular cysts, solid areas, bilateral lesions, ascites and intra-abdominal metastases.

> ### Learning point
>
> For patients with ovarian masses, the relative malignancy index (RMI) is used to predict the chance of malignancy. This index consists of the product of the serum CA125, ultrasound score (no characteristic features = 0, one feature = 1, more than one feature = 4) and menopausal status (premenopausal – 1, postmenopausal = 4). An RMI of over 200 has a sensitivity of up to 80% and specificity of up to 90% for ovarian cancer.

Fine needle aspiration or biopsy of ovarian masses is not recommended due to risk of tumour seeding. Neoadjuvant therapy is rarely used in ovarian malignancy as initial surgical debulking has been shown to improve survival. Optimal cytoreduction is defined as leaving residual disease < 1 cm. If this target has not been achieved during initial surgery, interval cytoreduction may be performed after three or four cycles of chemotherapy. Local radiotherapy is not useful in this situation and delaying definitive treatment for six months would not be appropriate.

CASE 2

D: Vemurafenib

This patient has stage IV malignant melanoma, a poor prognosis disease with a median survival time of seven months. However, two novel agents recently introduced have improved the prognosis of patients somewhat, as described below.

Vemurafenib is an orally available *BRAF* inhibitor suitable for patients with proven *BRAF* mutations (approximately 30% of cases). It acts to downregulate the mitogen activated protein kinase (MAPK) pathway. Disease progression may be associated with reactivation of the MAPK pathway and combination treatment with MEK inhibitors is under investigation as a second-line or combinatorial agent.

Ipilimumab is a human monoclonal antibody that blocks the action of CTLA4 and is suitable for patients who do not have a *BRAF* mutation.

Interferon and interleukin are traditional immunotherapy agents and have shown response rates of 15–20% in advanced melanoma. Dacarbazine chemotherapy is associated with response rates of up to 20%, but a proven benefit on overall survival has not been demonstrated.

CASE 3

B: 60 mg diamorphine s/c over 24 hours

Learning point

To convert oral morphine to subcutaneous diamorphine, the total dose over 24 hours should be divided by three (since subcutaneous diamorphine is three times as potent as oral morphine). This patient is receiving 120 mg (60 mg morphine sulfate BD) + 60 mg (20 mg oramorph TDS) = 180 mg. 180/3 = 60 mg diamorphine s/c over 24 hours. Oxycodone is twice as potent as oral morphine (ie 5 mg oxynorm = 10 mg oromorph).

Other commonly used agents in syringe drivers are midazolam (for agitation), hyoscine (for secretions) and cyclizine or haloperidol (for nausea).

CASE 4

E

Learning point

The blood tests show the classical metabolic disturbances of tumour lysis syndrome (TLS): hyperkalaemia, hyperphosphataemia, hyperuricaemia and hypocalcaemia. The clinical diagnosis of TLS involves finding laboratory evidence plus one or more of: creatinine greater than 1.5× the upper limit of normal, cardiac arrhythmia/sudden death, or a seizure.

Although the patients at highest risk of developing TLS are those with haematological malignancies including acute leukaemias, and high-grade non-Hodgkin's lymphomas, those with solid tumours sensitive to cytotoxic therapy including germ cell tumours and small cell lung cancer may also develop the syndrome.

Management of TLS which has developed despite allopurinol prophylaxis will follow local guidelines but typically involves aggressive intravenous hydration with close fluid balance monitoring, intravenous rasburicase and supportive measures to correct electrolytes such as insulin/dextrose pumps, calcium gluconate infusions and cardiac monitoring as necessary to treat hyperkalaemia. Occasionally haemodialysis may be required.

**CHAPTER 10
ANSWERS**

CASE 5

E: Antimetabolite; alkylating agent; anthracycline

Since it was first synthesised in 1956, fluorouracil (FU) has become one of the most important chemotherapeutic agents and is utilised in the treatment of many cancers including breast and colorectal cancer. It is synergistic with other agents such as platinum drugs, and is a radiosensitising agent. 5-FU forms a complex with the thymidylate synthase enzyme and therefore blocks DNA synthesis. Toxicities include diarrhoea and nausea.

Cyclophosphamide is an alkylating agent of the chloroethyl nitrogen mustard subgroup. These agents transfer ethyl groups onto DNA and cause cross linking and cell cycle arrest during G1-S transition. Cyclophosphamide is used in many high-dose chemotherapy regimens.

Doxorubicin is an anthracycline, a class of drugs which is derived from the fungal culture broth of *Streptomyces peucetius*. They may also be described as anti-tumour antibiotics, or topoisomerase II inhibitors (since this is their major cellular mechanism of action). Doxorubicin is widely used for lymphomas and breast cancer. An important side effect is cardiotoxicity related to cumulative dose.

Other classes listed have the following agents as members:

✦ Camptothecin: irinotecan, topotecan
✦ Taxanes: docetaxel, paclitaxel

CASE 6

A: Typical bronchial carcinoid tumour

Bronchial carcinoid tumours are a rare (2–3%) but important subtype of lung cancer. The prognosis and management are very different from that of bronchial adenocarcinoma or squamous cell tumours. The 5-year survival of typical bronchial carcinoid tumours is approximately 90%, compared to less than 10% for other non-small cell lung cancers. Atypical carcinoids are characterised by 2–10 mitoses/10 high-power fields, or the presence of necrosis. Large cell neuroendocrine carcinomas and small cell lung cancers have a mitotic index of greater than 10/10 high-power fields and may be poorly differentiated with significant necrosis.

The management of typical carcinoid tumours involves surgical resection where feasible. In advanced disease, somatostatin analogues and streptozocin-based chemotherapy are options.

CASE 7

B: Resting in a bed or chair more than 50% of the time

Performance status grading is a quick and straightforward way of communicating a patient's general functional ability. Traditionally, to treat a patient with palliative chemotherapy, a performance status of 2 or less was required in order that the benefits of treatment outweigh the risks of reduced quality of life or death. However, where symptoms are secondary to the malignancy itself, and it is considered likely to be a chemo-sensitive tumour, it may be appropriate to treat patients who have a performance status of up to 4 (for example in some haematological malignancies, testicular cancers etc). An alternative grading system is the Karnofsky performance score. The two systems are outlined in Tables 10.3 and 10.4.

Performance status
0 – You are fully active and more or less as you were before your illness
1 – You cannot carry out heavy physical work, but can do anything else
2 – You are up and about more than half the day and can look after yourself, but are not well enough to work
3 – You are in bed or sitting in a chair for more than half the day and you need some help in looking after yourself
4 – You are in bed or a chair all the time and need a lot of looking after

Table 10.3: Traditional performance status grading

Karnofsky performance status
100 – You do not have any evidence of disease and feel well
90 – You only have minor signs or symptoms but are able to carry on as normal
80 – You have some signs or symptoms and it takes a bit of effort to carry on as normal
70 – You are able to care for yourself but not able to carry on with all your normal activities or do active work
60 – You need help from time to time but can mostly care for yourself
50 – You need quite a lot of help to care for yourself
40 – You always need help to care for yourself
30 – You are disabled and may need to stay in hospital
20 – You are ill, in hospital and need a lot of treatment
10 – You are very ill and unlikely to recover

Table 10.4: Karnofsky performance status grading

CASE 8

C: Metastatic breast cancer: two years; stage 1 seminoma: no impact on survival; extensive stage small cell lung cancer: 6–12 months; metastatic small intestinal neuroendocrine tumour: ten years; metastatic prostate cancer: five years

Median survival times continuously improve with novel therapeutic strategies and optimal supportive care, but these figures give an approximate value at the time of writing.

Good prognostic factors in metastatic breast cancer include hormone receptor positivity, HER2 receptor negativity and metastases limited to bone. In stage 1 seminoma, the expected cure rate is over 95%, therefore no impact is made on median overall survival. For this reason, the long-term toxicities of any therapies planned (eg radiotherapy predisposing to secondary malignancy) are carefully considered. Extensive stage small cell lung cancer carries a particularly poor prognosis due to its high-grade, poorly differentiated nature. Initially responsive to chemotherapy, relapses are usually rapid and aggressive. Metastatic neuroendocrine tumours of the small intestine by contrast are most commonly well-differentiated, low-grade tumours and a median survival time of ten years may be expected with currently available treatment. Metastatic prostate cancer is common in men of increasing age and, although prognosis is affected by castration resistance status, overall a survival of approximately five years may be expected.

CASE 9

D: von Hippel–Lindau syndrome

Von Hippel–Lindau syndrome (vHL) is a rare autosomal dominant condition resulting from a mutation in the *VHL* tumour suppressor gene on chromosome 3. The syndrome predisposes to tumours including renal cell carcinomas, pancreatic neuroendocrine tumours and phaeochromocytomas, as well as central nervous system and retinal haemangioblastomas. In individuals found to have the vHL mutation, annual screening including abdominal ultrasound, urinalysis to detect haematuria, urinary cytology and urinary catecholamine measurement are used to detect malignancy early. Brain and spinal cord imaging are not routinely performed if there are no neurological symptoms.

Learning point

The other listed syndromes may be expected to present with the following disorders:

✦ MEN 1: pancreatic neuroendocrine tumours, hyperparathyroidism, pituitary tumours

✦ MEN 2: phaeochromocytomas, medullary thyroid cancers, hyperparathyroidism

✦ *BRCA2* mutation: breast cancer, ovarian cancer, prostate cancer, pancreatic cancer

✦ Neurofibromatosis: neurofibromas, schwannomas (including acoustic neuromas), café-au-lait spots

CASE 10

B: Nurse sitting up, oxygen, steroids (dexamethasone 16 mg per day with proton pump inhibitor), discuss with an oncologist

This patient has superior vena cava obstruction (SVCO) secondary to a presumed new diagnosis of lung cancer, and must be discussed with the oncology team. Initial management involves sitting the patient upright and providing supplementary oxygen aiming for saturations greater than 92%. Steroids should be administered at a dose of dexamatasone16 mg/day (oral or IV). If there is a high clinical suspicion of a new diagnosis of lymphoma, steroids may be witheld until a tissue diagnosis can be gained. This patient does not yet require intubation, and referral for bronchoscopy may be appropriate but not in the acute setting. Furosemide and bisoprolol have no role in the management of SVCO. This patient is likely to require the insertion of a SVC stent to relieve the symptoms of SVCO before starting palliative therapy for his malignancy.

CASE 11

C: Lung cancer

Lung cancer is the commonest cause of cancer-related mortality in the UK, accounting for 22% of cancer deaths.[1] The next commonest causes of cancer death are colorectal (10%), breast (7%) and prostate (7%) cancers. The incidence of lung cancer is decreasing (11% change 2000–2002 to 2009–2011); however, the lifetime risk is still high (1 in 14 for men, 1 in 18 for women).[2] Smoking causes 86% of lung cancer and is the most significant preventable cause of cancer in the world.

CASE 12

C: Active surveillance

This gentleman has low-risk prostate cancer (see Table 10.5).

Risk	PSA (ng/ml)		Gleason score		Clinical stage
Low	< 10	And	< 6	And	TI–TIIa
Intermediate	10–20	Or	7	Or	TIIb
High	> 20	Or	8–10	Or	> TIIc

Table 10.5: Assessment of risk in prostate cancer

Active surveillance is an option for patients with low-risk, early stage prostate cancer with operable disease who are unlikely to die from their tumour. Low-risk, early stage prostate cancer has a predicted 10-year survival of at least 90%.

Learning point

Surveillance involves monitoring prostatic-specific antigen (PSA) kinetics with tests every three to four months initially, regular digital rectal examination (every 6–12 months) and at 12 months a prostate re-biopsy. Alternative management would be radical prostatectomy (which is not routinely followed by adjuvant treatment), or radical radiotherapy (which is routinely followed by adjuvant hormonal therapy). Cytotoxic chemotherapy is only appropriate in the metastatic setting, and hormonal therapy is only used adjuvantly or in the metastatic setting.

CASE 13

A: Ultrasound guided liver biopsy

In this case, confirming the diagnosis suggested by the raised CA19-9 concentration (ie pancreatic cancer) will be most useful, and this would be best achieved by taking a biopsy of one of the large liver metastases. Endoscopy of the upper and lower gastrointestinal tract may be useful if the histology gained from biopsy is suggestive of an alternative malignancy. MRI scanning of the liver and PET scanning are not warranted in the first-line investigation of suspected metastatic pancreatic adenocarcinoma.

CASE 14

C: Give immediate intravenous broad spectrum antibiotics, rehydrate and monitor fluid balance

This patient has neutropaenic sepsis until proven otherwise.

Learning point

Intravenous broad spectrum antibiotics should be administered within 30 minutes in any case of suspected neutropaenic sepsis and blood results should not be awaited. This patient may well have a urinary tract infection, but intravenous broad spectrum antibiotics are required if the patient is at risk of neutropaenia. Antibiotic therapy should not be delayed to perform lumbar puncture (LP) if the patient is at risk of neutropaenia, even if clinically suspected. Furthermore LP may be relatively contraindicated as bone marrow suppression can be associated with a depressed platelet count and increased risk of haemorrhage.

Granulocyte colony-stimulating factor (GCSF) may be used in cases of high-risk neutropaenic sepsis but is not required routinely and does not replace the need for antibiotic therapy.

CASE 15

C: Discuss with oncology and neurosurgery teams, admit the patient, give analgesia, high-dose steroids and follow any further guidance from specialist teams

> ### Learning point
>
> Malignant spinal cord compression (MSCC) is a common complication of metastatic prostate cancer and a high index of suspicion is required when patients complain of back pain or any neurological symptoms (including weakness, sensory disturbance or bladder/bowel disturbance). The appropriate management includes hospital admission, analgesia, high-dose steroids (local protocols may vary but typically dexamethasone 16 mg daily with a proton pump inhibitor for gastro-protection), bed rest, bladder and bowel management, and thromboprophylaxis.

Patients with MSCC should not be discharged home, and chemotherapy or radiotherapy, although they may be appropriate, would not be the initial course of management. Palliative care referral is often appropriate in conjunction with planning more definitive management.

The technical feasibility of surgical management is to be considered in conjunction with consideration of the patient's quality of life and prognosis. If surgery is inappropriate, palliative radiotherapy to the area may induce tumour shrinkage and relieve pressure on the spinal cord. Steroids are used to reduce peri-tumoral oedema and may be weaned once definitive treatment is implemented.

CASE 16

D: Colonoscopy now

Learning point

The entire colon must be visualised since approximately 50% of patients will have a second adenomatous polyp at the time of initial diagnosis.

If colonoscopy confirms that no further polyps are present, surveillance colonoscopy should be repeated in five years; if three or more polyps are present at initial diagnosis, or if any polyp is 1 cm or greater in size, colonoscopy should be repeated in three years. Barium enema and CT scanning are not routinely used in the investigation of adenomatous colorectal polyps.

CASE 17

E: Bronchial squamous cell carcinoma

This man has hypercalcaemia in the absence of bony metastases. This is secondary to release of parathyroid hormone-related protein (PTHRP) which occurs in approximately 15% of cases of squamous cell lung cancer. Small cell lung cancer is associated with the syndrome of inappropriate antidiuretic hormone secretion (causing hyponatraemia) and Cushing syndrome, whereas bronchial carcinoid tumours can be associated with flushing and diarrhoea due to release of serotonin (in approximately 10% of cases). Mesothelioma and bronchial adenocarcinoma are not commonly associated with paraneoplastic syndromes.

CASE 18

D: Palliative care referral and a continuous subcutaneous diamorphine infusion, with documentation of a DNAR order in her notes

This elderly patient has advanced pancreatic cancer with an extremely poor prognosis; she requires appropriate terminal care and symptom control. Continuous subcutaneous infusions of analgesics reduce the need for multiple injections and are the more appropriate choice in this case. In addition to analgesics she may benefit from anticholinergic medication to reduce secretions, and if she becomes agitated, a neuroleptic or benzodiazepine. Communication with the next-of-kin is essential during terminal care, and the patient should be nursed in a side room if possible to allow privacy.

CASE 19

A: IV fluids and intravenous bisphosphonates

Hypercalcaemia is a common feature of metastatic malignancy affecting the bones. Its management depends on severity:

> **Learning point**
>
> ✦ Mild (asymptomatic, calcium < 3 mmol/litre): adequate oral hydration and stop any aggravating factors such as thiazide diuretics or calcium supplements.
>
> ✦ Moderate (asymptomatic or mildly symptomatic, calcium 3–3.5 mmol/litre): as for mild hypercalcaemia. If chronic, may not require immediate therapy, but if acute, treat as for severe hypercalcaemia.
>
> ✦ Severe (calcium > 3.5 mmol/litre): intravenous saline hydration to maintain urine output of 100–150 ml/hour and intravenous bisphosphonate (eg pamidronate 60–90 mg over two hours) to achieve prolonged control (onset of effect 2–4 days). Consider calcitonin 4 units/kg to achieve an acute reduction in calcium (12–48 hours). In extremely severe cases (Ca 4.5–5 mmol/litre or in patients with neurological symptoms), haemodialysis should be implemented.

Furosemide is not routinely administered in the absence of heart failure; however, it may be required to avoid fluid overload during hydration. Hydrocortisone is not utilised in hypercalcaemia related to solid malignancy but may be used when secondary to lymphomas or granulomatous disease. Oral bisphosphonates are not used in the management of acute malignant hypercalcaemia.

CASE 20

D: Subcutaneous LMWH for six months

Venous thromboembolism (VTE) is a common complication of malignancy and is associated with increased mortality. VTE is particularly common in certain solid tumours (eg tumours of the pancreas, kidneys and ovaries) and haematological malignancies (eg myeloma and lymphoma). Primary prophylaxis is not currently recommended for ambulatory patients.

Learning point

The European Society of Medical Oncology guidelines recommend the use of low-molecular-weight heparin (LMWH) for a total of six months.[3] For patients with ongoing active cancer (for example those receiving palliative chemotherapy), indefinite treatment should be considered due to the high risk of recurrence. A large clinical trial demonstrated that LMWH is more effective for reducing the risk of recurrent VTE in cancer patients than are coumarin derivatives (eg warfarin).[4] If anticoagulation is contraindicated (eg active bleeding, platelet count $< 50 \times 10^9$/litre) then a vena cava filter may be considered.

CASE 21

C: Colposcopy now

In the UK, cervical cancer screening is performed every three years between the ages of 25 and 49 and every five years from 50 to 64. Cervical dyskaryosis and cervical intra-epithelial neoplasia (CIN) are premalignant conditions. Mild dyskaryosis is detected in 5% of screening tests, moderate dyskaryosis in 1% and severe in 0.5%. Recent improvements in our understanding of human papilloma virus (HPV) have changed the recommendations for mild dyskaryosis, but for moderate–severe abnormalities, a direct referral for colposcopy is required.

Learning point

+ Borderline or mild dyskaryosis: if HPV negative, return to routine recall (LBC in three years), if HPV positive, refer for colposcopy.

+ Moderate dyskaryosis: refer for colposcopy.

+ Severe dyskaryosis: refer for colposcopy.

+ Inadequate sample: if persistent (three samples), refer for colposcopy.

+ Repeated abnormalities: if any abnormalities or inadequate results re-occur three times within a 10-year period, colposcopy should also be performed.

CASE 22

D: Smoking history

Mesothelioma is a malignancy of the pleura associated with asbestos exposure. The most important adverse prognostic factors are: poor performance status, non-epithelioid histology, male gender, low haemoglobin, high platelet count, high white cells, and high LDH. A history of smoking history does not carry any prognostic weighting in mesothelioma.

CASE 23

B: Osteosarcoma

High-grade osteosarcomas are most commonly diagnosed in teenagers and young adults (with a second peak in incidence over the age of 75 years). The commonest cancers in this age group are lymphomas, carcinomas (eg of thyroid, cervical or ovarian origin), and germ cell tumours. Chordomas are rare tumours which arise from the cellular remnants of the embryonic notochord and are found along the skull base and spinal cord. Malignant schwannoma (a malignant tumour of the peripheral nerve sheath) is a rare cancer that is frequently associated with neurofibromatosis. As a soft tissue tumour, it would not be expected to form a hard swelling like that of a bone tumour. Metastatic melanoma is rarer in this age group, and there is no history suggestive of osteomyelitis.

CASE 24

C: Female gender

Malignant melanoma is a skin cancer associated with exposure to ultraviolet light. An adverse prognosis is associated with a larger size and greater depth of invasion. Amelanocytic melanoma accounts for less than 5% of incidence and due to the lack of pigmentation, diagnosis is often delayed. Melanomas affecting mucosae (eg vulval, anal and oral) are also associated with a poor prognosis. The presence of ulceration is included in the TNM staging of melanoma and implies a minimum stage of IB.

CASE 25

D: $FEV_1 <$ 50% of predicted

Other contraindications include myocardial infarction within the last 30 days, recurrent laryngeal nerve involvement, a malignant pleural effusion, advanced mediastinal nodal disease or TNM stage > IIIB, the presence of distant metastatic disease. Overall, only approximately 10–20% of lung cancer patients are suitable for resection at the time of diagnosis. Age in itself should not be a contraindication. Hypercalcaemia may be due to a paraneoplastic syndrome and is not always indicative of metastatic disease.

CASE 26

D: Breast cancer

Radiotherapy has progressed significantly in recent years and 'mantle' radiotherapy (in which the cervical, thoracic and axillary lymph nodes were all irradiated in an extended field manner) is now rarely used.

Learning point

The long-term side effects of radiotherapy include secondary malignancies, in particular of the breast. For this reason, annual breast screening is recommended from eight years after treatment or the age of 25, which ever is later. There are also smaller risks of lung cancer, oesophageal cancer, thyroid cancer and melanoma. Cardiovascular disease is associated with previous radiotherapy, but not left ventricular hypertrophy in particular. Hypothyroidism and pneumonitis are also recognised long-term toxicities.

CASE 27

E: Clinical examination, mammography, FNA/biopsy

Triple assessment involves clinical examination, radiological assessment and pathological assessment. In postmenopausal women, mammography is the first-line radiological assessment of choice. In premenopausal women, because of a greater density of glandular tissue, the sensitivity of mammography is reduced and ultrasound is preferred. In practice, postmenopausal patients also undergo ultrasound to guide needle biopsy. Owing to its greater sensitivity and specificity, core biopsy is preferable to fine needle aspiration cytology.

CASE 28

E: Measurement of urinary 5-hydroxyindoleacetic acid

This patient has a small intestinal neuroendocrine tumour (NET) (carcinoid tumour). Diagnosis of this type of cancer is typically delayed (5–7 years on average) due to non-specific presenting symptoms. Symptoms of carcinoid syndrome include diarrhoea, wheezing, flushing and weight loss. Sigmoidoscopy and carcinoembryonic antigen (CEA) are useful in the investigation of suspected colorectal cancer, and although FDG PET scanning may be used in the staging of malignancy, it is rarely utilised for diagnosis. Furthermore, small intestinal NETs are frequently low-grade tumours with a low proliferative index, and do not demonstrate high uptake on FDG PET. Psychiatric evaluation is inappropriate at present; however, management of her low mood should not be ignored, particularly in the context of a new cancer diagnosis. Supportive counselling or therapy should be offered.

CHAPTER 10
ANSWERS

CASE 29

C: Stop and disconnect the pump, aspirate the line

The cytotoxic antimetabolite 5-fluorouracil (5-FU) and its orally bioavailable equivalent capecitabine cause coronary vasospasm in up 10% of patients, although life-threatening cardiotoxicity is seen in less than 1% of cases. 5-FU has a half-life of approximately ten minutes, and stopping the infusion is essential in a case such as this.

CASE 30

B: Immediate intravenous steroids

This patient has an intracranial malignancy causing raised intracranial pressure. It is likely this is a primary central nervous system malignancy such as glioblastoma multiforme, although further investigation to rule out a metastatic deposit would be required (once the patient's condition is more stable). The priority in managing this patient is to start high-dose steroids (eg dexamethasone 16 mg per day with a proton pump inhibitor for gastro-protection) to reduce peri-tumoral oedema and intracranial pressure. He does not require antibiotics unless there are features suggestive of infection, and lumbar puncture would be contraindicated due to the risk of coning. Palliative radiotherapy is likely to be required if surgery is not feasible.

CASE 31

C: Percutaneous endoscopic gastrostomy feeding

The management of head and neck cancers is complex and must be considered in a multidisciplinary setting. Dietician support is invaluable around the time of surgery or radiotherapy as maintaining adequate oral intake is impossible. Radiotherapy is associated with xerostomia, which may last several months or be permanent. The most appropriate choice for long-term nutritional support is a percutaneous endoscopic gastrostomy (PEG) tube. TPN is not recommended due to risks of infection and difficulty maintaining continuity in the community. Nasogastric tubes are prone to being dislocated and would be uncomfortable in this context. The use of a soft diet and artificial saliva would be appropriate after the patient has made some recovery from his treatment. Starving the patient for five days is not recommended.

References

1. Cancer Research UK. 2015. Lung cancer statistics. www.cancerresearchuk.org/cancer-info/cancerstats/types/lung

2. Cancer Research UK Statistical Information Team. Statistics on the risk of developing cancer, by cancer type and age. Calculated using 2008 data for the UK using the 'Adjusted for Multiple Primaries (AMP)' method (Sasieni P D, Shelton J, Ormiston-Smith N, et al. 2011. What is the lifetime risk of developing cancer?: The effect of adjusting for multiple primaries. Br J Cancer, 105:3, 460–465). www.cancerresearchuk.org/cancer-info/cancerstats/incidence/risk

3. Mandalà et al. 2011. Management of venous thromboembolism (VTE) in cancer patients: ESMO Clinical Practice Guidelines. Annals of Oncology, 22, Supplement 6, vi85–vi92

4. Lee A et al. 2003. Low-molecular-weight heparin versus a coumarin for the prevention of recurrent venous thromboembolism in patients with cancer. New England Journal of Medicine, 349, 146–153

CHAPTER 11

Ophthalmology

Katherine McVeigh and Tomas Burke

CASE 1

A 55-year-old man with a past medical history of rheumatoid arthritis, hypercholesterolaemia, hypertension and type 2 diabetes attends the diabetic retinopathy screening programme on an annual basis for monitoring of his background diabetic retinopathy. He was last seen there four months ago. He also attends the ophthalmology outpatient department for primary open angle glaucoma. He presents to the emergency clinic with a sudden painless reduction of vision in his right eye. Visual field testing of the right eye shows a new quadrantic defect in the infero-nasal visual field. What is the most likely diagnosis?

A. **Glaucoma progression**
B. **Diabetic papillitis**
C. **Retinal venous occlusion**
D. **Vitreous haemorrhage**
E. **Retinal detachment**

CASE 2

A 59-year-old man with no past medical history attends the emergency department with a sudden painless reduction of vision in his right eye. Clinical examination reveals visual acuity of 6/36. He has a subtle right relative afferent pupillary defect. Dilated fundoscopy reveals the appearance shown in Figure 11.1.

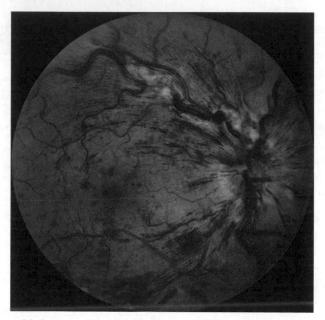

Figure 11.1

The left eye is normal. Of the following investigations, which is most likely to be abnormal in association with the ophthalmic condition that is present in this patient?

- A. **Blood pressure**
- B. **Lipid profile**
- C. **Blood glucose**
- D. **Protein C**
- E. **Factor V Leiden**

CASE 3

A 67-year-old lady of Philippino origin last saw her optician one year ago. She was noted to have moderate nuclear sclerotic cataracts bilaterally but was not keen to proceed with any surgical intervention at her review. She presents to the ophthalmology outpatient department with a 2-day history of a painful red right eye. Further questioning reveals that she has also been suffering with headaches, nausea and photophobia. She denies a history of vomiting and neck stiffness, although for the preceding two weeks she has noted intermittent painless haloes around lights in the evenings. Her medical systems review was non-contributory. On examination, her right pupil was noted to be greater in size than the left and was non-reactive to light or accommodation. The iris details were not clearly visible. Which of the following is most likely to lead to the correct the diagnosis?

A. **Gonioscopy of the anterior chamber angle**
B. **Temporal artery biopsy**
C. **Ultrasound B-scan**
D. **Applanation tonometry**
E. **Fluorescein angiography**

CASE 4

A 56-year-old male smoker, with a past medical history of inflammatory bowel disease, hypertension and hypercholesterolaemia, presents with a sudden painless loss of vision in the right eye for four hours. Examination reveals a visual acuity of hand movements in the right eye and 6/6 vision in the left eye. He had a right dense, relative afferent pupillary defect, and the appearance shown in Figure 11.2 was noted on fundoscopy.

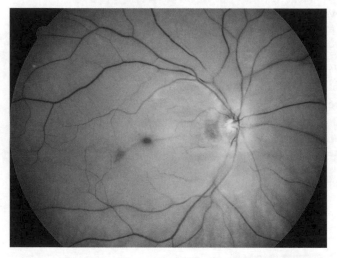

Figure 11.2

What is the most likely diagnosis?

    A. **Central retinal vein occlusion**
    B. **Cilio-retinal artery occlusion**
    C. **Central retinal artery occlusion**
    D. **Ocular ischaemic syndrome**
    E. **Ophthalmic artery occlusion**

CASE 5

A 58-year-old gentleman with an 8-year history of type 2 diabetes was referred to the ophthalmology outpatient department from the diabetic retinopathy screening service. Clinical examination with dilated fundoscopy revealed that he had background diabetic retinopathy in the left eye and proliferative diabetic retinopathy in the right, with evidence of gross optic disc and peripheral neovascularisation. He is awaiting panretinal photocoagulation laser to his left peripheral retina. What is the most appropriate investigation relevant to the immediate management of this patient?

- A. **Glycosylated haemoglobin concentration**
- B. **Fluorescein angiogram**
- C. **Full blood count**
- D. **Carotid Doppler ultrasound**
- E. **Optical coherence tomography**

CASE 6

A 32-year-old myopic lady, who wears monthly disposable contact lenses, presents to the emergency department. She has a red painful left eye with epiphora for the past 48 hours. There has been a moderate reduction in vision in her left eye, while the right eye is asymptomatic. Examination reveals a whitish opacity less than 1 mm in diameter in the stroma of the central cornea. There is some fluorescein uptake in the centre of the lesion. This lady has had a corneal scrape performed with a specimen sent to the microbiology laboratory for microscopy, culture and sensitivity. Conjunctival swabs have also been sent.

What is the next step in appropriately managing this patient?

- A. **Topical fuscidic acid**
- B. **Topical ofloxacin 0.3%**
- C. **Topical maxitrol (dexamethasone 0.1%, neomycin sulfate, polymyxin B sulfate)**
- D. **Topical chloramphenicol 0.5%**
- E. **Topical cefuroxime 5%**

CASE 7

A 55-year-old woman is referred to the glaucoma clinic due to raised intraocular pressures of 34 mmHg bilaterally. She has an extensive past medical history including type 2 diabetes, a recent myocardial infarction, chronic obstructive airways disease and renal stones. She also has depression for which she takes a monoamine oxidase inhibitor as previous selective serotonin reuptake inhibitors and tricyclic antidepressants were not proving effective. Past ocular history includes recurrent uveitis, which is currently under investigation. She reports a sensitivity to sulfonamides. What would be the most appropriate choice of topical agent to lower her intraocular pressure?

    A. **Prostaglandin analogue**
    B. **Beta blocker**
    C. **Alpha-2 agonist**
    D. **Carbonic anhydrase inhibitor**
    E. **Cholinergic agent**

CASE 8

You are reviewing a 35-year-old lady with type 1 diabetes in an outpatient clinic. She was originally referred by her GP with poorly controlled blood sugars and an HbA1c of 97 mmol/mol. She tells you that she is not on any other medications and that her general health is good. In passing, her husband mentions that she has had a few fainting episodes recently. She is sure that these are not due to hypoglycaemia because, in the past, when she has had hypoglycaemia she would experience a tremor and sweating before becoming faint. Her GP has referred her to a neurologist for investigation of these episodes. As she is leaving, you notice that her eyes are red and she tells you that this is because of some new eye drops she is taking from the eye clinic but she is unsure for what condition she is being treated.

For which of the following ophthalmic conditions is she currently receiving treatment?

    A. **Open angle glaucoma**
    B. **Acute anterior uveitis**
    C. **Infective keratitis**
    D. **Proliferative diabetic retinopathy**
    E. **Dry eye**

CASE 9

A 48-year-old lady with asthma is being routinely reviewed at the psychiatry clinic. She is in very good general health and only takes oral medication for depression and inhaled β-2 receptor agonists for her asthma. She suffers with periocular and facial eczema for which she uses a steroid ointment. She attends the ophthalmology clinic for management of primary open angle glaucoma, which had been well controlled and stable for ten years with latanoprost eye drops once daily to both eyes. She tells you that she has been at the ophthalmology clinic twice over the past four months and that there has been concern that the intraocular pressure (IOP) has been raised bilaterally and associated with progressive visual field loss. Reviewing the letters from the clinic you see that she is now taking three different eye drops to control her IOP (a prostaglandin F2 α-analogue, a carbonic anhydrase inhibitor and an α2-agonist). You note that she may require surgical intervention to control the IOP. She is very anxious about the thought of this.

Side effects of which of the following are likely responsible for progression of her glaucoma?

A. **Hydrocortisone 1% ointment**
B. **Topiramate**
C. **Paroxetine**
D. **Beta-2 receptor agonists**
E. **Amitriptyline**

CASE 10

In which of the following patients would driving be considered appropriate?

A. A 59-year-old heavy goods vehicle (HGV) driver with a Snellen visual acuity of 6/9 in his right eye and 6/18 in the left eye. No field defect was evident on his Esterman visual field.

B. A 47-year-old HGV driver with a Snellen visual acuity of 6/6 bilaterally and an Esterman visual field spanning 120 degrees on the horizontal field, 30 degrees above and below the horizontal meridian without any central defect of note.

C. An 82-year-old car driver with a past medical history of hypertension, hypercholesterolaemia and myocardial infarction, who suffered a microvascular sixth cranial nerve palsy four months ago that has now resolved. His Snellen acuity was 6/9 bilaterally.

D. A 74-year-old car driver who suffered with a homonymous quadrantanopia following a stroke 18 months ago which has remained relatively unchanged. He feels he has fully adapted to his field loss and his acuities were recorded as 6/9 bilaterally.

E. A 56-year-old car driver who suffers with proliferative diabetic retinopathy for which he has undergone extensive peripheral retinal photocoagulation laser treatment bilaterally. Snellen visual acuities were 6/6 bilaterally. Visual fields measured 100 degrees on the horizontal and 30 degrees above and below fixation.

CASE 11

A 49-year-old lady presents to the emergency department with vertical diplopia for two months. She feels that it is slowly getting worse. She is a smoker and reports that her eyes are quite gritty, especially in the morning when she wakes. She denies weight loss or gain, has a good appetite and has no other medical problems except for type 1 diabetes that she has had for 20 years. Clinical examination reveals limitation of upgaze on the left side. There is no proptosis. There is mild retraction of the upper and lower lids on the left side. Her visual acuities are 6/6 and she has normal optic nerve function bilaterally. She has mild conjunctival injection of the left eye and chemosis.

Which of the following is most likely to lead to the correct diagnosis?

A. Thyroid-stimulating hormone
B. Anti-acetylcholine receptor antibody
C. Antithyroid-stimulating hormone receptor antibody
D. A CT scan of brain
E. Electromyography

CASE 12

A 68-year-old lady has been treated for the past seven years with hydroxychloroquine for the management of systemic lupus erythematosus. She has a history of essential hypertension, but she is otherwise well and is asymptomatic. She takes 400 mg of hydroxychloroquine daily. Which of the following is most important to minimise the risk of ophthalmic side effects while taking the drug?

A. Monitoring of urea and electrolytes profile
B. Dark sun glasses with UV filters
C. High-dose macular pigments
D. Monitoring of full blood count
E. Monitoring of the blood glucose

CASE 13

A 58-year-old lady presents to the emergency department with a 2-week history of an increasingly painful, red right eye, worsening to a pain score severity of 9/10 over the past 48 hours. She tells you that her eye is extremely tender to touch and that her symptoms are exacerbated when she looks at bright lights or with ocular movement. She is not taking any regular medications and denies a history of trauma. She tells you that she has had on-going problems with sinusitis for the past number of months and an associated dry cough. Her GP has recently referred her to the otolaryngology service as she has associated reduced hearing on her right side. Urine microscopy is shown in Figure 11.3.

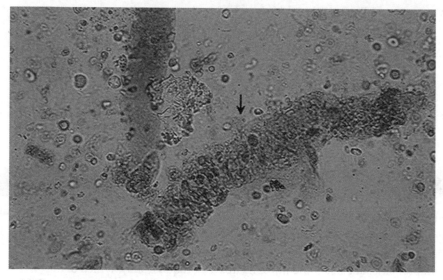

Figure 11.3

Which of the following is most likely to confirm the aetiology of her symptoms?

- A. **An MRI scan of orbits and sinuses**
- B. **Rheumatoid factor testing**
- C. **C-ANCA**
- D. **A chest X-ray**
- E. **Checking serum ACE level**

CASE 14

A 32-year-old asthmatic man presents to the emergency department complaining of reduced vision in his right eye over the past six months. He tells you that he was recently involved in a car accident. While driving he crashed into a car that he had not seen passing on his right side. He has a history of migraine headaches with visual symptoms, although he denies any attack in the past two months. Clinical examination reveals 6/6 vision bilaterally. Visual field tests reveal a right-sided superior quadrantanopia. An MRI of his brain and orbits showed established ischaemic changes in the parietal lobe on the left side.

Which of the following is the most appropriate next step in the management of this case?

A. **Ergotamine**
B. **Ibuprofen**
C. **Topiramate**
D. **Sumatriptan**
E. **Propranolol**

CASE 15

A 30-year-old man presents with intermittent diplopia over the past month. He has noted that his left upper eyelid droops in the evening. He denies headache and has no systemic symptoms. He has no significant medical history. Clinical examination reveals a 2 mm ptosis of the left upper eyelid. His pupils are equal and reactive. There is mild limitation of abduction in the left eye. Ocular movements in the right eye were normal. The ice-pack test was equivocal and a test for anti-acetylcholine receptor antibodies was negative. Which of the following is the most appropriate next investigation?

A. **MRI scan of brain and orbits**
B. **Tensilon® test**
C. **Anti-muscle-specific kinase antibody**
D. **Muscle biopsy**
E. **Single fibre-electromyogram**

CASE 16

An 85-year-old lady presented to the emergency department with intermittent episodes of reduced vision in her left eye and left-sided headache over the past week. The episodes of reduced vision lasted up to two minutes and happened once or twice per day over the preceding three days. The reduced vision had become permanent over the past 24 hours. She had experienced intermittent horizontal diplopia, worse on looking to the left, over the preceding two days also, but this has now resolved. Her standing erythrocyte sedimentation rate (ESR) was 92 mm/hour. Clinical examination revealed a visual acuity of 6/60 in the left eye (right eye 6/6). She has a left-sided relative afferent pupillary defect, but the pupils are of equal size. Her eye movements are normal bilaterally. The left optic nerve appears swollen and pale.

Which of the following clinical factors can most strongly predict the finding of an abnormal temporal artery biopsy?

A. **Jaw claudication**
B. **Diplopia**
C. **ESR 47 mm/1st hour**
D. **Temporal artery tenderness**
E. **Relative afferent pupillary defect**

CASE 17

A 43-year-old lady presents to the emergency department. She complains that in the last two days, her left eye has appeared smaller than her right eye. She denies any reduced vision, double vision or headache. She was involved in a minor road traffic accident three days ago but did not sustain any injuries. She has no past medical history. Clinical examination reveals a left-sided partial ptosis and anisocoria, with the left pupil 3 mm smaller than the right pupil in dark conditions and 2 mm smaller than the right pupil in light conditions. See Figure 11.4. Which of the following is most likely to confirm the diagnosis?

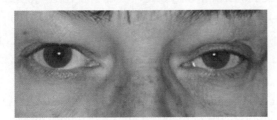

Figure 11.4

    A. Doppler ultrasound of the carotid arteries
    B. MRI scan of brain and orbits with gadolinium enhancement
    C. MR cerebral angiogram
    D. CT scan of thorax
    E. Apraclonidine 1% eye drops to both eyes

CASE 1

C: Retinal venous occlusion

Learning point

This patient has multiple risk factors for veno-occlusive disease including being over 50 years old, and having hypertension, diabetes and glaucoma. The most likely diagnosis is a branch retinal vein occlusion. These most commonly occur in the superotemporal quadrant of the ophthalmic vasculature, which is thought to be due to the increased number of venous arterial cross-overs in this quadrant. This is the explanation for the infero-nasal visual field defect.

It would be unusual for visual field changes in primary open angle glaucoma to progress suddenly. Usually, these patients are asymptomatic of their visual field loss until disease has become advanced. It is important to appreciate that the effects of the rheumatoid arthritis on a patient's hands may preclude them from instilling glaucoma drops appropriately. In the long term, this can lead to poor glaucoma control and subsequent visual field loss. Diabetic papillitis is a non-inflammatory optic neuropathy that can be uni- or bilateral. Ischaemia of the optic nerve is thought to play a role in its pathogenesis. Although it is more common in type 1 diabetes, it is known to be prevalent in older patients with type 2 diabetes. It is often asymptomatic, but can yield a progressive unilateral or bilateral loss of vision. Visual field testing reveals a central scotoma. Although vitreous haemorrhage and retinal detachment are recognised complications of diabetic retinopathy, and can cause visual symptoms, these are associated with proliferative changes, ie retinal neovascularisation. This gentleman was recorded as having background diabetic retinopathy at recent retinal screening which would make proliferative diabetic retinopathy unlikely, because such rapid deterioration is uncommon.

CASE 2

A: Blood pressure

This patient has suffered a central retinal vein occlusion (CRVO) in his right eye. Hypertension is the most likely associated systemic abnormality, followed by hyperlipidaemia and diabetes mellitus, respectively. Raised intraocular pressure and glaucoma are local risk factors. These conditions should be appropriately managed, with specialist input as required. According to the British Society of Haematology guidelines (2012), patients with RVO do not require investigation for hereditary thrombophilias.[1] On meta-analysis, only hyperhomocysteinaemia and anticardiolipin antibodies had significant associations with RVO. Therefore, testing for protein C deficiency or a factor V Leiden mutation is not advocated in this case.

CASE 3

D: Applanation tonometry

Learning point

This patient is experiencing an attack of acute primary angle closure glaucoma (APACG). Patients with smaller eyes, particularly those who are hypermetropes (long-sighted) and female, are more likely to have 'occludable angles' and be at risk of APACG. There is a further predisposition among Eskimos and people of south-east Asian descent. This patient's cataracts will result in a further narrowing of the anterior chamber drainage angles as the crystalline lens continues to enlarge in an antero-posterior direction throughout life as lens fibres are continually produced. For this reason, a patient who is pseudophakic (ie has had cataract surgery with insertion of a prosthetic intraocular lens) is at very low risk for developing APACG.

Examination classically reveals reduced vision, a red painful eye with a fixed, mid-dilated pupil. The presence of corneal oedema may be suggested by blurring of the iris details. The gold standard for measuring intraocular pressure (IOP) is applanation tonometry, although manual palpation of the globes can provide a crude assessment. Patients with APACG often present with systemic symptoms of nausea and vomiting.

Although gonioscopy of the anterior chamber angle can be a helpful tool in diagnosing a closed angle by allowing direct visualisation of the angle structures, this is very uncomfortable for the patient when the intraocular pressure is significantly raised, and marked corneal oedema will obscure the view. Corneal oedema occurs secondary to the effects of raised IOP on the corneal endothelial pump.

Ultrasound scanning can be useful in APACG; however, the scan of choice would be an anterior segment ('ultrasound biomicroscopy' (UBM)) scan rather than a B-scan, which images the posterior segment of the eye. UBM can reveal a closed angle.

This patient's symptoms are not in keeping with temporal arteritis, hence a temporal artery biopsy would not be particularly helpful. Fluorescein angiography is of no benefit in the diagnosis of APACG.

CASE 4

C: Central retinal artery occlusion

A central retinal artery occlusion (CRAO) typically presents with sudden painless loss of vision. This occurs due to an occlusion in the central retinal artery with secondary ischaemia of the inner retina. Clinically, a pale fundus with attenuated arterial vessels and an initial appearance of a 'cherry-red spot' in the macula are noted. It is important to enquire about any symptoms of giant cell arteritis as this is a potential cause of CRAO that should not be missed. The visual prognosis is poor and most patients present with vision of counting fingers or less. This may improve slightly in approximately one third of patients, regardless of whether treatment is provided. Complications include optic atrophy and neovascularisation, which most commonly occurs on the iris.

The presentation of ophthalmic artery occlusion is similar, although the occlusion occurs within both the retinal and choroidal circulations simultaneously. Vision tends to be reduced to light perception or less. The retina will appear white and there will not be an obvious cherry-red spot.

The cilio-retinal artery exists in only 20–30% of the population and, when present, supplies the central macula. As this vessel arises from the posterior circulation rather than the central retinal artery, patients with a CRAO who have a cilio-retinal artery supplying the macula can have sparing of their central vision. Cilio-retinal artery occlusion, on the other hand, will only affect the central vision. In ocular ischaemic syndrome, more marked ocular signs such as corneal oedema, anterior chamber inflammation, retinal haemorrhages and microaneurysms, would be expected. A central retinal vein occlusion would give the clinical appearance of a 'stormy sunset', with marked retinal haemorrhages in all four quadrants, cotton wool spots, venous dilation and tortuosity of vessels.

CASE 5

D: Carotid Doppler ultrasound

Learning point

The asymmetrical nature of the diabetic retinopathy suggests compromised ocular perfusion in the more severely affected eye and, hence, carotid doppler ultrasound should be performed to investigate for significant ($\geq$ 90%) carotid artery stenosis.[2]

Monitoring and tight control of vascular risk factors, including HbA1c, is crucial in preventing further potential long-term ocular complications. The Diabetes Control and Complication Trial noted that a reduction in the HbA1c in patients with type 1 diabetes from 9 to 7.2% was associated with a 76% reduction in retinopathy. The UK Prospective Diabetes Study demonstrated that, in type 2 diabetics, reducing the HbA1c from 7.9 to 7% can result in a 25% reduction of microvascular disease and associated complications.

According to the Royal College of Ophthalmologists guidelines,[3] patients with proliferative changes of diabetic retinopathy should be considered for a fluorescein angiogram (FFA), to determine the extent of retinal ischaemia. However, in patients who have obvious neovascular changes, eg new vessels with associated vitreous haemorrhage, panretinal photocoagulation laser treatment should be commenced as soon as possible (< 2 weeks), even before FFA, to avoid delaying treatment.

Full blood count (FBC) is useful to investigate for an anaemia which can cause a symmetrical retinopathy similar to diabetic retinopathy or exacerbate an underlying diabetic retinopathy. Therefore, FBC would not be the most appropriate investigation from the above list.

Optical coherence tomography (OCT) scans are predominately used in diabetic eye disease to quantify the oedematous changes associated with diabetic macular oedema. OCT has no role in the investigation of proliferative diabetic retinopathy.

CASE 6

B: Topical ofloxacin 0.3%

The most likely diagnosis is a contact lens-related microbial keratitis or corneal ulcer. However, it is important to remember that an infective keratitis may be fungal, viral or protozoal in nature. The common bacterial organisms include *Pseudomonas aeruginosa*, *Staphylococcus aureus*, *Staphylococcus epidermidis*, *Streptococcus* species and *Enterobacteriaceae*. A fluoroquinolone, such as levofloxacin or ofloxacin, or an aminoglycoside like gentamicin will provide the ideal gram-negative cover for *Pseudomonas*, which is the most common cause in contact lens wearers.[4] Since the fluoroquinolones are less toxic to the cornea, ofloxacin would be the monotherapy agent of choice.

In severe ulcers, patients with additional co-existent ocular surface disease or in immunocompromised individuals, these agents may be used in conjunction with cefuroxime. However, this second generation cephalosporin, and the bacteriostatic agents chloramphenicol and fuscidic acid, are not commonly used as monotherapy for treating contact lens-related corneal ulcers due to the spectrum of the organism covered. Systemic antibiotics should be considered in cases of potential corneal perforation or scleral involvement. Although steroids can be a useful adjunct in the management of microbial keratitis once the infective process is controlled, they are not used in the initial management due to localised immunosuppression, and hence maxitrol should be avoided in the immediate management of this case.

CASE 7

A: Prostaglandin analogue

Prostaglandin analogues are the most appropriate choice in this case.[5] They are a generally well-tolerated family of topical intraocular pressure (IOP)-lowering drugs, working by increasing the uveoscleral outflow of aqueous from the eye.

Beta blockers would not be appropriate in this circumstance owing to the patient's chronic obstructive airways disease. This class of drug is presumed to lower the IOP by reducing the rate of aqueous production in the eye by acting on the β receptors in the ciliary body. They come in non-selective (targeting both β1 and β2 receptors) and selective (targeting β1 receptors only) forms. Systemic β blockers will also lower intraocular pressure but are avoided from an ophthalmic perspective owing to the associated side effects.

Alpha-agonists act on the α2 receptors in the ciliary body to inhibit aqueous secretion in the eye and in some cases also increase uveoscleral outflow. They are the ideal choice for patients with contraindications to β blockers and are available in combination preparations with a β blocker. However, they would not be advisable in this case, as α-agonists are contraindicated in patients taking monoamine oxidase inhibitors.

Carbonic anhydrase inhibitors (CAI) may be used topically, orally or intravenously to reduce the IOP by reducing aqueous humour production in the ciliary body. Systemically, they also produce a weak diuresis. Preparations include brinzolamide, dorzolamide and oral/ intravenous acetazolamide. They are also available in combined forms with an adjunctive β blocker. They would be inappropriate in the above scenario as the patient has sensitivity to sulfonamides. If considering treatment with an oral or intravenous CAI, one should be aware of the common side effects which include hypokalaemia, hyponatraemia, renal stones, paraesthesia, nausea, impotence, malaise and depression. In addition to sulphonamide sensitivity, these agents are also contraindicated in patients with previously documented hypokalaemia, hyponatraemia, renal stones, use of thiazide diuretics and in pregnancy.

Cholinergic agents, such as pilocarpine, work on the muscarinic receptors of the ciliary muscle to increase outflow via the trabecular meshwork. This miotic agent is primarily used in the treatment of angle closure glaucoma and some secondary glaucomas, but is often poorly tolerated due to associated headaches.

Hyperosmotic agents such as glycerin or mannitol may also be considered for systemic use to lower the intraocular pressure. They work by increasing the plasma osmolality and hence draw fluid from the intraocular to the intravascular space. Side effects include diuresis, cardiac failure, urinary retention in men, nausea, headache, myocardial infarction and confusion. Caution should be taken in elderly patients, those with renal disease and diabetic patients due to the risk of ketoacidosis with glycerin. The use of these agents is contraindicated in patients with congestive cardiac failure and dehydration.

CASE 8

A: Open angle glaucoma

'Red eye', or conjunctival injection, is a common symptom in ophthalmic disease. Furthermore, many topical ophthalmic treatments can cause injection of the conjunctiva. In this patient, the adrenergic activity (tremor, palpitations, tachycardia, sweating etc), that usually occurs in response to hypoglycaemia, is being suppressed by the systemic absorption of the β blocker contained in the intraocular pressure-lowering eye drops that she is taking for glaucoma. Topical steroids and antibiotics are the treatments of choice for acute anterior uveitis and infective keratitis, respectively. These do not cause masking of adrenergic activity. Proliferative diabetic retinopathy is treated with panretinal photocoagulation laser. Eye drops have no role in its treatment. Dry eye is mainly treated with topical lubricants, the vast majority of which have no systemic side effects.

CASE 9

A: Hydrocortisone 1% ointment

> **Learning point**
>
> There have been a number of reports in the literature of patients experiencing worsening of their glaucoma due to the prescribed or surreptitious use of periocular or facial steroids that can cause raised IOP and cataract. Clinicians should exercise caution in prescribing these seemingly benign preparations in patients known to have glaucoma or in those with a family history of glaucoma.

As risk factors for glaucoma, medications deserve particular attention as they are a contributing factor in approximately one third of cases of angle closure. Attacks may be initiated by the use of any drugs with anticholinergic or sympathomimetic action such as selective serotonin reuptake inhibitors, monoamine oxidase inhibitors and tricyclic antidepressants, antihistamines and anti-spasmodics. Sulfa-containing medications may trigger an angle closure glaucoma attack by causing oedema of the ciliary body. In this case, we know the patient has open angles, and so topiramate, paroxetine and amitriptyline would not lead to an elevation of her IOP. While β blocker eye drops are used to control IOP, these medications are contraindicated in patients with asthma. Furthermore, β2 receptor agonists do not cause an increase in IOP.

CASE 10

C

A microvascular sixth nerve palsy should spontaneously begin to recover after six weeks. One must not drive when suffering with diplopia, but as long as the cranial nerve palsy has resolved, driving may be resumed. Alternatively, the use of prisms or a patch to relieve the diplopia would suffice as long as the Driver and Vehicle Licensing Agency (DVLA) feel the patient has appropriately adapted to the change.

Learning point

Amendments to the DVLA standards for driving were implemented in 2014.[6] The Esterman visual field remains the field of choice for testing the driving standards. It is performed binocularly. Standards state that category 1 drivers (cars, motorbikes) must have a minimum binocular visual acuity of 6/12 and the ability to read a licence plate at 20.5 m. The visual field must span 120 degrees on the horizontal, with 50 degrees either side of central and no significant defect within the central 20 degrees of fixation.

Category 2 drivers (HGV vehicles) must have a visual acuity of 6/7.5 in the better eye and 6/60 or better in the worse eye. The visual field must range 160 degrees horizontally, with 70 degrees either side of the midline, 30 degrees above and below midline and the absence of any significant defect within the central 30 degrees of fixation.

Therefore, patient A does not meet the required visual acuity for an HGV vehicle. Patient B's horizontal field measures only 120 rather than the required 160 degrees. All patients who have had a stroke/transient ischaemic attack (TIA) must not drive for one month. If the patient is a HGV driver, their licence will be refused or revoked for one year. Patient D has a stable visual field defect. Provided the vision and field remain static after a year and the driver is deemed to have adapted to any residual defect, they may be considered, under exceptional circumstances, for permission to drive. This would be subject to an on-road driving assessment, which patient D had not undertaken. Patient E has bilaterally constricted visual fields as a result of heavy retinal laser treatment and does not meet the Esterman field requirement to drive. For further information, see the DVLA's current medical guidelines for professionals – Vision appendix[7].

CASE 11

C: Antithyroid-stimulating hormone receptor antibody

This lady has symptoms and signs suggestive of thyroid eye disease (TED). This may occur with hyper-, hypo- or (rarely) euthyroidism. Therefore, thyroid-stimulating hormone (TSH) may be suppressed, raised or normal, in this condition. Antibodies to the TSH receptor are found in up to 95% of cases of TED and so this is the diagnostic test from the above list that is most likely to lead to the correct diagnosis.

Although a vertical diplopia can be associated with intracranial pathology, in the context of her other symptoms, TED is more likely. If it was felt that imaging was indicated, MRI is superior to CT for examining the posterior cranial fossa and identifying TED-associated orbital signs. Note that the swelling of the extraocular muscles in TED is confined to the muscle bellies, and this condition has a predilection for the inferior rectus.

Although myasthenia gravis can give any pattern of extraocular muscle weakness, in the context of the lid retraction, conjunctival injection and chemosis, TED is more likely. Therefore anti-acetylcholine receptor antibodies are a less favourable choice. Abnormalities have been reported on electromyography in patients with thyroid disease; however, the findings are non-specific.

CASE 12

A: Monitoring of urea and electrolytes profile

> ### Learning point
>
> It is recommended by the Royal College of Ophthalmologists that patients have a baseline check of renal function before commencing treatment with hydroxychloroquine.[8] Although the maximum dose of hydroxychloroquine should not exceed 6.5 mg/kg lean body weight (typically 200–400 mg daily), there have been reports of ocular toxicity at these doses, especially in the context of abnormal renal function.

The other choices listed are not known to have an effect on the development of hydroxychloroquine retinopathy.

Before commencing treatment and again at annual review, it is necessary to determine if a patient has any visual impairment that is not corrected with glasses. The reading performance with each eye, using appropriate reading correction, should be documented at baseline and review. If the patient can read small print, such as N8 or N6, then treatment with hydroxychloroquine can be commenced. If visual impairment is detected at baseline, then it is recommended that the patient attend an optometrist first, with ophthalmology referral by the optometrist if required.

Patients taking hydroxychloroquine are not routinely screened in ophthalmology clinics for the development of retinopathy and so patient counselling is crucial. If a change in vision is noted (particularly for reading, or patchy or distorted central vision), then the patient should seek advice from their prescriber +/– ocular review. Abrupt withdrawal of treatment may cause a flare-up of their inflammatory disease, and so this approach is not advocated in an unsupervised manner. Prescribers may wish to give patients an Amsler chart to perform self-monitoring of central visual function while taking the treatment. Patients developing hydroxychloroquine retinopathy may be asymptomatic or may develop central scotomata. Examination of the retina may reveal a bull's eye maculopathy. Unfortunately, there is no treatment. Cessation of therapy is advised to halt progression of vision loss; however, this may progress nonetheless.

CASE 13

C: C-ANCA

From an ophthalmic perspective, this lady has symptoms that are suggestive of scleritis. The pain is often described as severe and 'boring'. While redness of the eye is common, it may not be present if only the posterior sclera is involved, as in 'posterior scleritis'. Reduction of vision, painful eye movements and proptosis may all be seen with scleritis. The onset is usually gradual and recurrent episodes are common. With recurrent attacks, the sclera may become thinned and take on a 'bluish tinge'.

> ### Learning point
>
>
> Fifty per cent of patients with scleritis have an underlying systemic disease, as in this case. Commonly associated conditions include rheumatoid arthritis, ANCA-associated granulomatous vasculitis (ANCA-AGV, formerly known as Wegener's granulomatosis), relapsing polychondritis, systemic lupus erythematosus and sarcoidosis. Syphilis, tuberculosis, Lyme disease and, less commonly, bacterial or parasitic infections have also been implicated in the aetiology of scleritis.

In the context of this lady's otolaryngological and respiratory symptoms, a vasculitic process such as ANCA-AGV would be the most likely underlying systemic condition.

Imaging (MRI, chest radiography) may yield additional important clinical information about her extraocular symptoms, but it is the measurement of C-ANCA which is the most sensitive (92%) and specific (99%) test for diagnosing active ANCA-AGV.

While rheumatoid factor may be raised in ANCA-AGV, it is not sensitive or specific for the condition. Furthermore, while rheumatoid arthritis may be associated with scleritis, the constellation of symptoms in this case makes ANCA-AGV much more likely. Sarcoidosis can mimic the findings in ANCA-AGV, but the red cell casts detected on urine microscopy are suggestive of ANCA-AGV. Therefore, C-ANCA would be more appropriate than serum ACE in this case as a first-line investigation.

CASE 14

C: Topiramate

This patient has experienced permanent changes in the visual pathway secondary to ischaemia caused by migraine. This patient requires treatment that will prevent/reduce the number of future migraine attacks and the associated ischaemia. Preferred medications include propranolol, amitriptyline and topiramate. As propranolol, a β blocker, is contraindicated in this patient due to his co-existent asthma, topiramate is the most appropriate treatment from the choices listed. This patient is not currently experiencing an acute attack of migraine and so ergotamine, ibuprofen and sumatriptan would not be appropriate. While non-steroidal anti-inflammatory drugs may have some analgesic effects in migraine, they do not have any role in preventing further attacks. Sumatriptan and ergotamine are useful for aborting acute attacks of migraine, but do not have any role in reducing the frequency of attacks in the long term. Note that positron emission tomography (PET) scanning is useful in identifying hypoperfusion during attacks of migraine.

CASE 15

C: Anti-muscle-specific kinase antibody

This patient has symptoms and signs suggestive of ocular myaesthenia gravis. This is an uncommon autoimmune disease which causes fatiguable weakness. Generalised myasthenia presents with symptoms related to weakness of the limb, bulbar and respiratory muscles. Ocular myasthenia may occur in isolation or in conjunction with generalised myasthenia, and presents with ptosis and ophthalmoplegia which are variable and worse in the evening or when the patient is tired. Note that the pupil is never involved. Autoantibodies are generated against the post-synaptic acetylcholine receptors. The condition can occur at any age but has a bimodal distribution with peaks at approximately 20 and 60 years. It is more common in women and may be associated with other autoimmune diseases or thymoma.

Learning point

Anti-acetylcholine (ACh) receptor antibodies are present in up to 50% of cases in ocular myasthenia, lower than the 85% detected in generalised myasthenia gravis.[9, 10, 11]
Up to 47% of patients with generalised myasthenia gravis without anti-ACh receptor antibodies have antibodies to muscle-specific kinase.[12]

The ice-pack test requires application of an ice pack to the ptotic eyelid for a duration of two minutes. It is positive when there is a reduction in ptosis of ≥ 2 mm on the affected side. It has a sensitivity of up to 92% in myasthenia gravis.[13]

Although anti-muscle-specific kinase antibody has a lower sensitivity, it would be the most appropriate next step in the investigation of this patient, as both the Tensilon® (edrophonium) test and single fibre-electromyogram are procedures that have potential significant systemic side effects or are invasive, respectively. Muscle biopsy does not have a role in the diagnosis of myasthenia gravis. A MRI of the brain and orbits will appear normal in myasthenia gravis; however, this condition is known as the 'great mimic' and should always be considered when a pattern of extraocular muscle movement abnormalities 'does not fit' a particular pattern or when there is variability in diplopia or ptosis. Therefore, neuroimaging may be useful to exclude abnormalities (eg space-occupying, ischaemic or demyelinating lesions) when all other investigations do not allude to an underlying diagnosis.

CASE 16

A: Jaw claudication

> ### Learning point
>
> Giant cell arteritis (GCA) is the most common primary vasculitis of adults in the Western world. This lady fulfils four of the five criteria defined by the American College of Rheumatology for the classification of GCA.[14] These include age ≥ 50 years, new headache, temporal artery abnormalities, ESR ≥ 50 mm/1st hour and an abnormal temporal artery biopsy (TAB) showing vasculitis depicted by mononuclear cell infiltration or granulomatous inflammation, which is usually with multinucleated giant cells.

This lady has symptoms and signs suggestive of left-sided arteritic anterior ischaemic optic neuropathy secondary to GCA. The joint guidelines of the British Society of Rheumatology and the British Society of Health Professionals in Rheumatology (2010) identified a number of clinical features that are predictive of TAB positivity.[15] From most to least predictive, in terms of likelihood ratio, were temporal artery beading, temporal artery prominence, jaw claudication, diplopia and temporal artery tenderness.[16] The finding of a relative afferent pupillary defect has no predictive value relating to TAB. GCA causes abnormal eye movements by ischaemic effects either on the extraocular muscle or on the associated cranial nerve. In an effort to prevent the patient developing bilateral sequential optic neuropathy (risk up to 50% within 14 days), she must start systemic immunosuppression without delay.

CASE 17

C: MR cerebral angiogram

> ### Learning point
>
> This lady's symptoms and signs are suggestive of an acute left-sided Horner's syndrome. She has left-sided miosis and ptosis (the eye appears smaller due to drooping of the left upper eyelid causing narrowing of the palpebral aperture, ie pseudo-enophthalmos). Horner's syndrome is caused by damage to the sympathetic supply to the elevators of the eyelid (Müller's muscle) and the iris dilators (dilator pupillae). Ipsilateral conjunctival injection and facial anhydrosis are seen much less commonly, the latter suggestive of a lesion in the first- or second-order neurone. If the ipsilateral iris is paler ('hypochromic'), then the lesion is likely to be congenital.

In this case, the Horner's syndrome is most likely to have occurred secondary to internal carotid artery dissection following the minor trauma of the road traffic accident. An MR cerebral angiogram is the most appropriate investigation from the above list. Doppler ultrasound is a useful screening tool, but may not confirm the diagnosis, especially in internal carotid artery dissections without cerebral ischaemic events.[17] An MRI scan of brain and orbits with gadolinium would be useful if demyelination was suspected from the history. A CT thorax would be more appropriate to investigate the lung apices for a tumour involving the sympathetic chain should this be suspected from the history.

Finally, apraclonidine and cocaine eye drops can be used to confirm the diagnosis of Horner's syndrome. Cocaine will yield an immediate positive result whereby the unaffected pupil will dilate, while the affected pupil will not. Cocaine blocks the reuptake of noradrenaline and in the case of the affected eye, no noradrenaline is secreted. Apraclonidine, on the other hand, will result in a reversal of the anisocoria due to a marked dilation of the pupil on the affected side secondary to the development of a denervation hypersensitivity. This has been reported to take 5–8 days to develop.

References

1. British Committee for Standards in Haematology. 2012. Guidelines on the investigation and management of venous thrombosis at unusual sites. British Journal of Haematology, 159, 18–38

2. Dogru M et al. 1998. Modifying factors related to asymmetric diabetic retinopathy. Eye (Lond), 12, 929–933

3. The Royal College of Ophthalmologists. 2012 (updated July 2013). Diabetic Retinopathy Guidelines. www.rcophth.ac.uk/standards-publications-research/clinical-guidelines

4. The Royal College of Ophthalmologists. Autumn 2013. Focus, 'Microbial keratitis' www.rcophth. ac.uk/wp-content/uploads/2014/08/Focus-Autumn-2013.pdf

5. NICE. 2009. Glaucoma: Diagnosis and management of chronic open angle glaucoma and ocular hypertension. NICE clinical guideline 85. www.nice.org.uk/guidance/cg85/chapter/1-recommendations

6. DVLA. 2014. For medical practitioners: At a glance guide to the current medical standards of fitness to drive. www.gov.uk/government/publications/at-a-glance

7. DVLA. 2013. DVLA's current medical guidelines for professionals – Vision appendix. www.gov.uk/current-medical-guidelines-dvla-guidance-for-professionals-vision-chapter-appendix

8. The Royal College of Ophthalmologists. 2009. Hydroxychloroquine and Ocular Toxicity Recommendations on Screening. www.bad.org.uk/shared/get-file.ashx?id=774&itemtype=document

9. Lindstrom J et al. 1976. Antibody to acetylcholine receptor in myasthenia gravis: prevalence, clinical correlates, and diagnostic value. Neurology, 26, 1054–1059

10. Vincent A et al. 1985. Acetylcholine receptor antibody as a diagnostic test for myasthenia gravis: results in 153 validated cases and 2967 diagnostic assays. Journal of Neurology Neurosurgery and Psychiatry, 48, 1246–1252

11. Vincent A and Newsom-Davis J. 1982. Acetylcholine receptor antibody characteristics in myasthenia gravis. I. Patients with generalized myasthenia or disease restricted to ocular muscles. Clinical and Experimental Immunology, 49, 257–265

12. Niks E et al. 2007. Epidemiology of myasthenia gravis with anti-muscle specific kinase antibodies in the Netherlands. Neurology Neurosurgery and Psychiatry, 78, 417–418

13. Chatzistefanou K et al. 2009. The ice pack test in the differential diagnosis of myasthenic diplopia. Ophthalmology, 116, 2236–2243

14. Hunder G et al. 1990. The American College of Rheumatology 1990 criteria for the classification of giant cell arteritis. Arthritis and Rheumatism, 33, 1122–1128

15. The British Society of Rheumatology and the British Society of Health Professionals in Rheumatology. 2010. BSR and BHPR Guidelines for the management of giant cell arteritis. www.rheumatology.org.uk/includes/documents/cm_docs/2010/m/2_management_of_giant_cell_arteritis.pdf

16. Gerald W et al. 2002. Does This Patient Have Temporal Arteritis? JAMA, 287, 92–101

17. Arnold M et al. 2008. Ultrasound diagnosis of spontaneous carotid dissection with isolated Horner syndrome. Stroke, 39, 82–86

CASE 1

A 20-year-old woman, with a history of repeated self-harm by poisoning, presents 45 minutes following the ingestion of forty 500 mg tablets of paracetamol. She had an argument with her partner before the incident. On examination, she has a Glasgow Coma score of 15 and is maintaining her own airway.

Which of the following options is most appropriate in her immediate management?

- A. **Urgent referral to psychiatric services**
- B. **Consideration for use of activated charcoal**
- C. **Acetylcysteine infusion**
- D. **Gastric lavage**
- E. **Emetics**

CASE 2

You are called to see a 55-year-old man, admitted to the ward two days earlier for treatment of cellulitis. He has subsequently developed septicaemia. He now believes a fellow patient is trying to poison him and he has broken a chair to protect himself. There is no history of mental illness. The fellow patient and broken chair have been removed from the area. De-escalation techniques have failed. He is refusing oral medication and is threatening to attack the fellow patient.

Which of the following management options is most appropriate?

- A. **Intravenous lorazepam + intravenous haloperidol**
- B. **Intravenous lorazepam + intravenous olanzapine**
- C. **Intramuscular lorazepam + intramuscular chlorpromazine**
- D. **Intramuscular lorazepam + intramuscular haloperidol**
- E. **Intramuscular lorazepam + intramuscular olanzapine**

CASE 3

A 27-year-old man with schizophrenia presents to the emergency department with an acute onset, sustained muscle spasm in his neck. He is in pain and is holding his head in an abnormal posture. He is finding it difficult to speak and swallow. He attended the psychiatric outpatient clinic five days earlier, when he was prescribed a medication for auditory hallucinations. He has been compliant with this medication since.

Initial management should include:

A. **IV promethazine**
B. **IV procyclidine**
C. **Oral procyclidine**
D. **Oral promethazine**
E. **IV prothiaden**

CASE 4

A 35-year-old woman with a history of depression presents to the emergency department with profuse sweating, agitation, diarrhoea and a tremor. She has recently been suffering with migraines and has taken over-the-counter migraine relief tablets, within recommended limits, over the preceding two days. Examination reveals: heart rate 127 bpm, blood pressure 172/105 mmHg and temperature 39.5 °C. She is diaphoretic and restless, with a pronounced bilateral tremor. There is deep tendon hyperreflexia and both inducible and spontaneous muscle clonus, more pronounced in the lower limbs.

What is the most likely diagnosis?

A. **Neuroleptic malignant syndrome**
B. **Anticholinergic toxicity**
C. **Malignant hyperthermia**
D. **Serotonin syndrome**
E. **Meningitis**

CASE 5

A 23-year-old man presents at the emergency department in an agitated state. He believes insects are crawling over his body and that he is having a heart attack. Friends are in attendance, who allege his drink was spiked at a party they attended four hours previously. On examination, he is hyperactive, sweating and agitated. The heart rate is 132 bpm, blood pressure 179/102 mmHg and temperature 37.5 °C. He is flushed in appearance and the pupils are dilated bilaterally. The physical examination otherwise is unremarkable.

What is the most likely cause?

A. **Amphetamine toxicity**
B. **Schizophrenia**
C. **Serotonin syndrome**
D. **Morphine toxicity**
E. **Methadone toxicity**

CASE 6

A 35-year-old man, with a known diagnosis of schizophrenia, is brought to hospital by his community psychiatric nurse. He is agitated and intermittently responds to unseen stimuli. He is complaining of stiffness in his arms and legs, and has found it difficult to get out of bed for the past two days. He is perspiring profusely. The patient had attended the psychiatric outpatient clinic six days previously, where his medications were changed. On examination, he is disorientated to time and place. The heart rate is 127 bpm, blood pressure 145/92 mmHg and temperature 40.7 °C. He is diaphoretic. Cardiovascular, respiratory and gastrointestinal system examinations are largely unremarkable. There is pronounced muscular rigidity affecting all four limbs.

What is the most likely cause of his presentation?

A. **Encephalitis**
B. **Malignant hyperthermia**
C. **Serotonin syndrome**
D. **Toxic encephalopathy**
E. **Neuroleptic malignant syndrome**

CASE 7

A 60-year-old man presents with a progressive decline in global cognitive function, with associated impairment in function. Following investigation, he is diagnosed with Alzheimer's dementia. Which of the following is *not* associated with the development of Alzheimer's dementia?

A. *ε4* gene mutation on chromosome 19
B. *PSEN-1* gene mutation on chromosome 14
C. *DEM-4* gene mutation on chromosome 13
D. *APP* gene mutation on chromosome 21
E. *PSEN-2* mutation on chromosome 1

CASE 8

A 23-year-old girl presents to the emergency department on three separate occasions. She believes she is having a heart attack before each attendance, but her symptoms subside by the time of her arrival. Symptoms last approximately 15 minutes, with no obvious trigger, and include palpitations, shortness of breath and chest pain. She states that she does not 'feel real' during the episodes and thinks she is losing her mind. No physical explanation is found for her symptoms.

Her symptoms are most in keeping with:

A. Generalised anxiety disorder
B. Agoraphobia
C. Fear of hospital
D. Panic disorder
E. Obsessive compulsive disorder

CASE 9

An 18-year-old woman with anorexia nervosa is admitted to the medical ward. She has not eaten in two weeks and has a BMI of 14 kg/m^2.

Which is the least likely serum endocrine disturbance?

    A. **Elevated growth hormone**
    B. **Low cortisol**
    C. **Low luteinising hormone (LH)**
    D. **Low follicle-stimulating hormone (FSH)**
    E. **Low oestrogen**

CASE 10

You are called to assess a 27-year-old woman who presents to the emergency department following a failed attempted suicide, by hanging. She is intoxicated with alcohol. She is unemployed and lives alone.

Which is a recognised risk factor for completed suicide?

    A. **Recent new relationship**
    B. **Alcohol abstinence**
    C. **Female sex**
    D. **No history of prior attempts**
    E. **Physical illness**

CASE 11

A 32-year-old man with schizophrenia attends for a routine medical assessment. He reports a history of childhood encephalitis. He read on the internet that this can be associated with schizophrenia development in later life.

Which is **not** a known risk factor associated with schizophrenia?

A. **Rural upbringing**
B. **Afro-Caribbean race**
C. **History of childhood encephalitis**
D. **Family history of schizophrenia**
E. **History of birth asphyxia**

CASE 12

A 15-year-old young man attends the emergency department with severe anxiety, agitation and auditory hallucinations. He admits to smoking cannabis two hours earlier. There is an 18-month history of regular cannabis misuse.

Which of the following is correct? The relative risk of him developing schizophrenia in later life is:

A. **The same as the general population**
B. **A two-fold increase**
C. **A two-fold reduction**
D. **A four-fold increase**
E. **A four-fold reduction**

CASE 13

A patient becomes angry and irritable during the course of a medical interview. He is annoyed that you declined to prescribe diazepam for his back pain and states he will 'wreck the place' if he is not listened to.

Which of the following is the most appropriate course of action?

A. Tell the patient you are angry with him for behaving in this way
B. Move the patient into the waiting area, where other patients can assist
C. Use physical contact to reassure the patient
D. Seat the patient near to the door, so that he may escape easily, if feeling trapped
E. Avoid fixed eye contact

CASE 14

A 42-year-old man complains of abdominal cramps, muscle aches and insomnia, 24 hours after admission to hospital for treatment of a groin abscess. Excessive lacrimation, rhinorrhoea, diaphoresis, piloerection and yawning are noted on examination. His pupils are dilated bilaterally.

Which of the following is most likely?

A. Alcohol withdrawal
B. Amphetamine withdrawal
C. Opiate withdrawal
D. Cannabis withdrawal
E. Caffeine withdrawal

CASE 15

A 55-year-old man presents to the neurology clinic with abnormal movements. His wife reports that he has become depressed and anxious over the past six months. His father had similar difficulties and died aged 60. Last week, he broke the television in frustration as he could not operate the remote control.

The most likely diagnosis is:

A. Depression
B. Lewy body dementia
C. Huntington's disease
D. Vascular dementia
E. Pick's disease

CASE 16

A 52-year-old man is transferred to the rehabilitation ward following treatment for an ST elevation myocardial infarction. Over the subsequent months, he reports low mood, loss of interest, reduced self-esteem and thoughts of life not worth living. He is diagnosed with a depressive illness.

Which is the most appropriate first-line antidepressant in this instance?

A. Amitriptyline
B. Citalopram
C. Sertraline
D. Mirtazepine
E. Moclobemide

CASE 17

A 37-year-old patient is transferred from the psychiatric ward with mild chest pain, shortness of breath and a temperature of 39.4 °C. On examination, he is tachycardic (heart rate 142 bpm), with evidence of mitral regurgitation and peripheral oedema. Following investigation, a diagnosis of myocarditis is made.

Which of the following medications is the most likely causative agent?

A. **Promethazine**
B. **Chlorpheniramine**
C. **Prochlorperazine**
D. **Chlorpromazine**
E. **Clozapine**

CASE 18

A 32-year-old man attends the day procedure unit for gastroscopy. He reports a constant churning feeling in his stomach over the past four years, which worsens when he is under stress. He states he was always 'a worrier' as a child, but since the birth of his children, he has become much more tense. He worries excessively about everyday problems, which other people tend to ignore. You notice he has a fine tremor and he is sweating during the interview. The gastroscopy and other investigations to date have been within normal limits.

The most likely diagnosis is:

A. **Generalised anxiety disorder**
B. **Agoraphobia**
C. **Fear of hospital**
D. **Panic disorder**
E. **Obsessive compulsive disorder**

CASE 1

B: Consideration for use of activated charcoal

The initial management of most poisoning cases is medical. Consider the administration of activated charcoal (50 g for adults; 1 g/kg body weight for children) if more than 150 mg/kg paracetamol has been taken within the last hour. There is normally no indication to start acetylcysteine without a paracetamol blood concentration (taken at four hours), provided the result can be obtained and acted upon within eight hours of ingestion.[1] Late presentations and staggered overdoses may well require treatment without a blood result, since interpretation of levels is problematic. Emetics, gastric lavage, cathartics, whole bowel irrigation and multiple doses of activated charcoal are not recommended.[2]

CASE 2

D: Intramuscular lorazepam + intramuscular haloperidol

> **Learning point**
>
> In the acutely disturbed patient, rapid tranquillisation and physical intervention should only be considered once de-escalation and other strategies have failed. If the patient refuses oral medication, intramuscular agents should be considered.

Intramuscular lorazepam +/– intramuscular haloperidol is a reasonable next step. Intramuscular lorazepam should not be given within one hour of intramuscular olanzapine. Intravenous medications should only be used in exceptional circumstances and following discussion with senior clinicians. Intramuscular chlorpromazine is not recommended. For further reading, see reference[3].

CASE 3

B: IV procyclidine

Acute dystonias (uncontrolled muscle spasms) are a recognised adverse effect of antipsychotic medications, as are other extrapyramidal symptoms (pseudo-parkinsonism, akathisia (restlessness) and tardive dyskinesia (abnormal involuntary movements, particularly orofacial)). Acute dystonias can occur within hours of an increase in dose or commencement of an antipsychotic agent. They occur commonly in young, male, neuroleptic naive patients who are prescribed high-potency antipsychotics (eg haloperidol). Treatment is with anticholinergic agents (eg procyclidine) by oral, IM or IV routes depending on severity of symptoms. In this instance IV procyclidine is appropriate, due to swallowing difficulties.

CHAPTER 12
ANSWERS

CASE 4

D: Serotonin syndrome

Learning point

Serotonin syndrome is a potentially life-threatening illness resulting from increased serotonergic transmission in the central nervous system. It is a clinical diagnosis, made in a patient who has been exposed to a serotonergic agent and who exhibits typical clinical features – classically, the triad of mental state changes, autonomic instability and neuromuscular abnormalities. Clinically, it can be differentiated from the other conditions described above by the presence of neuromuscular activation – increased muscle tone, ataxia, tremor, hyperreflexia, myoclonus and clonus (more pronounced in the lower limbs).

Selective serotonin reuptake inhibitors are most commonly implicated in the pathogenesis (implied in the history above, for the treatment of depression) with toxicity in this instance being precipitated by self-administration of triptan medication.

CASE 5

A: Amphetamine toxicity

Amphetamine toxicity is associated with symptoms affecting the cardiovascular (chest pain, palpitations), gastrointestinal (diarrhoea, dry mouth, anorexia and nausea/vomiting) and neurological systems (mental state changes, dyskinesias and formication – the sensation of insects crawling on the skin). In addition, there may be hypertension (which could give rise to stroke), tachycardia (with risk of other arrhythmias), flushing, diaphoresis and mydriasis. Morphine and methadone toxicity are more commonly associated with miosis. Serotonin syndrome would be a differential diagnosis, although the history and symptoms in this instance make the diagnosis less likely.

CASE 6

E: Neuroleptic malignant syndrome

Learning point

Neuroleptic malignant syndrome (NMS) is a potentially life-threatening medical emergency associated with the use of neuroleptic medications. It is characterised by mental state changes, autonomic instability, muscular rigidity and fever. It has a reported mortality of approximately 15%. Although elevated serum creatine kinase (CK) is *not* essential for the diagnosis, increasing levels correlate with severity and prognosis. CK levels are typically greater than 1000 U/litre in confirmed cases.

While neuroleptic medications (particularly high-potency, first-generation antipsychotics such as haloperidol and chlorpromazine) are usually implicated in the pathogenesis of NMS, it can also be associated with agents with no known dopaminergic action.

Treatment involves stopping the causative medication, initiating supportive measures (eg cooling blanket/ice baths for hyperthermia) and considering dantrolene, bromocriptine or amantadine therapy.

Although it shares some of the clinical features of serotonin syndrome (mental state changes, autonomic instability etc), this condition can be clinically differentiated by the absence of myoclonus, hyperreflexia and ataxia (NMS is more typically associated with sluggish responses, such as bradykinesias and rigidity).

CASE 7

C: *DEM-4* gene mutation on chromosome 13

The two presenilin genes (*PSEN-1* and *PSEN-2*), along with the *APP* mutation on chromosome 21, are independent risk factors for early onset Alzheimer's dementia (AD). They are among some of the rarer risk factors for AD development. The apolipoprotein E (*APOE*) gene is the gene most frequently implicated in late onset Alzheimer's dementia. *APOE ε4* in particular confers a four-fold increase of developing AD (compared to the general public) with a ten-fold risk in homozygotic individuals (ie those in whom the allele is present on both homologous chromosomes). The *DEM-4* gene is *not* associated with AD.

CASE 8

D: Panic disorder

Panic disorder is characterised by recurrent episodes of severe, unprovoked, overwhelming anxiety symptoms. Their pattern of occurrence is unpredictable, due to lack of identifiable triggers. Episodes start abruptly and typically last between 5 and 20 minutes. There is cross-system symptomatology, including autonomic arousal symptoms (tachycardia, diaphoresis, tremor, dry mouth), cardiac/respiratory/gastrointestinal symptoms (chest pain, dyspnoea, a choking sensation, nausea, abdominal pain) and neurological symptoms (fear of dying/losing control, light-headedness and derealisation/depersonalisation).

Learning point

Panic disorder can only be diagnosed when other physical causes have been excluded.

CASE 9

B: Low cortisol

Anorexia nervosa is a condition commonly affecting young woman (1 : 10 male : female ratio). It is characterised by deliberate/self-induced weight loss (BMI 15% below normal or less), marked distortion of body image (patients commonly perceive themselves as 'fat') and a pathological desire for thinness. There is usually evidence of a widespread endocrine disorder involving the hypothalamic–pituitary–gonadal axis. Typically, serum LH, FSH, progestogens and oestrogens are reduced, with resulting amenorrhoea. Growth hormone and cortisol are typically elevated.

CASE 10

E: Physical illness

Learning point

Known risk factors for completed suicide include male sex, marital status (increased risk in single, divorced and widowed people), alcohol/drug dependence, social isolation, unemployment, diagnosed mental illness and previous suicide/self-harm attempts. Concurrent physical illness is also a recognised risk factor.

Decisions about referral, discharge and admission to hospital for patients who have self-harmed should be based on a comprehensive assessment, including a risk assessment.

CASE 11

A: Rural upbringing

The lifetime prevalence of schizophrenia is estimated at 0.5 to 1%. Schizophrenia is a neurodevelopmental disorder and has recognised associations with Afro-Caribbean and South Asian races, birth asphyxia, childhood encephalitis, intrauterine infections, first standing at later than 12 months, cannabis misuse and family history of schizophrenia (particularly in first degree relatives). In addition, there is a strong association with urban birth and upbringing, with an estimated relative risk of 2.2 in this population, compared with rural counterparts.[4]

CASE 12

B: A two-fold increase

Overall, cannabis use appears to confer a two-fold risk of later schizophrenia or schizophreniform disorder.[5]

CASE 13

E: Avoid fixed eye contact

The NICE guidelines for the management of violence advocate de-escalation techniques before other interventions.[3]

> ### Learning point
>
> Staff should avoid provocational gestures, including prolonged eye contact and confrontational statements. Preferably, one staff member should assume control of the situation, giving clear advice or instructions to the patient. Where possible, other patients in the vicinity should be facilitated to leave and extra support from other staff should be sought. Staff should try to establish a rapport with the patient, offering realistic options and acknowledging the patient's concerns. Interviews should be conducted where staff can easily exit the room, if under escalating threat of violence.

**CHAPTER 12
ANSWERS**

CASE 14

C: Opiate withdrawal

Opioid withdrawal syndrome is not life-threatening, but can be extremely unpleasant. It presents as a flu-like illness, with excessive sneezing, lacrimation, rhinorrhoea and abdominal cramping. The classic piloerection or 'goose bumps' associated with opioid withdrawal gives rise to the term 'cold turkey'. It is also characterised by nausea, vomiting, diarrhoea, yawning, dilated pupils and muscle cramps. Onset of symptoms is variable, depending on the half-life of the implicated opioid drug, eg heroin withdrawal symptoms typically commence 6–24 hours following the last dose.

CASE 15

C: Huntington's disease

Huntington's disease (HD) is an hereditary disorder of the central nervous system characterised by a classic triad of movement problems, cognitive deficits and psychiatric manifestations. There is an autosomal dominant pattern of inheritance. HD is caused by an expansion of a CAG triplet in the huntingtin gene on chromosome 4. Patients usually present in the fifth or sixth decade with typical involuntary/choreiform movements. Common psychiatric associations are depression, anxiety, psychosis, violence and aggression.

CASE 16

C: Sertraline

Depression is a common co-morbidity following acute myocardial infarction (MI). It is associated with increased mortality during this period. First-line pharmacological treatment for depression, in general, is a selective serotonin reuptake inhibitor, eg citalopram/sertraline. This group of antidepressants are generally better tolerated than tricyclics, monoamine uptake inhibitors and other classes. In a statement in 2011, the MHRA issued caution when prescribing citalopram in patients at risk of Torsade de Pointes (including patients with previous MI). This is in relation to its effects on prolonging the QT interval. As such, it is not recommended in this instance. There is good evidence supporting the effectiveness and tolerability of sertraline in patients who develop a major depressive illness post MI.

CASE 17

E: Clozapine

While infections and autoimmune disease are commonly implicated in the aetiology of myocarditis, iatrogenic causes can be overlooked. Clozapine, an antipsychotic medication used in treatment-resistant schizophrenia, is a known cause of myocarditis. It has also been linked to agranulocytosis and pulmonary embolism. Strict initiation guidelines and monitoring protocols are implemented in the UK for the use of clozapine.

CASE 18

A: Generalised anxiety disorder

Generalised anxiety disorder is characterised by a persistent state of anxiety or apprehension in everyday situations, with no obvious trigger. There is cross-system symptomatology, including autonomic arousal symptoms (tachycardia, diaphoresis, tremor, dry mouth), cardiac/respiratory/gastrointestinal symptoms (chest pain, dyspnoea, a choking sensation, nausea, abdominal pain) and neurological symptoms (fear of dying/losing control, light-headedness and derealisation/depersonalisation). Patients can also complain of muscle tension and an inability to relax.

CHAPTER 12 ANSWERS

Learning point

Physical disorders (including hyperthyroidism) and substance misuse (eg amphetamines) should be excluded before the diagnosis is made.

References

1. The National Poisons Information Service/TOXBASE®. 2015. Information on the management of paracetamol overdose

2. NICE. 2004. Self harm: The short-term physical and psychological management and secondary prevention of self-harm in primary and secondary care. NICE clinical guideline 16. www.nice.org.uk/guidance/cg16

3. NICE. 2005. Violence: The short-term management of disturbed/violent behaviour in in-patient psychiatric settings and emergency departments. NICE clinical guideline 25. www.nice.org.uk/guidance/cg25

4. Mortensen et al. 1999. Effects of family history and place and season of birth on the risk of schizophrenia. New England Journal of Medicine, 340, 603–608

5. Arseneault et al. 2004. Causal association between cannabis and psychosis: examination of the evidence. The British Journal of Psychiatry, 184, 110–117

CASE 1

A 50-year-old man presents to the emergency department with a significant cough which has been persistent for several weeks. He has been producing small amounts of dirty sputum. He thinks there may have been some blood in this recently and is unsure if he has lost weight. He admits to drinking heavily and is homeless. On examination you notice he is unkempt, looks unwell and is very thin. The respiratory rate is 20 breaths/min, oxygen saturation 94% on room air, pulse 90 bpm, blood pressure 105/74 mmHg. He is apyrexic. There are no palpable cervical lymph nodes. You notice tar staining on his fingers but no finger clubbing. There is reduced air entry at the right upper zone with some crackles. A chest X-ray is shown in Figure 13.1.

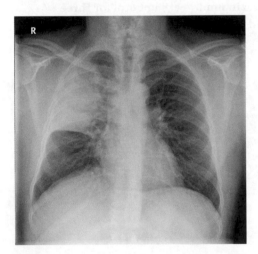

Figure 13.1

What is the best first-line investigation for this man?

    A. **Sputum sent urgently for culture examination for acid fast bacilli**

    B. **CT scan of chest with contrast**

    C. **Bronchoscopy**

    D. **Mantoux test**

    E. **HIV test**

CASE 2

A 36-year-old lady who is 30 weeks pregnant presents with a swelling at the side of her neck. She has had this for two months. It is increasing in size and is tender. She is originally from Thailand and has been living and working in the UK for six years. Her husband is from the UK. She is a non-smoker. She complains of tiredness, intermittent sweats and feeling unwell for several weeks. She blamed her symptoms on her pregnancy. The obstetric team feel the pregnancy is progressing satisfactorily, but the baby is measuring slightly small for dates. A biopsy is taken from the mass. It showed caseating granulomata and is Ziehl–Neelsen positive. The organism is confirmed at culture to be *Mycobacterium tuberculosis* and is sensitive to first-line drugs.

What is the correct treatment regimen?

A. **Rifampicin alone for six months**
B. **Rifampicin + isoniazid for six months**
C. **Rifampicin + isoniazid + pyrazinamide + ethambutol for two months, then rifampicin alone for four months**
D. **Rifampicin + isoniazid + pyrazinamide + ethambutol for two months, then rifampicin and isoniazid for four months**
E. **Rifampicin + isoniazid + pyrazinamide + ethambutol for three months, then rifampicin and ethamutol for three months**

CASE 3

A 66-year-old lady has been referred by her GP to the emergency department. She has a 2-day history of cough and fever and is bringing up green sputum. She has no chest pain or haemoptysis. She is an ex-smoker of ten years, with a 20 pack/year history. She has never complained of chest symptoms previously. On examination she is flushed. Her respiratory rate is 32 breaths/min, oxygen saturation 94% on room air, pulse rate 98 bpm, blood pressure 105/78 mmHg and temperature 38.2 °C. On auscultation of the chest there was reduced air entry at the right lung base with coarse crackles; this area was dull on percussion. There was nil else of note on examination. Her chest X-ray is shown in Figure 13.2.

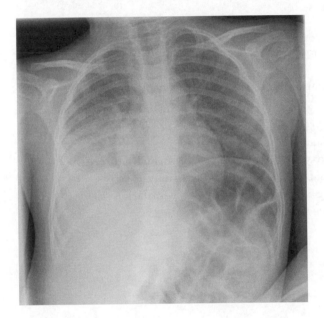

Figure 13.2

Blood tests show: Haemoglobin 132 g/litre, White cells 14×10^9/litre, Neutrophils 12×10^9/litre, Platelets 274×10^9/litre, C-reactive protein 80 mg/litre, Sodium 136 mmol/litre, Potassium 4.1 mmol/litre, Urea 9.2 mmol/litre, Creatinine 90 µmol/litre.

What additional investigation should be carried out?

    A. **Sputum examination for acid fast bacilli (AFB)**

    B. **Urinary antigens (legionella and pneumococcus)**

    C. **CT scan of thorax**

    D. **Spirometry**

    E. **Arterial blood gas (ABG) analysis**

CASE 4

A 68-year-old man is brought to the emergency department. His family called an ambulance as he had become increasingly unwell. He complained of worsening dyspnoea over a few days with associated cough and green spit. On arrival of the ambulance crew, his oxygen saturation is 74%, respiratory rate 28 breaths/min, temperature 37.5 °C, pulse rate 90 bpm, blood pressure 110/70 mmHg. He was given high-flow oxygen and the oxygen saturation improved to 97%. On arrival at the emergency department he is drowsy, but rousable to voice. The respiratory rate is 24 breaths/min, pulse rate 102 bpm and blood pressure 114/74 mmHg. Chest examination reveals reduced air entry throughout, a prolonged expiratory phase and expiratory wheeze.

Arterial blood gas analysis on 10 litre/min oxygen via a non-rebreather mask showed: pH 7.29, PaO_2 16 kPa, $PaCO_2$ 9.3 kPa and bicarbonate 28 mmol/litre.

What is the most appropriate next step in his management?

- A. **IV furosemide, IV glyceryl trinitrate infusion, start continuous positive airways pressure**
- B. **Doxapram IV infusion**
- C. **Reduce inspired oxygen, give nebulised bronchodilators, give steroids and repeat the arterial blood gas analysis**
- D. **Refer to intensive care for intubation and ventilation**
- E. **Start non-invasive ventilation**

CASE 5

A 72-year-old man with a history of chronic obstructive pulmonary disease (COPD) and alcohol abuse has been on the ward for five days. He was treated for an infective exacerbation of COPD with steroids, nebulised bronchodilators and oral antibiotics. He also received IV Pabrinex® and oral chlordiazepoxide as treatment for his alcohol withdrawal. Earlier in the day he was found to be drowsy and an arterial blood gas (ABG) analysis on room air showed: pH 7.29, PaO_2 6.9 kPa, $PaCO_2$ 10.1 kPa, bicarbonate 30 mmol/litre. He was started on non-invasive ventilation (NIV) with settings as follows: inspiratory positive airways pressure (IPAP) 14 cm H_2O, expiratory positive airways pressure (EPAP) 4 cm H_2O and an oxygen flow rate of 3 litre/min.

You review his ABG one hour after initiation of NIV: pH 7.28, PaO_2 8.1 kPa, $PaCO_2$ 9.9 kPa, bicarbonate 32 mmol/litre.

What is the most appropriate next step in management?

A. **Increase IPAP**
B. **Increase EPAP**
C. **Increase oxygen flow rate**
D. **Intubation and ventilation**
E. **Stop NIV and palliate his symptoms**

CASE 6

A 55-year-old man has been referred by his GP after his wife requested a consultation. He has complained of excessive tiredness, and his wife reports loud snoring and occasions where he seems to stop breathing. He is otherwise well. He has a history of a tonsillectomy as a child and hypertension for which he is currently taking irbesartan. He drives a car. He smokes ten cigarettes per day. His weekly alcohol intake is approximately 20 units, mainly at weekends. On examination, his body mass index is 31 kg/m² with collar size 41 cm (16.5 inches). He has a mild overbite. His Epworth sleep score is 13/24. Heart sounds are normal with no murmurs. There is no ankle oedema. An overnight oximetry test had been completed before clinic attendance showing: mean oxygen saturation 93%, minimum saturation 86%, duration of recording 7 h 34 min, oxygen desaturation index 6.6 dips per hour (> 4%), total dips 48, heart rate fluctuations 25 per hour (> 6 bpm).

What is the most significant reading from the overnight oximetry?

    A. **Mean saturations**
    B. **Heart rate fluctuations per hour**
    C. **Minimum saturations**
    D. **Oxygen desaturation index dips per hour**
    E. **Length of recording**

CASE 7

A 63-year-old lady is referred with a 4-week history of cough, dirty sputum, intermittent haemoptysis and one stone (6.35 kg) of weight loss. She is on her second course of antibiotics. She smokes 20 cigarettes per day, with a 40 pack/year history. She has a history of hypertension and angina, and her exercise tolerance is one quarter mile.

Her investigations are as follows:

+ Spirometry: FEV_1 1.7 (80% predicted), FVC 2.3 (90% predicted), ratio 73%, transfer factor 65%.

+ Chest X-ray: left lower lobe soft tissue mass.

+ CT scan of thorax with contrast: mass at the left lower lobe 4.5 cm × 2 cm. Left hilar node 1.5 cm, sub-carinal node 1.5 cm. No metastatic disease seen.

+ Bronchoscopy: evidence of tumour past the origin of the left lower lobe bronchus.

+ Pathology: in keeping with non-small cell lung carcinoma, squamous in origin.

+ PET CT scan: left lower lobe mass, SUV max 7.5. Left hilar node is fludeoxyglucose avid, the sub-carinal node had no uptake.

Her case is discussed at the lung cancer multidisciplinary meeting. What other investigation is likely to be requested before treatment can be started?

A. **Endobronchial ultrasound with biopsy of sub-carinal node**
B. **CT scan of brain**
C. **Shuttle walk test**
D. **Cardiopulmonary exercise stress test**
E. **Cardiac angiography**

CASE 8

A 68-year-old man with a 60 pack/year smoking history was referred to clinic. He complains of a cough that has been present for more than six weeks, and has an abnormal chest X-ray. He also complains of fatigue and weight loss. His performance status is 1. A CT scan was carried out showing a right lower lobe mass, with adjacent right hilar lymphadenopathy (see Figure 13.3).

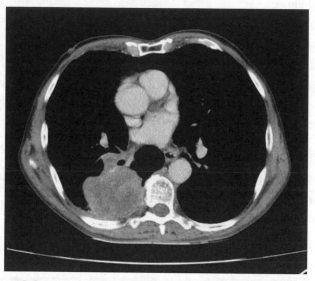

Figure 13.3

Bronchoscopy was performed, and small cell lung cancer was confirmed from biopsy samples. He was referred to the oncology team. A CT scan of brain was carried out and showed no focal abnormality.

What is the treatment plan most likely to be proposed for this man?

- A. **Chemotherapy alone**
- B. **Chemotherapy + radiotherapy to chest**
- C. **Chemotherapy + chest radiotherapy + prophylactic cranial radiotherapy**
- D. **Surgery**
- E. **Palliative care alone**

CASE 9

A 35-year-old lady with a long history of asthma has been referred back to clinic. She complains of an increase in symptoms with a wheeze and cough at night. She has had occasional sputum. Eight weeks ago a chest X-ray showed a patch of consolidation. She was given oral antibiotics and steroids and made a good improvement. She states that she is taking three puffs of her combination inhaler twice per day; in addition she is using her short-acting β agonist four to five times per day. There have been no obvious environmental changes to account for the deterioration in her condition. On examination there is equal air entry bilaterally, no crackles and generalised expiratory wheeze. A chest X-ray was repeated and there was no consolidation or focal changes.

Which action is least helpful?

A. **Check total IgE**
B. **Check inhaler compliance with GP records**
C. **IgG aspergillus precipitins**
D. **Sputum culture with fungal testing**
E. **CT scan of chest**

CASE 10

An 18-year-old man is brought to the emergency department with an acute onset of dyspnoea and wheeze. He has a history of asthma and is on regular inhalers. He has had viral symptoms for two days. On arrival, you find that his airway is patent and oxygen is being delivered at 10 litre/min via a non-rebreather mask. He is unable to complete sentences. There is audible wheeze and poor air entry bilaterally. Oxygen saturation is 94%. Respiratory rate is 28 breaths/min. The pulse rate is 108 bpm and blood pressure is 110/68 mmHg. The capillary refill time is two seconds. He is alert. Capillary blood glucose is 4.9 mmol/litre, and his pupils are equal and reacting to light. A blood gas analysis reveals: pH 7.38, PaO_2 11.2 kPa, $PaCO_2$ 4.0 kPa. He is given salbutamol and ipatropium bromide by nebuliser, 40 mg prednisolone orally and 2 g magnesium sulfate intravenously. A repeat blood gas analysis reveals: pH 7.36, PaO_2 9.1 kPa, $PaCO_2$ 5.1 kPa.

What is the most appropriate next step in management?

A. **Continue with current management and repeat ABG in one hour**
B. **Give IM adrenaline**
C. **Start an IV salbutamol infusion**
D. **Load with IV aminophylline**
E. **Refer to the intensive care unit**

CASE 11

A 25-year-old lady presents with cough, shortness of breath, fever and headache. She has no history of chest disease, is on no regular medications and is a non-smoker. She works as an accountant. On examination, her respiratory rate is 24 breaths/min, oxygen saturation 93% on room air, pulse rate 92 bpm, blood pressure 114/72 mmHg and temperature 37.5 °C. On auscultation there are basal inspiratory squeaks and crackles, but no wheeze. White cells 12×10^9/litre, neutrophils 11×10^9/litre, eosinophils 0.3×10^9/litre, C-reactive protein 30 mg/litre. The biochemistry was otherwise within normal limits. Her chest X-ray shows infiltrates bibasally, but worse on the left. She is given oral antibiotics and discharged with a diagnosis of a community-acquired pneumonia (CURB65 0). She presents two months later with similar features. She had developed acute dyspnoea associated with cough and fever. The respiratory rate is now 28 breaths/min, oxygen saturation 91% on room air, pulse rate 96 bpm, blood pressure 118/76 mmHg and temperature 37.6 °C. There are inspiratory squeaks and crackles on auscultation. Her chest X-ray is shown in Figure 13.4, as is an image from her CT scan.

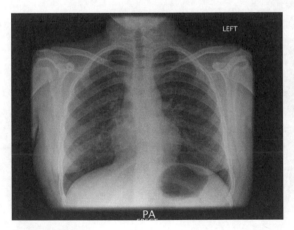
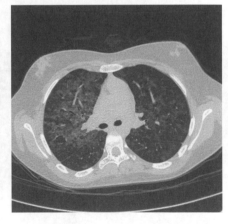

Figure 13.4

Lung function testing shows: FEV$_1$ 1.4 (77% predicted), FVC 1.7 (80% predicted), ratio 82% predicted, and transfer factor 60% predicted. Bronchoscopy shows normal anatomy, no endobronchial lesions and bronchial washings are predominantly lymphocytic (50%). What is the most likely diagnosis?

    A. **Non-specific interstitial pneumonia**
    B. **Acute presentation of sarcoidosis**
    C. **Atypical pneumonia**
    D. **A drug reaction**
    E. **Hypersensitivity pneumonitis**

CASE 12

A 30-year-old man presents with chest pain and shortness of breath for four hours. He has no history of lung disease. He is a smoker of ten cigarettes per day and admits to smoking cannabis occasionally. On examination he shows increased work of breathing. The respiratory rate is 26 breaths/min, oxygen saturation 93% on room air (100% on 10 litre/min oxygen), pulse rate 102 bpm and blood pressure 116/62 mmHg. Chest examination demonstrates reduced breath sounds on the left with reduced expansion and hyper-resonance on the same side. His chest X-ray is shown in Figure 13.5.

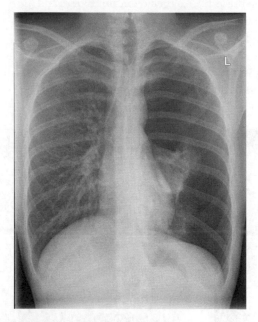

Figure 13.5

What management option should be considered first?

    A. **Oxygen to ensure saturations > 92%**

    B. **Aspirate with large-bore cannula**

    C. **12 G chest drain, Seldinger technique**

    D. **28 G chest drain, blunt dissection**

    E. **CT scan of chest**

CASE 13

A 55-year-old man is referred to clinic for management of his chest symptoms. He has no documented spirometry. He complains of dyspnoea, especially on exertion, cough and sputum mainly in the mornings. His exercise tolerance is half a mile on flat ground when he feels well. He has recently finished a course of antibiotics and steroids. In the last year he has had approximately three courses of each with no hospital admissions. He has been prescribed a long-acting muscarinic antagonist and a combination long-acting β-2 agonist with inhaled corticosteroid. On examination, the respiratory rate is 16 breaths/min, oxygen saturation on room air 95% and blood pressure 132/78 mmHg. Chest examination reveals fair air entry and some expiratory wheeze. ECG shows sinus rhythm. His chest X-ray shows hyperinflated lungs with no consolidation or mass seen.

What pattern are you likely to see on spirometry?

    A. FEV_1 4L (90% predicted)
    B. FEV_1/FVC ratio 84%
    C. Increase in FEV_1 of 250 ml post salbutamol
    D. FEV_1/FVC ratio post bronchodilator 64%
    E. FEV_1 60% predicted, FVC 70% predicted

CASE 14

An 18-year-old lady with cystic fibrosis has been admitted to the ward for treatment of an exacerbation. Her baseline FEV_1 is 65% predicted, but this has fallen to 52%. Her sputum chronically cultures *Pseudomonas aeruginosa* which is multi-resistant; she has also cultured *Stenotrophomonas maltiphilia*. Her weight has dropped by 2 kg in three months, and her body mass index is now 16 kg/m². She has impaired glucose tolerance. She can be poorly compliant with airway clearance and nebulisers. She is studying for her A level examinations. An arterial blood gas analysis on room air revealed: pH 7.37, PaO_2 9.6 kPa, $PaCO_2$ 4.5 kPa. Her current treatment regimen includes IV piperacillin-tazobactam and tobramycin, nebulisers including DNase, dietary supplements, pancreatic enzyme supplements, vitamins and a proton pump inhibitor. She is anxious and asks about needing a lung transplant. What would be most concerning for a transplant team at this point in this patient?

A. **Body mass index**
B. **Lung function**
C. **Culture of *Stenotrophomonas maltophilia***
D. **Impaired glucose tolerance**
E. **Poor compliance to nebulised treatments**

CASE 15

A 66-year-old man is referred with an unresolved chest infection. He has had dyspnoea on exertion, and a dry cough lasting more than eight weeks. He has taken two courses of antibiotics with little improvement. He feels unwell with malaise and myalgia, and he has lost 2 kg in eight weeks. He is a non-smoker, has no past medical history and takes no regular medications. On examination, there is no finger clubbing, respiratory rate is 20 breaths/min, oxygen saturation 93% on room air, pulse rate 88 bpm, blood pressure 138/72 mmHg and temperature 37.2 °C. A few scattered crackles are heard on chest examination. Urinalysis is normal. Blood tests reveal: white cells 12×10^9/litre, neutrophil count 10×10^9/litre, C-reactive protein 48 mg/litre, ESR 36 mm/1st hour. Routine biochemical testing is unremarkable. Spirometry is mildly restrictive in nature. His chest X-ray shows patchy bilateral infiltrates. Sputum culture shows no growth. There is no clinical or radiological improvement with a further course of antibiotics. A high-resolution CT scan of the chest shows areas of consolidation, with air bronchograms and areas of ground glass change in basal and subpleural areas. Bronchoscopy shows no endobronchial lesions and mixed inflammatory cells (lymphocytes, neutrophils and eosinophils) are seen on analysis of lavage fluid.

What is the most likely diagnosis?

- A. **Eosinophilic pneumonia**
- B. **Cryptogenic organising pneumonia**
- C. **Bronchoalveloar carcinoma**
- D. **Pulmonary vasculitis**
- E. **Lymphoid interstitial pneumonia**

CASE 16

A 69-year-old lady is referred with recurrent chest infections. She states that she has had two or three infections every year for many years and recently she has had an infection that required two courses of antibiotics to resolve. She describes a chronic cough with daily sputum which can vary in colour from clear to very green, but has never had haemoptysis. She also describes feeling more breathless on exertion over the last year. She is an ex-smoker, having stopped 25 years ago. She previously smoked 20 cigarettes per day for 20 years. Her GP sent a sputum sample during her last infection, which grew *Moraxella catarrhalis*.

A high-resolution CT scan of chest has been carried out, and is shown in Figure 13.6.

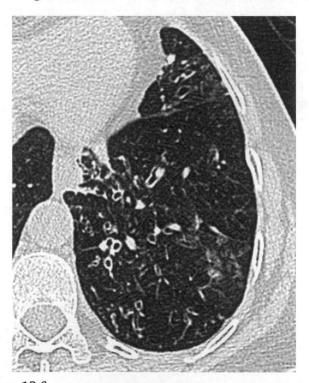

Figure 13.6

What would be the most effective management intervention?

    A. **Immunoglobulin infusion**

    B. **Long-term regular antibiotic therapy**

    C. **Nebulised colomycin**

    D. **Chest physiotherapy with airway clearance at home**

    E. **Surgery**

CASE 17

A 64-year-old lady with a history of advanced breast cancer with known bone metastases is seen in the oncology clinic complaining of dyspnoea and right-sided chest pain, with no cough or spit. A chest X-ray is arranged and it shows a moderate right-sided pleural effusion. She is referred to the respiratory team; a bedside ultrasound shows a significant, simple effusion to a depth of 10 cm. A pleural aspiration is carried out and 500 ml of slightly blood-stained fluid is removed. Analysis shows: pH 7.3, protein 40 g/litre, LDH elevated, gram stain negative, cytology is awaited. A repeat chest X-ray shows a reduced but significant effusion. The lady remains breathless and oxygen-dependent. A decision is made to insert an intercostal drain. If cytology confirms a malignant effusion, what would be the best long-term option for the management of the pleural effusion?

A. **Palliative care after drain removal**
B. **Pleurex catheter**
C. **A successful pleurodesis**
D. **Repeated pleural aspirations when symptomatic**
E. **Surgical pleurectomy**

CASE 18

A 74-year-old man presents with dyspnoea on exertion, dry cough and reduced exercise tolerance over a number of months. He was previously fit and well. He is an ex-smoker and is a retired solicitor with no occupational exposures. He describes no systemic symptoms. On examination he has finger clubbing, oxygen saturation 92% on room air and there are fine end-inspiratory crepitations. FEV_1 2.8 (65% predicted), FVC 3.2, FEV_1:FVC ratio 88% and transfer factor 55% predicted. He has been referred for CT scanning. What pattern on CT are you most likely to see?

A. **Predominantly ground glass change with minimal honeycombing**
B. **Predominantly subpleural, bibasal honeycomb change**
C. **Thick-walled airways with centrilobular nodules**
D. **Patchy ground glass change with air trapping and small nodules**
E. **Consolidative change with air bronchograms**

CASE 1

A: Sputum sent urgently for culture examination for acid fast bacilli

This man most likely has pulmonary tuberculosis (TB). His risk factors include his homelessness, alcohol abuse and apparent poverty. Other risk factors for TB may include country of origin, HIV status and co-existing medical conditions (eg diabetes, renal disease, chemotherapy, anti-TNF therapy and malnutrition).

Although this man has very little sputum, usually patients will be able to produce samples under supervision from a physiotherapist, nurse or doctor. Chest physiotherapy +/– sputum induction would be the next option. Most people with a lung cavity will be able to produce sputum and will be smear positive with a high bacillary load, therefore respiratory personal protective equipment should be used.

If the patient could not produce a sputum sample, bronchoscopy would be the next investigation with washings sent for acid fast bacilli examination, Ziehl–Neelsen staining and culture to assess for the presence of *Mycobacterium tuberculosis* and the antimicrobial sensitivities. However, this procedure is not without risk to the patient and also to the endoscopy staff owing to the high risk of exposure, so is best only being done if there is no alternative.

Sputum sent for routine culture will not identify *M. tuberculosis*.

A CT scan of chest may be helpful, and may be required; however it will not give a definite diagnosis as a differential diagnosis would be lung carcinoma.

Learning point

The Mantoux test is a skin prick test where tuberculin is given intradermally. The result is read at 48 hours. It needs to be interpreted in the context of the clinical picture, ethnic origin and BCG vaccination history. A Mantoux < 5 mm is negative, but one can find a negative Mantoux with active TB, particularly if there is significant immunoparesis or disseminated disease. A Mantoux of 5–15 mm can either indicate infection with TB (either latent or active), or reflect previous BCG exposure. A Mantoux > 15 mm suggests that a patient has or has had TB infection in the past. This could be latent, active or previously treated. The Mantoux test cannot give sensitivities of the organism. Since it is unable to distinguish between latent and active disease, the test is not helpful in this case.

If this gentleman proved to be smear positive for acid fast bacilli on sputum analysis or from the washings taken at bronchoscopy, he would need to be isolated in a negative pressure room. If at home, isolation in the home is advised. An initial PCR test will confirm if the organism is from the *M. tuberculosis* complex, and will give information on the presence or absence of the commonest rifampicin resistance mutation. Rifampicin resistance at PCR is strongly predictive of multi-drug-resistant disease, as isolated rifampicin resistance is rare in the UK. Culture is also key to confirming which member of the *M. tuberculosis* complex is present. If a multi-drug-resistant strain is seen, the patient is no more infectious, but will require more complex treatment for a longer duration with close monitoring, as compliance is vital. They may need a combination of up to five drugs for 12–24 months. Homeless patients on TB treatment should have directly observed therapy (DOT), usually arranged through a TB nurse specialist depending on local provision.

CASE 2

D: Rifampicin + isoniazid + pyrazinamide + ethambutol for two months, then rifampicin and isoniazid for four months

This lady has lymph node *M. tuberculosis*. Full culture results and sensitivities should be sought but treatment should be initiated at the time of confirmation. Treatment regimens can be adjusted if required as cultures can take 8–10 weeks.

The standard treatment is rifampicin + isoniazid + pyrazinamide + ethambutol for two months, changing to rifampicin and isoniazid for a further four months if fully sensitive to first-line drugs and when there are no issues with compliance.

Learning point

There is no change to the treatment regimen in pregnancy; however, this person also needs Vitamin B6 (pyridoxine) for the duration of treatment in pregnancy and while breastfeeding, as she is at higher risk of peripheral neuropathy. Additionally, there is a theoretical risk of isoniazid-related neuropathy in breast-fed babies, so vitamin B6 is also given to mothers who are breast-feeding. The agents are not known to be teratogenic. The outcome in the first trimester of pregnancy is the same as if she was not pregnant. In the second and third trimesters, the outcome is variable. Treatment is advised, as active disease is more harmful to baby and mother. Mothers who are breastfeeding should be advised that the drugs are again safe as there are low concentrations in the milk.

Lymph node disease commonly increases in size on treatment and patients should be advised that this is common and not a sign of treatment failure. Patients starting on anti-tuberculous treatment should be warned of the potential side effects, especially nausea. Rifampicin will turn body fluids an orange/red colour. More concerning effects would be vomiting, jaundice and abdominal pain – if these occur, patients should be advised to stop treatment and attend urgently for assessment including liver function testing. There is reduced efficacy of the oral contraceptive pill. Visual acuity should be measured before starting treatment and during the course owing to the potential effects of ethambutol. Patients should be advised to seek medical advice if there is any deterioration in vision. They should be assessed for the cause of visual deterioration and, if confirmed to be ethambutol related, this would be stopped. Care should also be taken to check for possible drug interactions.

CASE 3

B: Urinary antigens (legionella and pneumococcus)

Urinary antigens is the correct answer, as she has a severe pneumonia.

Learning point

The British Thoracic Society guideline states that patients with moderate and severe community-acquired pneumonia (CAP) should have microbiological tests including blood cultures, sputum for culture and sensitivity, pneumococcal urinary antigen and, in high-severity (CURB65 3–5) CAP, legionella urinary antigen.[1]

This lady has a community-acquired pneumonia with a CURB65 score of 3 (urea > 7 mmol/litre, respiratory rate > 30 breaths/min and age > 65 years; no documented confusion and blood pressure is > 90 mmHg systolic and > 60 mmHg diastolic).

There is no suspicion of TB from the history, so sputum AFB would not be requested at this point, but there should be a low threshold to test for this if there are atypical symptoms or signs. A CT scan is not required at this point as there are no red flag symptoms for cancer and no mass lesion on the chest X-ray. A chest X-ray should be carried out after six weeks to ensure complete resolution, and if there were persisting changes or worrying features, a CT scan should be requested at that stage. Spirometry may be most useful after recovery from the acute infection. This lady may have underlying chronic obstructive pulmonary disease with her significant smoking history. An ABG analysis is not indicated as part of the initial plan as saturations on room air are satisfactory. However, this should be carefully monitored. A drop in saturation of 3% should prompt reassessment, most likely including ABG testing. This may also be helpful in assessing acid–base balance.

continued

**CHAPTER 13
ANSWERS**

Learning point

The definition of CAP comprises symptoms of an acute lower respiratory tract illness, with new focal chest signs on examination, at least one systemic feature (sweats, fevers, shivers, aches, temperatures) and no other explanation of the illness. Everyone admitted to hospital with suspected CAP should have a chest X-ray as soon as possible. A patient with a CURB65 score of 3 or more should be reviewed by a senior doctor at the earliest opportunity, and if they have a score of 4 or 5, they should be assessed as to their need for critical care. Antibiotics should be administered within four hours. Empirical antibiotic regimens should be followed according to local protocol. The decision regarding an oral or intravenous route of administration of antimicrobials should be decided based on the severity of the illness.

CASE 4

C: Reduce inspired oxygen, give nebulised bronchodilators, give steroids and repeat the arterial blood gas analysis

This man has hypercapnic respiratory failure. He most likely has underlying chronic obstructive pulmonary disease (COPD), and has had high-flow oxygen therapy.

The British Thoracic Society guideline for non-invasive ventilation (NIV) states that medical management should be maximised initially. This should include controlled oxygen therapy to maintain oxygen saturation between 88 and 92%, nebulised salbutamol, nebulised ipratroprium, oral prednisolone 30 mg and an antibiotic agent when indicated. Therefore, answer C is correct. If there is no significant improvement, further intervention should be initiated, which would most likely be with NIV.

Clinically this picture does not fit with an exacerbation of heart failure and answer A is therefore not correct. Doxapram is a central nervous system stimulant which can be used as a respiratory stimulant to increase tidal volume and respiratory rate with an expected associated fall in $PaCO_2$ and rise in PaO_2. However, it is very toxic and less effective than NIV, so is rarely used in clinical practice.

If medical management fails in this man, NIV may be the next treatment option to consider; however, if there were concerns about airway patency or if he was deteriorating, the intensive care unit team should be involved. An assessment of functional and pre-morbid state should be made early so that decisions regarding escalation of care and ceiling of treatment can be made. Before starting NIV, a plan should be in place as to what to do if NIV fails. Oxygen therapy is vital – severe hypoxia will cause death more rapidly than hypercarbia. However, in patients with known and suspected hypercarbia, start oxygen therapy at low concentrations and increase gradually to achieve adequate oxygenation. Blood gas analysis should be carried out to ensure $PaCO_2$ and pH levels are satisfactory.

CASE 5

A: Increase IPAP

This man has type two respiratory failure, on the basis of his background of COPD, and he has been over-sedated causing decompensation. After one hour of NIV treatment his blood gas shows little improvement.

Learning point

There are multiple reasons why this may be the case. A common problem often concerns patient compliance, as treatment is uncomfortable and some cannot tolerate the mask. Other issues include air leakage due to a poorly fitting mask or the equipment not being set up properly. Someone experienced in NIV should generally set up and initiate treatment. If there are no issues with the machine or mask, then machine settings may need to be adjusted. An IPAP of 18–20 cm H_2O should be the aim to achieve therapeutic response. Increasing EPAP will improve oxygenation as will increasing the entrained oxygen. In this case, his oxygenation has improved so EPAP and oxygen do not need to be adjusted at this point. If the entrained oxygen concentration is too high, the $PaCO_2$ may continue to be driven up. Target oxygen saturation on NIV should be 88–92%.

If improvement is not made on NIV, intubation and ventilation is a potential treatment option. However, in this case NIV has not been optimised and an increase in IPAP should be attempted.

At the initiation of NIV, decisions should be made in regard to whether escalating care or treatment withdrawal is more appropriate in the event of treatment failure. In this case it is too early to withdraw treatment. An assessment of premorbid and functional state is required to make a fair and accurate assessment, as well as discussions with the family and the patient involved.

CASE 6

B: Heart rate fluctuations per hour

This overnight oximetry recording is non-diagnostic for obstructive sleep apnoea syndrome (OSAS), but is suspicious on the basis of heart rate fluctuation and clinical history. Further investigation will be required. A limited polysomnography (PSG) test should be organised to confirm or rule out OSAS. This study looks at chest wall and abdominal wall movement, air flow and snoring, limb movements as well as oxygen saturation and heart rate. A full PSG (which includes electroencephalography) is not always required – it is more labour-intensive to carry out and report.

Learning point

To diagnose OSAS, look at the oxygen desaturation index (ODI): > 5/hour is abnormal, 15–30/hour is moderate and > 30/hour is severe. The patient in this question has an ODI of 6.6, which is abnormal, but not diagnostic. The fluctuation in heart rate may indicate arousal or partial arousal from sleep in keeping with hypopnoeas, which are not picked up as full apnoeic episodes. This is the most significant finding from this overnight oximetry test. Mean and minimum oxygen saturation can add more information, but are not diagnostic in OSAS.

Obstructive sleep apnoea syndrome is the repetitive collapsing of the upper airway with associated arousal from sleep to reactivate muscle strength to resolve hypoxia and hypercapnia. Hypopneas are incomplete obstructions causing fragmented sleep, which therefore causes daytime sleepiness. OSAS is where the patient is sleepy during the day also.

If proven on limited PSG, treatment will include advice regarding lifestyle measures, weight loss, reducing alcohol (especially at night), smoking cessation, adjusting medications (especially sedatives) and generally improving sleep hygiene. Mandibular advancement devices may be helpful in some cases. These are devices to bring the bottom jaw forward to help in keeping the pharynx open. They are poorly tolerated in many cases.

For significant OSA with sleepiness, continuous positive airways pressure (CPAP) is used. It uses room air under pressure to splint open the oropharynx to reduce arousals, reduce sleep fragmentation, improve sleep quality and therefore reduce daytime sleepiness. It can be highly effective and improve quality of life significantly. Some people find CPAP difficult to use, and compliance can be an issue.

continued

Patients with OSAS should be told never to drive if sleepy and they should notify the Driver and Vehicle Licensing Agency and their motor insurance company. When treated, they should be safe to drive. Untreated OSAS can cause significant morbidity including poor concentration, accidents, memory problems and increased cardiovascular risk.

CASE 7

D: Cardiopulmonary exercise stress test

This lady has a T2a, N1, M0 squamous cell lung carcinoma. She has been fully assessed and appropriately discussed at a lung cancer multidisciplinary meeting. These meetings should include respiratory physicians, thoracic surgeons, oncologists (clinical and medical), a pathologist, a radiologist with an interest in thoracic imaging and a palliative care team including a lung cancer specialist nurse.

Potentially this lady has curative disease by means of surgery; however, it has to be established if she is fit enough to undergo this surgery.

Endobronchial ultrasound guided biopsy of the sub-carinal node would be required if the PET CT findings were indeterminate. In this case, however, the report shows no uptake and the node is therefore not likely to be involved. A CT scan of brain would not routinely be requested unless there were specific indications. The shuttle walk test can be helpful as a functional assessment tool, but cannot assess cardiac function.

Learning point

A cardiopulmonary exercise stress test measures VO_2 max as well as other parameters. It looks at oxygen consumption, carbon dioxide production and cardiac function. It will determine if the patient's limiting factor is their pulmonary or cardiac function, and will be most helpful in assessing if this lady will be fit for curative surgery.

If she is not fit for curative surgery, assessment would be made to see if she would benefit from radical radiotherapy with potentially curative intent.

A cardiac angiogram may be required if there were concerns regarding her ECG during cardiopulmonary exercise stress testing. This may indicate that a patient is not fit for surgery.

A lung cancer nurse should be available at every stage of the diagnosis and treatment for both patients and carers. Smoking cessation should be encouraged at every stage; however, surgery should not be postponed for this reason.

In non-small cell adenocarcinomas, epidermal growth factor receptor and anaplastic lymphoma kinase testing may be carried out. If positive, targeted chemotherapy agents may be used with good response. These therapies are biological agents used in the palliative treatment of lung cancer, but would not influence treatment choice in the radical setting.

CASE 8

C: Chemotherapy + chest radiotherapy + prophylactic cranial radiotherapy

This man has limited stage small cell lung cancer. Small cell cancer accounts for 10–15% of lung cancers and has either limited or extensive staging. Limited stage disease is confined to the ipsilateral hemithorax; extensive stage is disease anywhere else. Anyone with confirmed small cell lung cancer should be referred to an oncologist urgently and should be seen within a week.

Learning point

The treatment approach will depend on fitness and co-morbidities. If fit (performance status 0–1), combined chemotherapy and radiotherapy would be used. Chemotherapy would be a cisplatin-based combination for four to six cycles. Concurrent radiotherapy would be offered if the tumour, at diagnosis, was suitable to be encompassed within a radical radiotherapy field. Radiotherapy is commenced with the second cycle of chemotherapy to allow time for radiotherapy planning.

For extensive stage disease, a platinum-based chemotherapy regimen would be used for a maximum of six cycles if fit. Prophylactic cranial irradiation should be offered to most of those with limited disease unless they have progressed on first-line treatment, and in those with extensive disease, if the performance status is 2 or less and they have had a good response to chemotherapy. It is advised at the completion of chemotherapy, and has been shown to improve survival by 5.4%.

Survival without treatment is very poor – approximately 6–12 weeks. With treatment, in limited disease, median survival is 18–20 months.

This man would most likely have combined chemotherapy, radiotherapy and prophylactic cranial irradiation.

Small cell lung cancer is associated with a number of paraneoplastic syndromes. The syndrome of inappropriate antidiuretic hormone presents with hyponatraeima. Symptoms are non-specific. Patients are usually euvolaemic. Tests include urinary electrolytes (sodium usually > 40 mmol/litre), urinary osmolality (> 100 mOsmol/kg) and serum osmolality (< 275 mOsmol/kg). Management in the first instance is to fluid-restrict. Other treatments can be considered if this is unsuccessful.

Other paraneoplastic manifestations include: ectopic ACTH production with Cushing's syndrome, Eaton–Lambert myasthenic syndrome, cerebellar syndrome and limbic encephalitis.

Lymphangitis carcinomatosis is seen in all types of lung cancer (and other cancers) when pulmonary lymphatics are infiltrated with tumour. It causes dyspnoea and cough. The chest X-ray may show fine linear shadowing throughout both lung fields. It can resemble pulmonary oedema, and can be more readily diagnosed on CT scanning. Treatment with steroids and diuretics can help with symptoms, but is usually short-lived. It is often a sign of very advanced disease.

Performance scales are important in assessment in lung cancer and there are two scales commonly used. Please refer to Chapter 10, Oncology and Palliative Medicine – performance scales.

CASE 9

E: CT scan of chest

> ### Learning point
>
> Her deterioration in symptoms could be for a variety of reasons and she should be fully investigated. Checking that asthma is the correct diagnosis is appropriate.

A peak flow diary may be helpful, but at clinic, reversibility testing with a short-acting β-2 agonist may be more reliable. $FEV_1 > 15\%$ (200 ml) after salbutamol (inhaled or nebulised) is diagnostic.

Checking compliance is important – this can be done by checking GP prescription records. Her inhaler technique should also be assessed.

As the chest X-ray and examination are unremarkable, there is no immediate indication for a CT scan. Other factors potentially causing deterioration here would include aspergillus sensitisation. Aspergillus is a commonly encountered fungus with a wide range of effects. Asthmatics with an IgE response to aspergillus can develop precipitins (IgG antibodies). Spores can grow within airways causing mucous plugging and flitting areas of consolidation. This would be treated with inhaled steroids, and possibly a course of oral steroids, to reduce the inflammatory response and prevent progression. IgE levels in asthma are often raised, and are associated with atopy, allergic rhinitis and eczema. These patients may have positive skin prick testing to common allergens. Eosinophil counts can be raised in asthma, especially if there is associated eczema, but a total eosinophil count of $> 1 \times 10^9$ is unusual, and should raise the possibility of an alternative diagnosis.

Allergic bronchopulmonary aspergillosis is probably a progression of the previously described reaction with inflammatory airway damage and resulting bronchiectasis in a central pattern in the upper lobes. As well as deteriorating asthma symptoms, patients may have mucous plugging, dark mucous, blood and sputum eosinophilia, and possibly haemoptysis (not a feature of the case described). The chest X-ray may show flitting infiltrates, bronchiectatic change and mucous impaction. This requires treatment involving steroids, at high doses, and itraconazole (> 4 months with liver function test monitoring). Response and relapse should be monitored with IgG precipitins to aspergillus. Other forms of aspergillus disease include invasive aspergillus pneumonia, semi-invasive aspergillosis, aspergilloma and hypersensitivity pneumonitis secondary to aspergillus spores.

CASE 10

E: Refer to the intensive care unit

> ### Learning point
>
>
>
> This man presented with acute severe asthma and, despite appropriate treatment, he deteriorates and develops features of life-threatening asthma. These include: a peak expiratory flow rate < 33% predicted/best, oxygen saturation < 92%, PaO_2 < 8 kPa, silent chest, reduced respiratory effort, a normal $PaCO_2$, cyanosis, cardiac arrthymias, confusion, exhaustion and coma.

The correct answer is to refer to ICU – early referral is preferable for assessment even if he does improve and does not need to go. IV salbutamol is not included in the management of acute severe asthma as the evidence for its use is unclear. It is mentioned as a treatment option for children > 2 years as a single IV bolus in the British Thoracic Society (BTS) guidelines. If the nebulised route is unreliable, the intravenous route can be considered, and usually the IV route is reserved for those patients who are in extremis or who are already ventilated, although there is little evidence to support this practice. IV aminophylline is not in the BTS guideline. It is unlikely to show any additional bronchodilation over the treatments already mentioned. Aminophylline also has significant side effects including vomiting and arrhythmias. If required, it should be used in an intensive care unit setting. IM adrenaline would be used in anaphylaxis, but is not commonly employed in life-threatening asthma. The BTS/Scottish Intercollegiate Guidelines Network (SIGN) guideline on the management of asthma includes a section on specific management of adolescents, 10–19 years old.[2] This is a guide to specific problems in this age group including problems with communication and confidentiality regarding patients and their parents, associations with anxiety and depression, the transition to adult asthma services, issues with inhaler technique and compliance in school, and the need to develop age-appropriate self-management plans.

Follow-up of this man after discharge from hospital should include further education regarding his condition, asthma nurse follow-up, asthma clinic attendance and the provision of a self-management plan with specific pointers as to when to increase medications and when to seek help. Any psychosocial issues should also be addressed. Patients with severe asthma and adverse psychosocial factors are at risk of death.

The stepwise management of asthma as described in the BTS/SIGN guideline should be followed.

continued

CHAPTER 13 ANSWERS

Exhaled nitric oxide is a helpful measurement in asthma and is being increasingly used in clinical practice. It is highly sensitive, and more work is required to elucidate the role of this tool. < 25 parts per billion (ppb) is considered normal; > 50 ppb is highly predictive of eosinophilic airway inflammation and a positive response to corticosteroid therapy.

Omalizumab is a humanised monoclonal antibody which binds to circulating IgE, markedly reducing levels of free serum IgE. In adults and children over six years of age, it is licensed in the UK for those patients on high-dose inhaled steroids and long-acting β-2 agonists who have impaired lung function, are symptomatic with frequent exacerbations and have allergy as an important cause of their asthma. Omalizumab is given as a subcutaneous injection every two to four weeks depending on dose. This is usually prescribed by a tertiary asthma centre.

CASE 11

E: Hypersensitivity pneumonitis

This lady has acute hypersensitivity pneumonitis (HP), previously known as extrinsic allergic alveolitis, which can be acute, chronic or subacute, and is caused by the inhalation of organic antigens.

Learning point

There are a wide range of causative agents. In the acute form, symptoms can develop four to eight hours post exposure to the antigen. The chronic form typically presents with progressive dyspnoea, dry cough and weight loss. Investigation hinges on radiology. On plain X-ray, in acute HP, there can be diffuse infiltrates with tiny nodules. Alternatively, the chest X-ray can be normal. In chronic HP, reticular change is predominant in the upper and mid-zones; however, high-resolution CT scanning of the chest will be most useful. In acute HP there may be ground glass change, with poorly defined nodules and increased lucency on expiratory views representing air trapping. Pulmonary function testing typically shows a restrictive pattern with a reduced transfer factor. Blood testing typically shows neutrophilia, not eosinophilia. IgG precipitins can be found in up to 90% of cases. Bronchoalveolar lavage often shows a lypmhocytosis, but this is not diagnostic. To make a diagnosis there needs to be a history of exposure, clinical features and CT findings.

Finding the causative agent can be difficult. A detailed history is required, including details of home circumstances, and places where the patient has stayed and visited. Duck and goose down duvets or pillows, pets, chemical exposures (paints), mouldy hay and contaminated water are all known to be causes, among others. Management is mainly in avoiding the trigger, if known. Treatment is required when patients are unwell; this usually involves steroids and there is normally a good response. Acute HP does not necessarily progress to the chronic form, and patients with chronic HP do not always have acute episodes.

This is not a typical picture for non-specific interstitial pneumonia (NSIP). This patient is younger than the typical NSIP patient (40–50 years) and the presentation is more acute than would be expected – usually six months to three years of symptoms. A high-resolution CT scan would show ground glass change and fine reticulations with minimal honeycombing. Sarcoidosis is a multisystem disease with a range of presentations and severity. Patients often have lymphadenopathy and parenchymal infiltrates, and can progress to fibrosis. This case is not typical for sarcoidosis. Atypical pneumonia is unlikely. This disease would be expected to produce more focal signs on chest X-ray and CT. It is unlikely to cause air trapping, ground glass change and a significant reduction in transfer factor. However, it would be a differential diagnosis and could be ruled out after investigation (sputum culture, urinary antigen analysis and respiratory viral panel). A drug reaction could explain some of these symptoms and results; however, no history has been given in this regard. 'Pneumotox' is a useful online resource for checking known drug reactions that may cause lung disease.

CASE 12

B: Aspirate with large-bore cannula

This man has a significant pneumothorax and is symptomatic. On chest X-ray it is measured as > 2 cm at the level of the hilum (this is the measurement commonly used in the UK; in other countries, different measurements may be used to assess the size of a pneumothorax).

Pneumothoraces can be subdivided into primary, secondary and traumatic (including iatrogenic). Spontaneous primary pneumothoraces (SPP) are more common in tall, thin, younger men with no underlying lung disease. Tobacco smoking is a risk factor, as is cannabis smoking. Patients with secondary pneumothoraces are generally older, with a smoking history and with evidence of underlying lung disease on examination or on chest X-ray. Causes include chronic obstructive pulmonary disease, asthma, interstitial lung disease, tuberculosis, *Pneumocystis jiroveci* pneumonia (PJP), cystic fibrosis, Langerhans' cell histiocytosis and others.

Learning point

In SPP, if a patient is asymptomatic, management may be the administration of high-flow oxygen and observation with repeat X-rays. If the patient is symptomatic, aspiration should be the first intervention. This is performed using an aseptic technique, with local anaesthetic, a large-bore cannula and a three-way tap. If symptoms improve and on X-ray the size of the pneumothorax has decreased, further intervention may not be required. If the size of the pneumothorax remains unchanged and symptoms remain, a chest drain will be required.

Chest drains are associated with significant morbidity and potential mortality. They are usually placed in the 'triangle of safety' – the triangle bordered by the anterior border of the latissimus dorsi, the lateral border of the pectoralis major muscle, a line superior to the horizontal level of the nipple, and an apex below the axilla. Smaller drains (8–14 G) are usually sufficient in SPP. Larger drains (24–28 G) should be used in trauma cases, secondary pneumothoraces, with severe subcutaneous emphysema, and in mechanically ventilated patients with pneumothoraces.

Be aware of tension pneumothoraces. Patients present with respiratory distress, agitation, hypotension, raised jugular venous pressure and tracheal deviation away from the affected side with reduced air entry on the same side. Treatment is to decompress with a large-bore cannula inserted into the second intercostal space, mid-clavicular line on the side of the pneumothorax, followed by a chest drain.

continued

CT scanning is helpful in assessing the size of a pneumothorax, looking for underlying lung disease and for guiding placement of chest drains in complex cases.

Recurrence is common. In SPP, the recurrence rate varies between 16 and 54%. In secondary pneumothoraces, there is also variability, but recurrence can be as high as 80% for Langerhans' cell histiocytosis. Mortality in secondary pneumothoraces is approximately 10%.

High-flow oxygen can be given unless contraindicated. Oxygen may reduce the partial pressure of nitrogen in the blood and encourages removal of air from the pleural space. It may help resolution of pneumothoraces, although there is no evidence for this. This approach can limit a patient's mobility, which could be detrimental. A balance should be sought.

If there is a persistent air leak for > 48 hours, suction should be considered. If a small drain is being used, a large-bore drain should be considered and thoracic surgical referral made. The thoracic surgical team should also be involved if a patient has recurrent pneumothoraces or if they work in a profession at risk, eg a pilot or diver.

In the context of a patient with HIV, PJP treatment should be given empirically. Chest drain insertion and surgical referral should be made early.

In cystic fibrosis, pneumothorax is associated with severe lung disease and is treated as a secondary pneumothorax. Patients will most likely need a chest drain +/- antibiotics. Again surgical referral should be made early and discussion with the local transplant team should take place if this is likely to be a future consideration, as some pleural procedures make transplantation more difficult.

Catamenial pneumothorax is the name given to pneumothoraces whose onset is associated with menstruation and are usually recurrent. This phenomenon may be due to pleural endometriosis. Treatment usually requires surgical intervention and hormone therapy.

Diving is not advised at all unless a definitive surgical procedure has been carried out. Flying is not advised until there is clear evidence of resolution, and guidelines state it is prudent to leave flying for a week after this.

CASE 13

D: FEV$_1$/FVC ratio post bronchodilator 64%

This man clinically has chronic obstructive pulmonary disease (COPD) and obstructive lung function would be expected as in answer D. Spirometry should be interpreted by appropriate personnel. It is a measurement of the volume of expired air against time. Many other measurements are possible in the lung function lab.

> ### Learning point
>
> For diagnosis the main measurements are FEV$_1$ and FVC. The FEV$_1$ is the amount of air blown out in the first second after maximal inspiration (following maximal exhalation). FVC is the maximum amount of air blown out in a forced manoeuvre. The proportion of FEV$_1$ against FVC is a clinically useful index of air flow limitation: < 70% is diagnostic of COPD. FEV$_1$ is then used to assess severity – mild is > 80% predicted, moderate is 50–80% predicted, severe is 30–50% predicted, and very severe < 30% (GOLD guideline).[3] Measurements should be taken post bronchodilators.

In asthma, reversibility after bronchodilators is considered diagnostic if there is an increase of > 200 ml in FEV$_1$.

Restrictive lung disease shows a reduction in both FEV$_1$ and FVC with a maintained ratio. Serial measurements of spirometry are often more useful than one isolated result, especially in the context of an acute exacerbation.

The management of an acute exacerbation includes increased bronchodilators, often in nebulised form, antibiotics if sputum is purulent, oral steroids (as effective as intravenous preparations), oxygen if required, arterial blood gas analysis to look for respiratory failure, physiotherapy and mucolytic agents.

Overall management of COPD includes stopping smoking (this is vitally important at every stage) and engaging in physical activity. Avoidance of air pollution at work, outside and in the home is also important.

Inhaled therapy is important and options for therapy have increased greatly in recent years. Bronchodilators and inhaled corticosteroids (ICS) are recommended. If FEV$_1$ is > 50% predicted, choose a long-acting β-2 agonist (LABA) or a long-acting muscarinic antagonist (LAMA). If FEV$_1$ is < 50% predicted, use a LABA/ICS combination or LAMA. If patients are short of breath on a single agent, consider using a LABA/ICS and LAMA together.

continued

Other factors to consider are involvement of the multidisciplinary team, including respiratory nurses, physiotherapists, dieticians, occupational therapists, social workers and the palliative care team in advanced disease. Long-term oxygen therapy or ambulatory oxygen, theophyllines, inhibitors of phosphodiesterase type four, mucolytic agents and vaccinations should all be considered in appropriate patients. In COPD, antioxidants, antitussive agents and prophylactic antibiotics are not part of treatment plans routinely.

The other important intervention available is pulmonary rehabilitation. These programmes have been shown through meta-analysis and randomised control trials to provide benefit to patients. They are cost-effective and potentially reduce disability, improve quality of life and restore independence. They improve functional exercise and health status. No improvement in exacerbation rate has been shown, but patients with exacerbations have shorter hospital stays. Patients perform better on walk testing and there is a subjective reduction in dyspnoea. After the programme has finished (usually after six to eight weeks), there is some carry over with the improvements felt, but patients require a maintenance programme or repeat course to maintain benefit. Any patient with chronic lung disease should be referred; before this, their medical management should be maximised and patients should be well motivated. Those with long-term oxygen therapy are not excluded. Those felt to be unsuitable include patients with unstable angina, severe heart valve disease, cognitive impairment or locomotor problems. Classes involve physical exercise, education, psychological support, smoking cessation advice and nutritional advice. Many find meeting others in a similar position beneficial.

CASE 14

A: Body mass index

At this point the most concerning feature is that of her low body mass index (BMI).

> ### Learning point
>
> Ideally for transplant, BMI should be > 17 kg/m² (and < 30 kg/m²). FEV_1 is down from baseline values and would be expected to improve again with appropriate treatment of the exacerbation. Transplantation should be considered if FEV_1 < 30% predicted or if > 30% but with a rapid decline over a short period of time. Young women with a rapid deterioration have a poor prognosis and therefore should be considered early for transplant assessment. Respiratory failure (PaO_2 < 7.3 kPa and $PaCO_2$ > 6.7 kPa) is associated with a < 50% survival at two years without transplantation. *Stenotrophomonas maltophilia*, although often resistant, is not a contraindication to transplantation. The presence of *Burkholderia cenocepacia* on culture would be worrying. Patients with this are not transplantable, and they have been shown to do poorly after surgery. These patients generally do less well and have worse outcomes overall. Other subgroups can do better and may be transplanted.

B. cenocepacia is one strain of a group of *B. cepacia* complex. Infection control measures are vital to separate *B. cepacia*-affected and non-*B. cepacia*-affected patients to prevent cross infection. This means separate clinics and wards.

Impaired glucose tolerance is not a contraindication to transplantation; however, uncontrolled diabetes or diabetes causing target organ damage can prevent a patient getting a transplant. Other conditions that make transplantation difficult or impossible would include osteoporosis, uncontrolled hypertension and coronary artery disease.

Transplant assessment also looks at compliance with therapy, motivation, social support, mental illness and emotional state, as all these factors can affect the post-operative period and beyond. Often these can be modified if required. Non-compliance with tablet medications is taken more seriously than with time-consuming nebulisers and airway clearance measures.

In cystic fibrosis (CF), many other issues should be addressed. 70% of CF patients have the F508del/F508del mutation, although many other mutations exist. As a result there is a spectrum of disease severity. Respiratory factors: it is important to maintain lung function and monitor sputum cultures. Nutritional factors: often patients need nutritional support,

continued

either with supplements or enteral feeding; weight should be monitored and advice may be needed regarding enzymes and vitamins. Gastrointestinal factors: there is annual screening for liver cirrhosis and portal hypertension. Endocrine factors: at the age of 30 years, approximately 50% of patients will have CF-related diabetes. Patients should have yearly screening.

Other factors include the assessment of psychosocial wellbeing and fertility advice (often women can be sub-fertile and men may have absent vas deferens). As therapies improve, more patients with CF are becoming pregnant, which raises other management difficulties. To address all of these areas, the attention of a full multidisciplinary team is required.

Treatment of exacerbations should be based on the most up-to-date sputum analysis results or on the last course of effective antibiotics for that patient. Generally, antibiotics are given at higher doses and for longer courses than would normally be the case. Nebulised antibiotics can also be used, often in monthly cycles to try to avoid antibiotic resistance. Intravenous access can be difficult so mid/long lines or tunnelled central lines should be considered. Antibiotic resistance can develop as multiple courses are required, and allergic reactions can develop; antibiotic desensitisation can be undertaken. Physiotherapy is important in management, and airway clearance at home helps patients keep well. Anti-mucolytic nebulisers (eg DNase) are used to cleave DNA from dead neutrophils, reducing sputum viscosity and helping clearance. These are not effective for all patients.

Management of other systemic manifestations are important, eg gastro-oesophageal reflux disease, pancreatitis, liver cirrhosis, portal hypertension, osteoporosis, arthropathy, vasculitis and nasal problems.

One genotype, G551Dl (4–5% of patients), now has a targeted gene therapy called ivacaftor, which has been shown to improve lung function and reduce exacerbation rates.

CHAPTER 13
ANSWERS

CASE 15

B: Cryptogenic organising pneumonia

This is most likely to be cryptogenic organising pneumonia (COP), previously known as bronchiolitis obliterans organising pneumonia (BOOP, one of the idiopathic interstitial pneumonias).

Learning point

COP causes plugging of alveolar spaces with granulation tissue. It can be idiopathic (cryptogenic) or secondary to a variety of other causes, eg infection, drug reactions, radiotherapy, connective tissue disease and many others. It can take weeks to diagnose and is often mistaken for a slow-to-resolve chest infection. Transbronchial biopsy can be helpful in diagnosis. It may show plugging of the alveolar spaces with granulation tissue; the lung architecture is preserved in most cases. Treatment is with steroids at high doses for prolonged courses. Most patients see a dramatic improvement, and if not, the diagnosis should be reconsidered. Prognosis is generally good; however, on weaning down steroid doses, relapse can be common. Steroid-sparing agents, such as azathioprine and cyclophosphamide are often used.

Eosinophilic pneumonia can be acute or chronic. The acute form has a short presentation over a few days. Patients become unwell with fever, cough and dyspnoea; they are often hypoxic. X-rays show interstital or alveolar infiltrates. Lavage shows very high eosinophil counts. There are typically no eosinophils in peripheral blood. Treatment is with steroids. Chronic eosinophilic pneumonia has a longer duration of onset with pronounced systemic symptoms. Patients can have haemoptysis, night sweats, asthma-like symptoms, cough, sputum and dyspnoea. There is sputum eosinophilia, but blood levels can be normal. X-rays show peripheral dense opacities with ill-defined margins. Treatment is also with steroids.

Pulmonary vasculitis is rare and features can be non-specific – they often mimic other conditions. This condition should be suspected if there is weight loss, raised inflammatory markers, and a lack of response to regular treatments. Granulomatosis with polyangiitis (previously known as Wegener's granulomatosis) is associated with ENT symptoms in 90% of cases. Patients often present with haemoptysis, pleuritic chest pain and a purpuric rash. Urinalysis can show haematuria and proteinuria. There are often cavitating lesions on chest imaging. Goodpasture's disease is also commonly associated with haemoptysis and abnormal urinalysis. Pulmonary haemorrhage and ground glass change can be seen on CT imaging.

continued

A bronchoalveolar carcinoma is an adenocarcinoma and can present with patches of apparent consolidation. COP can also present atypically with an isolated area of abnormality that is often presumed to be a malignant lesion. Biopsy and radiological follow-up is required in these cases to ensure appropriate treatment. The typical history in lymphoid interstitial pneumonia is much longer, over many months or years with cough and dyspnoea. It is a very rare condition that is characterised by diffuse lymphoid infiltrates. Malignant transformation is recognised. High-resolution CT scanning shows predominantly ground glass change, often with reticulations and occasionally honeycombing. Lavage shows non-clonal lymphocytosis. It may progress in one third of cases to extensive fibrosis.

CASE 16

D: Chest physiotherapy with airway clearance at home

This is a typical history and CT scan for a patient with bronchiectasis, which is irreversible, abnormal dilatation of bronchi with chronic airways inflammation associated with sputum production, recurrent infections and airways obstruction. There are extensive causes and associations to be considered when assessing these patients.

Learning point

Investigation should aim to confirm the diagnosis and look for the cause or associated conditions, as many of these are potentially treatable. Investigations may include: sputum analysis – culture and tests for acid fast bacilli, pulmonary function testing, measurement of immunoglobulins, aspergillus precipitins, cystic fibrosis genotyping in appropriate patient groups, autoantibodies, skin prick testing, bronchoscopy and swallow imaging. A high-resolution CT scan (HRCT) along with the clinical history is usually diagnostic. On HRCT, typical findings include airway dilation and thickening with a lack of tapering of bronchioles. The 'signet ring sign' is common – when the thickened dilated bronchi are larger than the accompanying vascular bundle.

Aims of management involve treating any underlying causes, preventing infective episodes and dealing with any infective episodes effectively. Physiotherapy is a key element of management. This may involve patients clearing their own airways, active cycle of breathing, postural drainage, cough augmentation or acapella devices. Nebulised drugs and oral mucolytic agents can also be used.

Knowledge of sputum microbiology is important to assess for antibiotic resistance and so that targeted antibiotic therapy can be used. Patients with bronchiectasis may need higher doses of antibiotics than normal, and these are often continued for 10–14 days. There is often a typical order of progressive bacterial colonisation starting with *Staphylococcus aureus*, *Haemophilus influenza*, *Moraxella catarrhalis* and then *Pseudomonas* species. An attempt to eradicate these when present is important. Infection with *Pseudomonas* may cause more frequent and severe exacerbations, worsening of symptoms and a faster decline of lung function. Commonly, oral ciprofloxacin is used as first-line agent with nebulised colomycin. Patients with *Pseudomonas* who are unwell often need courses of intravenous antibiotics – usually an anti-pseudomonal penicillin and an aminoglycoside.

Self-management plans are important, and give patients a degree of control of their disease. Patients should be advised to have annual influenza and pneumococcal vaccinations (as should all patients with chronic lung diseases).

Immunoglobulin infusions may be indicated if a specific deficiency is identified. This treatment is usually managed in conjunction with an immunologist.

Long-term antibiotics may be indicated if a patient has more than three exacerbations requiring antibiotics per year. These can be nebulised or oral. Azithromycin is often used three days per week; studies have shown that it improves exacerbation frequency, spirometry and sputum microbiology.

Nebulised colomycin is used in the management of *Pseudomonas* infection.

In the past, surgery was used as a treatment option to remove the affected lobe; this is not common practice now but may be done in rare cases.

CASE 17

C: A successful pleurodesis

Malignant pleural effusions are common and are seen with lung, breast and ovarian cancers as well as lymphomas and mesothelioma. Diagnosis is made on cytology testing of a pleural fluid sample. The clinical picture of exudative fluid with high LDH is very suspicious for a malignant effusion. Immunostaining can take some time but is useful to see if the effusion has the same pattern as the original disease. In undiagnosed cancers it may give pointers to the primary disease. Cytology has a sensitivity of 60%. If the first sample does not give clear answers, there is value in sending more fluid; however, further samples are unlikely to help.

Ultrasound is now used routinely to assist safe aspiration and drain placement. A respiratory physician or radiologist can assist with this, and real-time assessment is preferable. Ultrasound is more accurate than CT for assessing the size of an effusion and it is better in identifying loculations.

Learning point

A malignant effusion is a poor prognostic sign associated with reduced survival. Discussion with the oncology team is helpful in assessment of prognosis and to decide if further treatment will be possible and appropriate. If prognosis is very poor (eg less than one month expected survival), repeated aspirations as required for symptom control may be best as the morbidity and potential mortality of a chest drain may not be beneficial. Repeated aspirations for someone with a longer prognosis may cause the effusion to become more complex, with the development of a pleural infection or loculations. Lung beneath an effusion can become trapped and when fluid is removed the pleural surfaces cannot oppose. This can be difficult to manage.

Pleurodesis is when a chemical sclerosant, commonly sterile talc, is infiltrated into the pleural space via a chest drain to cause an inflammatory reaction. This results in the pleural surfaces sealing together, so preventing re-accumulation of the pleural fluid. If there is trapped lung, pleurodesis can be attempted if > 50% of the lung is opposed, but is less likely to be successful. Surgical pleurectomy in advanced cancer would not be indicated.

Palliative care should be undertaken throughout, but if symptoms are felt to be secondary to the effusion, then drainage of fluid is required as medication will not be effective alone. Long-term drains, for example, Pleurex drains, can be used in certain patients if pleurodesis is not possible or has been unsuccessful and fluid is re-accumulating. They can be sited by experienced physicians, radiologists and surgeons. Patients can be mobile and may go home with these in situ; trained staff can drain fluid away regularly. There are risks associated, including infection and complications if they become dislodged.

In this lady, successful pleurodesis would be the best outcome for symptom relief and quality of life.

The general classification of pleural effusions is based on pleural protein +/− LDH concentrations. Transudates have protein < 30 g/litre, exudates > 30 g/litre. In borderline cases (25–35 g/litre or when serum protein is abnormal), Light's criteria can be applied. Fluid is deemed to be exudative if pleural fluid protein:serum protein ratio is > 0.5, or if the pleural fluid LDH:serum LDH ratio is > 0.6, or if the pleural fluid LDH is > two thirds the upper limit of the normal serum LDH.

Transudates are typically secondary to an organ failure – liver, kidneys or heart most commonly. Treatment of the underlying condition is vital. Intercostal drains are not usually indicated.

Exudates can be malignant, due to an infective cause, secondary to rheumatological disease, chylothorax, drugs and many aetiologies. The underlying cause again should be sought and managed. Therapeutic aspiration or drain +/− pleurodesis can be used.

Haemothorax is diagnosed when the haematocrit of the fluid is > 50% that of the peripheral blood.

> ### Learning point
>
> In simple parapneumonic effusions, fluid is exudative with a clear appearance and normal fluid markers. These effusions will often resolve spontaneously with treatment of the infection. A complicated parapneumonic effusion is when fibrin has been made and septae can be formed. The fluid is infected but not purulent. It may be cloudy, the pH is < 7.2, glucose < 2.2 mmol/litre, LDH > 1000 U/litre and culture may be positive. These patients need a chest drain. Empyema is frank pus in the pleural cavity. It can be multiloculated, culture may be positive and a drain is required. It can cause complications by forming a thick pleural peel, which may require surgical decortication. Antibiotic treatment for these infections should be guided by culture and the microbiology team.

A milky, turbid effusion is typical of a chylothorax. Chylomicrons are present and the triglyceride concentration is typically > 110 g/dl. It is caused by damage to the thoracic duct and leakage of lymph fluid, usually due to malignancy, lymphoma, trauma, thoracoplasty or lymphangioleiomyomatosis (LAM).

CASE 18

B: Predominantly subpleural, bibasal honeycomb change

This is a typical presentation of idiopathic pulmonary fibrosis (IPF), previously known as cryptogenic fibrosing alveolitis or usual interstitial pneumonia. It is one of the idiopathic interstitial pneumonias that come under the broad description of interstitial lung disease. The cause of IPF is unknown. It is a progressive condition and there is no cure; 50% die within three years. The CT appearances should be reported or reviewed by a radiologist with an interest in chest radiology. A picture of predominantly subpleural, bibasal honeycomb change is typical. Any atypical features may lead to a different diagnosis. The other patterns described are typical of other conditions: A – non-specific interstitial pneumonia (NSIP), C – respiratory bronchiolitis-associated interstitial lung disease (RB-ILD), D – hypersensitivity pneumonitis, E – pneumonia.

There are many causes of fibrosis and other causes should be sought with blood investigations and discussion at a multidisciplinary meeting. IPF does not necessarily need a tissue diagnosis, and consensus at a multidisciplinary meeting looking at the clinical picture, pulmonary function tests and CT appearances, preferably at a regional centre, is adequate. IPF patients have been shown to do badly after biopsy.

Learning point

Management of IPF is mainly supportive, including oxygen supplementation if required, pulmonary rehabilitation, education and specialist nurse support. Transplantation if appropriate, and end-of-life care, should be discussed also. There has been extensive research into proposed treatment. Unfortunately, many treatments have been shown to do harm, eg azathoprine, prednisolone, N-acetylcysteine, warfarin, co-trimoxazole, mycolphenalate and sildenafil. N-acetylcysteine alone is being investigated – the benefits are unclear but it has been shown to do no harm. Pirfenidone has been recently approved by NICE as a potential therapy. In trials it was shown to reduce the risk of disease progression and it has been shown to improve FVC modestly in mild to moderate disease. Issues with it include gastrointestinal upset and photosensitivity, and its great cost, despite the modest improvements in disease and quality of life. Other companies are developing new drugs for IPF – most recently Nintedanib.

Non-specific interstitial pneumonia is a spectrum of diseases ranging from a cellular inflammatory form that responds well to steroids and has a good prognosis, to the fibrotic form which is more like IPF. It generally affects younger patients and is often associated with other conditions. High-resolution CT (HRCT) scans show predominantly ground glass change. Pulmonary function is restrictive with a reduced transfer factor. A biopsy is often needed and treatment is with steroids.

Acute interstitial pneumonia is a rapidly progressive disease with diffuse alveolar damage, profound hypoxia and respiratory failure. There is no treatment and it is fatal in > 50% of cases. Survivors will have chronic lung disease.

Respiratory bronchiolitis-associated interstitial lung disease (RB-ILD) is an idiopathic condition seen in younger male smokers and can be asymptomatic. It involves the accumulation of pigmented macrophages in bronchioles. On HRCT there are centrilobular nodules, ground glass change and thick-walled airways, often with emphysema. If patients can stop smoking, prognosis can be very good.

Desquamative interstitial pneumonia is also seen in smokers and may be a progression from RB-ILD. HRCT shows ground glass change and histology is similar to RB-ILD. Biopsy is generally needed to confirm diagnosis. Management includes smoking cessation +/– steroids. It can have a relapsing and remitting course.

Other causes of fibrosis include connective tissue diseases (rheumatoid arthritis, systemic lupus erythematosis, systemic sclerosis and ankylosing spondylitis), drugs (eg amiodarone and chemotherapy agents), radiotherapy, inorganic pneumoconioses (asbestos, coal and silicosis), hypersensitivity pneumonitis, sarcoidosis, vasculitis and eosinophilic conditions.

References

1. British Thoracic Society. 2009. Guideline for the management of community acquired pneumonia in adults. www.brit-thoracic.org.uk/media/113217/Annotated-BTS-Guideline-for-the-management-of-CAP-in-adults-2015-web.pdf

2. British Thoracic Society/Scottish Intercollegiate Guidelines Network. 2014. British guideline on the management of asthma. www.brit-thoracic.org.uk/document-library/clinical-information/asthma/btssign-asthma-guideline-2014

3. Global Initiative for Chronic Obstructive Lung Disease (GOLD). 2015. Global Strategy for the Diagnosis, Management and Prevention of COPD. www.goldcopd.org

Rheumatology

Auleen Millar

CASE 1

A 59-year-old school caretaker presents with increasing shortness of breath with a noticeable reduction in his exercise tolerance over a six-month period. He had previously been diagnosed with Raynaud's disease by his GP and recently had been referred for swallowing difficulties. There was no other medical or drug history.

On examination, skin changes were noted in both hands with thickening that extended to the upper arms and trunk. The respiratory rate was 24 breaths/min. Chest auscultation was unremarkable. The jugular venous pressure was elevated with prominent V waves and there was mild pedal oedema. On praecordial auscultation there were two heart sounds with a loud pulmonary component of the second sound, and a systolic murmur loudest on inspiration at the lower left sternal edge.

A skin biopsy showed fibrosis and blood investigations revealed the presence of anti-topoisomerase antibodies.

What is the gold standard investigation of choice to confirm the cause of the patient's shortness of breath?

A. **Pulmonary function testing with spirometry and transfer factor**
B. **Echocardiography**
C. **Right heart catheterisation**
D. **ECG**
E. **Exercise stress test**

CASE 2

A 64-year-old lady with a history of hypertension and hypercholesterolaemia is admitted with sudden unilateral loss of visual acuity in the right eye associated with a right-sided headache and temporal tenderness. She recently complained of bilateral jaw pain, shoulder tenderness with early morning stiffness and had noted some weight loss. Her full blood count reveals: haemoglobin 98 g/litre, MCV 84 fl, platelets 680×10^9/litre and normal white cells. Inflammatory markers are elevated: ESR 112 mm/1st hour, C-reactive protein 60 mg/litre. Liver and renal function tests are within normal limits. Fundoscopy reveals a pale optic disc. A CT scan of brain is reported as normal.

The most likely diagnosis is:

A. **Cortical blindness from a vertebro-basilar stroke**
B. **Acute ischaemic optic neuropathy**
C. **Cerebral abscess**
D. **Central retinal artery occlusion**
E. **Disseminated malignancy with brain metastasis**

CASE 3

Regarding patients on long-term glucocorticoids, which of the following options is most correct?

A. **They are at risk of ketosis**
B. **They may develop tertiary adrenal insufficiency**
C. **They may develop low serum sodium and high serum potassium concentrations**
D. **They can develop anterior sub-capsular cataracts**
E. **They can develop osteoarthritis**

CASE 4

Which of the following ophthalmic conditions is *not* associated with rheumatoid arthritis?

    A. **Keratoconjunctivitis sicca**

    B. **Episcleritis**

    C. **Scleritis**

    D. **Anterior uveitis**

    E. **Ulcerative keratitis**

CASE 5

A 64-year-old male smoker presents with shortness of breath and haemoptysis. He describes a six-month history of nasal crusting with intermittent nose bleeds.

Initial investigations reveal: White cells 18×10^9/litre (70% neutrophils, 3% eosinophils), Platelets 750×10^9/litre, Coagulation screen: normal, Creatinine 390 µmol/litre, Creatinine kinase: normal, ESR 70 mm/1st hour, C-ANCA 1:160 with antibodies to PR3, ANA 1:80, Anti-ds-DNA: negative, Rheumatoid factor: negative, Urinalysis: protein +++, blood ++.

Chest X-ray: several cavitating pulmonary nodules.

What is the most likely diagnosis?

    A. **Microscopic polyangiitis**

    B. **Granulomatosis with polyangiitis**

    C. **Eosinophilic granulomatosis with polyangiitis**

    D. **Polyarteritis nodosa**

    E. **IgA vasculitis**

CASE 6

A 43-year-old woman has been diagnosed with psoriatic arthritis. She was commenced on sulfasalazine three weeks ago. She presents feeling unwell with a fever and a maculopapular rash. Blood investigations show a high leukocyte count with an eosinophilia. Her liver transaminases are elevated. On examination, cervical lymphadenopathy is present.

What is the most likely cause of her rash?

A. Sulfonamide allergy
B. Drug rash with eosinophilia and systemic symptoms
C. Paradoxical flare of skin psoriasis
D. Hypereosinophilic syndrome
E. Streptococcal infection

CASE 7

A 26-year-old man presents with a 12-week history of pain and stiffness in his hands and right heel. On examination, there is swelling over several metacarpo-phalangeal joints bilaterally and at both wrists. On his left hand, the third and fourth distal interphalangeal joints are swollen and tender. Nail pitting is also present. There is a focal area of tenderness on the plantar aspect of his right heel. His X-rays are shown in Figure 14.1.

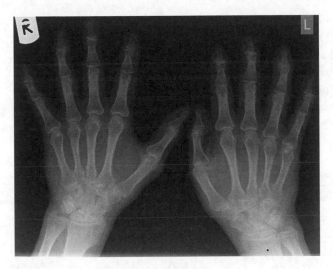

Figure 14.1

What is the most likely diagnosis?

   A. **Seropositive rheumatoid arthritis**
   B. **Seronegative rheumatoid arthritis**
   C. **Psoriatic arthritis**
   D. **Polyarticular gout**
   E. **Inflammatory osteoarthritis**

CASE 8

A 79-year-old man presents with a hot swollen knee. This is his third such attack in the past year. He has a past medical history of ischaemic heart disease, type 2 diabetes and renal impairment with an eGFR of 45 ml/min per 1.73 m². Serum urate is 0.42 mmol/litre. Joint aspirate confirms monosodium urate crystals. The joint fluid culture was negative and an intra-articular injection of corticosteroid was given with resolution of his symptoms.

What is the next most appropriate step to take?

A. **Allopurinol 100 mg once daily**
B. **Sulfinpyrazone 100 mg once daily**
C. **Allopurinol 100 mg on alternate days**
D. **Colchicine 500 μg twice daily**
E. **Febuxostat 80 mg once daily**

CASE 9

A patient presents with features in keeping with ankylosing spondylitis. Which of these genetic factors is most commonly associated with this condition and can be requested routinely in clinic?

A. **HLA-B27**
B. **HLA-B51**
C. **HLA-DRB1**
D. **CTLA4**
E. **PTPN22**

CASE 10

A 32-year-old man presents with the acute onset of an inflammatory polyarthropathy. His only other past medical history is a diagnosis of lupus pernio. On examination he has widespread active synovitis. Blood results show that he is rheumatoid factor and anti-cyclic citrullinated peptide antibody negative. X-rays of his hands are shown in Figure 14.2.

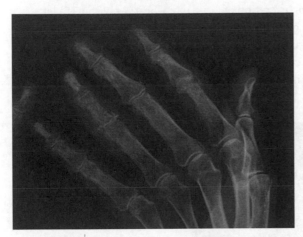

Figure 14.2

The next most appropriate investigation is:

    A. **Anti-nuclear antibody**
    B. **Anti-double-stranded DNA antibody**
    C. **Chest X-ray**
    D. **X-ray other symptomatic joints**
    E. **Ultrasound scan of the joint**

CASE 11

A 36-year-old Lithuanian woman presents with shortness of breath and chest pain. She speaks very little English but you discern that she has had a diagnosis of 'arthritis' for years. She has an erythematous rash over her face and hands with evidence of a destructive polyarthropathy in her hands. Her ESR is 70 mm/1st hour, creatinine is 98 µmol/litre and urinalysis shows +++ of protein. A 24-hour urine collection shows protein excretion of 1.5 g/day. Chest X-ray shows a left-sided pleural effusion with a globular heart. Subsequent echocardiography reveals a small circumferential pericardial effusion. Analysis of the pleural aspirate shows an exudate with high glucose and low LDH. Microscopy is negative for bacteria including acid fast bacilli. Immunology results are awaited. Hand X-rays are shown in Figure 14.3.

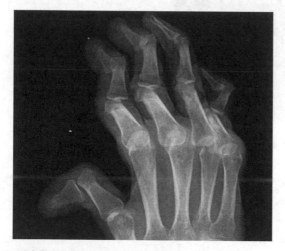

Figure 14.3

What is the most likely diagnosis?

- A. **Rheumatoid arthritis**
- B. **Psoriatic arthritis**
- C. **Systemic lupus erythematosus**
- D. **Primary Sjögren syndrome**
- E. **Chronic Lyme disease**

CASE 12

A 68-year-old man with chronic rheumatoid arthritis complains of fatigue. Blood tests reveal haemoglobin of 81 g/litre, with haematocrit of 0.26. Serum iron is low. Liver and renal function tests are normal. He is on treatment with anti-tumour necrosis factor therapy and low-dose methotrexate. He occasionally takes non-steroidal anti-inflammatory drugs.

What is the least likely cause of his anaemia?

A. **Impaired iron release from macrophages**
B. **Gastrointestinal bleeding**
C. **Decreased production of erythropoietin**
D. **Impaired intestinal iron absorption**
E. **Haemolysis**

CASE 13

A 32-year-old previous intravenous drug user is referred because of joint pains. He describes early morning stiffness that improves with mobilisation. On examination he has tenderness of multiple metacarpo-phalangeal joints and over both wrists. He has a vasculitic rash on his lower legs. His rheumatoid factor is high but anti-cyclic citrullinated peptide (CCP) antibodies are negative. Anti-nuclear antibody (ANA) is positive with a titre of 1:160. ANCA screening is negative. Complement testing shows a normal C3 but a markedly reduced C4 level. Liver function tests and renal function are normal. Tests for hepatitis A and B viruses and HIV are negative. Anti-hepatitis C antibodies were detected.

Which of the following is most correct?

A. **A diagnosis of rheumatoid arthritis considering the clinical symptoms and positive rheumatoid factor – a negative anti-CCP does not exclude this diagnosis**
B. **Systemic lupus erythematosus is likely due to the positive ANA and low complement levels**
C. **The positive hepatitis C viral test is not relevant to the diagnosis but may cause problems with immunosuppressive disease-modifying therapy for an inflammatory arthritis**
D. **Given the low C4 and significantly elevated rheumatoid factor, a sample for cryoglobulins should be sent**
E. **Despite the normal ANCA, a diagnosis of vasculitis should be suspected first and a skin biopsy is required**

CHAPTER 14
QUESTIONS

CASE 14

A 42-year-old man is admitted with haemoptysis. His past medical history includes a previous admission for aseptic meningitis and a dural sinus thrombosis. On examination he has a follicular rash on both thighs, oral aphthous ulceration and a single scrotal ulcer. The most appropriate investigation to confirm the cause of the haemoptysis is:

A. Pulmonary angiography
B. Chest X-ray
C. Anti-nuclear antibodies, lupus anticoagulant and anticardiolipin antibodies
D. Ventilation perfusion scan
E. Helical CT scan of chest

CASE 15

A 17-year-old boy is admitted with a 2-week history of general lethargy. He complains of a sore throat, generalised myalgia, arthralgia and chest pain that is worse on lying flat. On examination he has a faint erythematous rash, a pericardial rub and a palpable splenic edge. He is pyrexic at 39.1 °C.

Investigations reveal: Haemoglobin 108 g/litre, White cells 22.9 × 10⁹/litre with predominant neutrophilia, Platelets 503 × 10⁹/litre, ESR 114 mm/1st hour, C-reactive protein 298 mg/litre, ALP 107 U/litre, GGT 134 U/litre, AST 46 U/litre, ALT 42 U/litre, Ferritin 9134 μg/litre, Iron 8.2 μmol/litre, Troponin T 124 ng/litre.

ECG confirms ST changes in keeping with pericarditis, and echocardiography shows a 2 cm pericardial effusion with a global wall motion abnormality.

The most appropriate management is:

A. Serial ECGs after initial non-steroidal anti-inflammatory drugs
B. Serial echocardiography after initial non-steroidal anti-inflammatory drugs
C. Myocardial perfusion scan
D. Gadolinium enhanced cardiac MRI scan
E. Coronary angiography

CASE 16

A 52-year-old man presents complaining of fatigue and weakness after several falls at home. He also describes some recent difficulty swallowing and reports weight loss of 10 kg over the past six months. Past medical history includes type 1 diabetes and hypertension. He is a lifelong smoker. Apart from his insulin regimen, medications include simvastatin 40 mg daily and ramipril 10 mg daily. On examination, he has periungual erythema, a livedo rash on his arms, and an erythematous rash on his anterior chest wall and upper back in a V-shaped distribution. He states that the latter rash is aggravated by sunlight. He is unable to rise from a seated position without using his arms and he cannot hold his arms at shoulder height for more than a few seconds.

Initial results show: Haemoglobin 11.1 g/litre, MCV 84 fl, ESR 64 mm/1st hour, C-reactive protein 56 mg/litre, Bilirubin 14 μmol/litre, AST 120 U/litre, ALT 38 U/litre, GGT 30 U/litre, ALP 34 U/litre, CK 4200 U/litre.

Which of the following investigations would be most likely to confirm the diagnosis?

A. **Barium swallow**
B. **CT scan of chest, abdomen and pelvis**
C. **Electromyography**
D. **MRI scan**
E. **Muscle biopsy**

CASE 17

A 69-year-old woman with a history of rheumatoid arthritis presents with abdominal swelling. She was diagnosed at the age of 32 years, and has been treated with multiple disease-modifying therapies which have all been stopped either due to side effects or lack of efficacy. She declined treatment with biologic agents owing to concern about adverse effects, and has been treated for the last number of years with oral prednisolone. She has failed to attend several recent outpatient appointments. She is rheumatoid factor positive and anti-cyclic citrullinated peptide (anti-CCP) antibody positive, and has significant deformities due to her history of high disease activity. She now presents with shortness of breath. On examination she has significant pitting oedema and clinical evidence of a right-sided pleural effusion. Pleural aspiration is consistent with a transudate. Blood pressure is 170/96 mmHg. Urinalysis shows 3+ protein and further tests reveal nephrotic range proteinuria, elevated creatinine and low serum albumin. Tests for viral hepatitis are negative. The most likely cause of her current condition is:

A. **Renal artery stenosis**
B. **Proteinuria due to previous gold or penicillamine treatment**
C. **New onset of lupus nephritis**
D. **AA amyloidosis**
E. **Henoch–Schönlein purpura**

CASE 18

A 43-year-old man with a history of rheumatoid arthritis was recently commenced on adalimumab fortnightly in combination with methotrexate. He presents to the emergency department after six months of treatment with shortness of breath. He had recently developed a malar rash which flares with sunlight exposure. He complains of malaise, low-grade fevers and weight loss. His GP had sent an anti-nuclear antibody screen (which was normal pre-treatment) because of the nature of the facial rash. This showed that he was anti-histone antibody positive. His chest X-ray is shown in Figure 14.4.

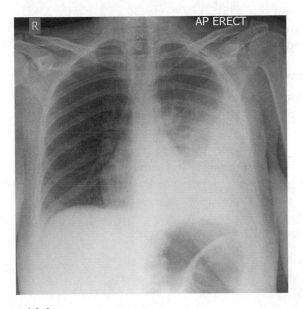

Figure 14.4

Which of the following is the most likely cause of his symptoms?

   A. **Pneumonia due to immunosuppression**
   B. **Tuberculosis**
   C. **A malignant pleural effusion**
   D. **Drug-induced side effects**
   E. **New onset of idiopathic connective tissue disease**

CASE 19

A 35-year-old woman with a recent diagnosis of systemic lupus erythematosus presents on the acute medical take with shortness of breath. Medications include the oral contraceptive pill and hydroxychloroquine 200 mg twice daily. She is a smoker of ten years and past medical history includes a previous fracture of her right arm and a miscarriage at nine weeks' gestation. She complains of back pain and right-sided chest pain, worse on inspiration. On examination she has a livedo reticularis rash on her arms and legs. Her respiratory rate is 22 breaths/min and oxygen saturations are 97% on room air. A chest X-ray is reported as normal.

Blood results show: Haemoglobin 12.2 g/litre, White cells 2.4×10^9/litre, Neutrophils 1.2×10^9/litre, Lymphocytes 0.98×10^9/litre, Platelets 92×10^9/litre, PT 10.1 s, APTT 29.4 s, Fibrinogen 1.4 g/litre, C-reactive protein 8 mg/litre.

Which of the following is the most likely diagnosis?

A. **Osteoporotic vertebral collapse**
B. **Serositis secondary to lupus**
C. **Tietze syndrome**
D. **Hughes syndrome**
E. **Community-acquired lower respiratory tract infection**

CASE 20

A 43-year-old Afro-Caribbean woman with a 1-year history of systemic lupus erythematosus presents with acute confusion. Her family have noticed increasing confusion over the past few days. Before this the patient had complained of increasing lethargy, bruising and nose bleeds. On examination the lady is disorientated in place and time. She has evidence of widespread purpura and is pyrexic (temperature 37.9 °C). Her blood pressure is 182/98 mmHg, and pulse rate 110 bpm.

Blood tests reveal: Haemoglobin 5.2 g/litre, Reticulocytes 14%, White cells and differential white cell count normal, Platelets 32×10^9/litre, ESR 110 mm/1st hour, Urea 22 mmol/litre, Creatinine 160 µmol/litre, eGFR 42 ml/min per 1.73 m^2, Bilirubin 42 µmol/litre, AST 88 U/litre, ALT 80 U/litre, PT and APTT normal, LDH 1600 U/litre, Coombs' test negative, Blood film: schistocytes, Urinary albumin/creatinine ratio 60, Tests for hepatitis viruses negative, Tests for Epstein–Barr virus and cytomegalovirus negative, Anti-double-stranded DNA antibody titre 80 IU/ml, Complement C3 and C4 – reduced.

The most appropriate management is:

- A. **IV rituximab**
- B. **IV cyclophosphamide**
- C. **Plasmapheresis**
- D. **Haemodialysis**
- E. **Bone marrow aspiration**

CASE 21

A 42-year-old woman presents to the ear, nose and throat team with severe nasal pain. She has a history of sinusitis and asthma. Examination reveals an obvious mass in the right nasal passage, and CT scanning confirms extensive soft tissue opacity involving the frontal, ethmoid, maxillary and sphenoid sinuses consistent with severe sinonasal polyposis. Blood results show:

✦ ESR 41 mm/1st hour

✦ C-reactive protein 26 mg/litre

Peripheral blood eosinophilia is noted. Urinalysis reveals +++ protein and +++ blood. During surgery for a nasal polypectomy, she has a cardiac arrest. A representative image from her echocardiogram is shown in Figure 14.5. Analysis of the fluid from the pathology shown demonstrates an exudate, with histiocytes/mesothelial cells and numerous eosinophils ++++. Pathology from the polypectomy shows necrotic areas with vascular and perivascular inflammation, with giant cells and histiocytes, and infiltration by a large number of eosinophils and plasma cells.

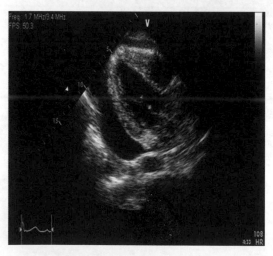

Figure 14.5

Which of the following is the most likely diagnosis?

A. **Brugada syndrome**

B. **Anaphylaxis**

C. **Viral infection**

D. **Eosinophilic granulomatosis with polyangiitis (EGPA)**

E. **Hypereosinophilic syndrome**

CASE 22

What is the likelihood that a first degree relative of a patient with rheumatoid arthritis will share the diagnosis?

A. **2–10 times the population prevalence of the disease**
B. **The same as the general population**
C. **0.5–1.5% risk of developing the disease**
D. **60–80% risk of developing the disease**
E. **100% risk of developing the disease**

CASE 23

A 32-year-old woman presents with a new diagnosis of rheumatoid arthritis (RA). She is rheumatoid factor positive and anti-cyclic citrullinated peptide (anti-CCP) antibody positive. After a baseline chest X-ray she is commenced on methotrexate 15 mg weekly and folic acid. At subsequent reviews, despite titration of her methotrexate, she has ongoing high disease activity with a disease activity score of 5.2 and nausea with higher doses of methotrexate. What is the next most appropriate management step?

A. **Start anti-tumour necrosis factor (TNF) therapy**
B. **Stop methotrexate and start sulfasalazine**
C. **Stop methotrexate and start leflunomide**
D. **Switch to subcutaneous methotrexate only**
E. **Switch to subcutaneous methotrexate and consider the addition of a second disease-modifying anti-rheumatic drug (DMARD)**

CHAPTER 14 QUESTIONS

CASE 24

A 65-year-old woman with long-standing rheumatoid disease presents complaining of numbness in her right leg and difficultly walking. She had a severe flare of her disease recently and required an intramuscular steroid injection in her right buttock one week ago. On examination she has sensory loss over the right lateral calf and foot with a normal knee jerk and absent ankle jerk. Which of the following is the most likely explanation for her current presentation?

A. **Rheumatoid vasculitis with mononeuritis multiplex**
B. **Sciatic nerve injury after gluteal injection**
C. **Common peroneal nerve trauma**
D. **Meralgia paraesthetica**
E. **Piriformis syndrome**

CASE 1

C: Right heart catheterisation

The diagnosis is scleroderma. Anti-topoisomerase antibodies are a type of anti-nuclear antibody. Their presence indicates the potential for diffuse systemic involvement with an early incidence of pulmonary fibrosis, diffuse gastrointestinal disease, oliguric renal failure or, as in this case, pulmonary arterial hypertension (PAH). Patients with limited cutaneous scleroderma and anti-centromere antibodies are generally considered at greater risk of PAH than patients with diffuse disease.

In the presence of PAH, pulmonary function tests will show normal spirometry but a reduced transfer factor. Although spirometry might alert physicians to the presence of early pulmonary fibrosis or pulmonary hypertension, this test will not be sufficient to confirm the presence of pulmonary hypertension with certainty.

> ## Learning point
>
> Echocardiography is usually performed yearly in all patients with scleroderma to help identify mild to moderate PAH before patients become symptomatic. There are, however, some limitations to its use in evaluating pulmonary hypertension. PAH is suspected in patients with a pulmonary artery pressure (PAP) greater than 25 mmHg; however, the full haemodynamic definition includes having a mean PAP greater than 25 mmHg, a mean pulmonary capillary wedge pressure < 15 mmHg (to exclude PAH due to left heart disease) and a pulmonary vascular resistance of > 3 Woods units. Therefore, right heart catheterisation (RHC) should be performed in all cases in which PAH is suspected. It not only confirms the diagnosis, but also eliminates other cardiac causes and assesses the degree of right heart dysfunction. Another important role of RHC is vasoreactivity testing to identify patients who may benefit from long-term therapy with calcium channel blockers.

An ECG in patients with pulmonary hypertension may show signs of right ventricular strain such as right axis deviation, but will not confirm the diagnosis. Exercise stress testing is generally indicated when there is a clinical suspicion of ischaemic heart disease. The clinical picture does not correlate with this.

CASE 2

B: Acute ischaemic optic neuropathy

The most likely diagnosis is giant cell arteritis (GCA) with acute ischaemic optic neuropathy secondary to occlusion of the posterior ciliary arteries.

Learning point

The American College of Rheumatology diagnostic criteria for GCA are:

1. Age at disease onset ≥ 50 years of age.

2. New headache: new onset of or new type of localised pain in the head.

3. Temporal artery abnormality: temporal artery tenderness to palpation or decreased pulsation unrelated to arteriosclerosis of cervical arteries.

4. Increased ESR: ≥ 50 mm/1st hour by the Westergren method.

5. Abnormal artery biopsy: biopsy specimen with an artery showing vasculitis characterised by a predominance of mononuclear cell infiltrate or granulomatous inflammation, usually with multinucleated giant cells.

Giant cell arteritis is diagnosed if at least three of these five criteria are present.[1]

Bilateral shoulder and/or pelvic girdle pain and stiffness can also be seen in polymyalgia rheumatica with or without GCA. Anaemia, thrombocytosis and weight loss are widely described in both conditions. Patients may also present with fever, sometimes as high as 38 °C, and may fulfil criteria for pyrexia of unknown origin.

Regarding cortical blindness secondary to a vertebro-basilar stroke, the signs and symptoms of vertebro-basilar ischaemic events include cortical blindness, cranial nerve palsies, cerebellar ataxia, vertigo and involvement of the sensory or pyramidal tracts which are absent in this case. It should still be considered as a possible diagnosis, as involvement of the vertebro-basilar arteries in GCA can cause cortical blindness due to vertebro-basilar stroke. The intracranial arteries in GCA are typically spared.

Cerebral abscess, although possible with raised inflammatory markers and visual loss, would be rare in the absence of additional neurology and has been virtually excluded with a normal CT scan.

Central retinal artery (CRA) occlusion will cause sudden painless loss of vision. A 'cherry-red spot' can be seen on fundoscopy with a surrounding pale retina. Although GCA can cause visual loss secondary to CRA occlusion, this is rare and the classical signs on fundoscopy were not present in this patient. If not directly linked to GCA, central retinal occlusion would not be associated with the inflammatory response, anaemia and weight loss.

CASE 3

B: They may develop tertiary adrenal insufficiency

Chronic glucocorticoid use may cause atrophy of the fasciculata and reticularis zones of the adrenal glands, with resulting adrenal insufficiency. This is termed tertiary adrenal insufficiency. Ketosis is very rare as the gluconeogenic and glycogenic effects of glucocorticoids offer protection from ketosis – they do not cause type 1 diabetes. The outer glomerulosa zone is not influenced by glucocorticoid treatment unlike in autoimmune adrenal insufficiency, and therefore changes in the biochemical profile are not seen. Although they are known to cause cataracts, a posterior sub-capsular cataract is most common. Steroids will increase the risk of osteoporosis, not osteoarthritis.

CASE 4

D: Anterior uveitis

Rheumatoid arthritis (RA) is a systemic autoimmune inflammatory condition that causes an erosive inflammatory arthropathy. It can also have important extra-articular manifestations. Ophthalmic involvement can have potential sight-threatening consequences, so early detection and treatment is paramount.

Learning point

Keratoconjunctivitis sicca (dry eyes) can be found in many autoimmune rheumatological conditions. It can be the presenting symptom in conditions such as primary Sjögren's syndrome, or can occur in other autoimmune conditions as a secondary Sjögren's syndrome. It is the most common ophthalmic pathology in RA, and may occur due to ocular surface inflammation and subsequent compromise of tear secretion.

Episcleritis is usually benign and involves inflammation of the episclera. In contrast, scleritis is generally more severe, involving inflammation throughout the entire thickness of the sclera. Severe pain is a prominent feature and the condition requires immediate ophthalmic attention.

Ulcerative keratitis is also associated with RA and can have devastating consequences. It can lead to rapid corneal keratolysis or corneal melt, perforation of the globe and loss of vision.

Anterior uveitis is most commonly associated with HLA-B27 and seronegative inflammatory disease such as ankylosing spondylitis and Behçet's disease.

CASE 5

B: Granulomatosis with polyangiitis

Granulomatosis with polyangiitis (GPA) (previously known as Wegener's granulomatosis) affects small and medium-sized arteries. Other forms of vasculitis that affect vessels of similar size include eosinophilic granulomatosis with polyangiitis (Churg–Strauss syndrome) or microscopic polyangiitis (MPA). Polyarteritis nodosa (PAN) is said to predominantly affect medium-sized arteries.

> ### Learning point
>
> There are multiple classification criteria; however, the 1990 American College of Rheumatolgy criteria for the diagnosis of granulomatosis with polyangiitis are shown below:[2]
>
> 1. Nasal or oral inflammation: development of painful or painless oral ulcers or purulent or bloody nasal discharge.
> 2. Abnormal chest radiograph: chest radiograph showing the presence of nodules, fixed infiltrates or cavities.
> 3. Urinary sediment: microhaematuria (> 5 red cells per high-power field) or red cell casts in the urinary sediment.
> 4. Granulomatous inflammation on biopsy: histological changes showing granulomatous inflammation within the wall of an artery or in the perivascular or extravascular area.
>
> Patients are diagnosed with GPA if at least two of these four criteria are present. This approach yields a sensitivity of 88.2% and a specificity of 92%.

Anti-nuclear cytoplasmic antibody (ANCA) does not form part of these criteria, but a 2011 revision of the Chapel Hill Consensus Conference (CHCC) definitions for vasculitis now includes ANCA in the criteria and focuses less on vessel size.[3]

The most frequent manifestation in GPA is involvement of the upper airways, with over 75% of patients affected, but lung and renal manifestations are also common. Apart from GPA, Goodpasture's disease and MPA are potential causes of pulmonary renal syndrome. IgA vasculitis, although it affects the kidneys in the form of an IgA nephropathy, and other systems such as the bowel, joints and skin, does not present with airways disease.

continued

CHAPTER 14 ANSWERS

Granulomatosis with polyangiitis (GPA), MPA and eosinophilic granulomatosis with polyangiitis (EGPA) are also known as ANCA-associated vasculitides. In GPA, C-ANCA and anti-PR3 are useful clinical tools, although rarely patients with GPA can have a positive P-ANCA with MPO specificity – a feature preferentially seen in MPA and EGPA. PAN is not associated with ANCA positivity.

In this clinical scenario, with evidence of pulmonary renal syndrome and a positive C-ANCA, the most likely diagnosis is GPA.

CASE 6

B: Drug rash with eosinophilia and systemic symptoms

The patient has classical features of 'drug rash with eosinophilia and systemic symptoms' (DRESS), which is a rare but potentially severe reaction to sulfasalazine. It is a form of delayed drug hypersensitivity syndrome, and can develop on first exposure to a drug and within eight weeks of initiating therapy. Sulfonamides and several aromatic anticonvulsants including phenytoin, phenobarbital and carbamazepine are the most common culprits, although other drugs have been implicated. The exact pathogenesis remains unclear. Treatment includes withdrawal of the offending drugs. In some cases, steroids can be considered. A mortality of 10% has been reported.

CASE 7

C: Psoriatic arthritis

The presence of erosions in the distal interphalangeal (DIP) joints is not seen in either seropositive or seronegative rheumatoid arthritis, which classically spares the distal interphalangeal joints, affecting mainly the metacarpo-phalangeal and proximal interphalangeal joints in a symmetrical pattern. Seronegative arthropathies typically have an asymmetrical distribution and patients can also develop enthesitis, which is suggested in this history with symptoms in keeping with plantar fasciitis. The most likely type of seronegative arthropathy is psoriatic arthritis, given the finding of nail pitting. Some patients present with only the nail findings in conjunction with joint involvement.

The history is not in keeping with gout given the duration of the symptoms, although it must be remembered that polyarticular gout is an important differential diagnosis in a patient with asymmetrical involvement, and a thorough history for risk factors and examination for tophi is important.

The patient is too young to consider osteoarthritis (OA), although in patients with DIP swelling, this must be considered. Patients with a strong family history of nodal OA may also develop symptoms at an early age.

CASE 8

A: Allopurinol 100 mg once daily

The current attack is treated; however, two or more attacks of gout in a 12-month period should be an indication for urate-lowering therapy. Sulfinpyrazone is contraindicated in renal failure. At a GFR of 45 ml/min per 1.73 m², allopurinol can be used safely at a dose of 100 mg/day with monitoring of renal function and may be titrated according to eGFR. Colchicine is used to treat acute attacks and carries risks with long-term use. It is not a treatment used in the long-term prevention of gout.

CHAPTER 14 ANSWERS

CASE 9

A: HLA-B27

HLA-B27 (human leukocyte antigen B27) is a class I surface antigen encoded by the B locus in the major histocompatibility complex (MHC) on chromosome 6 and presents antigenic peptides to T cells.

Learning point

Although 90% of people with ankylosing spondylitis (AS) are HLA-B27 positive, not all people with HLA-B27 develop AS. HLA-B27 has other disease associations: it is implicated in other types of seronegative spondyloarthropathy such as psoriatic arthritis and reactive arthritis, eye disorders such as acute anterior uveitis and iritis, and ulcerative colitis-associated spondyloarthritis.

HLA-B51 is associated with Behçet's disease, HLA-DRB1 with anti-cyclic citrullinated peptide antibody positive rheumatoid arthritis (RA), CTLA4 with systemic lupus erythematosus (SLE), PTPN22 with a number of autoimmune diseases including RA, SLE and Graves' disease.

CASE 10

C: Chest X-ray

The patient has sarcoidosis. This is a potentially multisystem inflammatory disease, and patients can present in a variety of ways.

> ### Learning point
>
>
> The respiratory system is most commonly involved, and disease there can be described in four stages:
>
> Stage 0 – no intra-thoracic involvement
>
> Stage I – bilateral hilar adenopathy
>
> Stage II – pulmonary parenchyma involved
>
> Stage III – pulmonary infiltrates with fibrosis
>
> Stage IV – end-stage lung disease with pulmonary fibrosis and honeycombing

The skin is the second most commonly involved organ. Lupus pernio is pathognomonic of sarcoidosis. Presentation with erythema nodosum, bilateral hilar lymphadenopathy on chest X-ray and arthralgia is known as Löfgren syndrome, which has a relatively good prognosis.

The presence of sarcoid in the bones typically correlates with cutaneous lesions and progressive disease. The hand X-rays show a lace-like or reticular pattern of destruction in the metaphyses.

Although X-rays of other joints may show further osseous involvement, a chest X-ray is the next most important investigation to help confirm the diagnosis and an important initial investigation to assess the extent of pulmonary involvement. Musculoskeletal ultrasound may be useful to examine the extent of synovitis and antibody tests can be useful as part of the diagnostic work-up.

CASE 11

C: Systemic lupus erythematosus

The patient has systemic lupus erythematosus (SLE). The hand X-rays show a Jaccoud's arthropathy. This is a non-erosive deforming arthropathy. Although the X-ray displays osteopenia and subluxation at multiple joints, there is a lack of the erosions that would be seen in chronic rheumatoid, psoriatic arthritis or arthritis associated with chronic Lyme disease. Patients with primary Sjögren syndrome can experience arthralgia without any evidence of significant synovitis or X-ray changes, although erosive changes have been reported in some patients with more severe disease. Systemic rheumatoid can cause pleural and pericardial effusions. The effusions in SLE are usually exudates (ie protein content > 3 g/100 ml) with high glucose concentrations and low LDH levels, whereas infections and rheumatoid arthritis are associated with low glucose effusions. Although Sjögren syndrome can have systemic manifestations, the more common pulmonary manifestations would be complications from dryness of the airways and, more rarely, interstitial lung disease. Cardiac complications are also rare but can include pericarditis, and renal involvement can be seen in the form of an interstitial nephritis.

CASE 12

E: Haemolysis

Patients with rheumatoid arthritis can develop anaemia for a variety of reasons. Pro-inflammatory cytokines can inhibit erythropoietin production in the kidney and can induce hepcidin, which inhibits iron absorption and iron release by macrophages. Patients are also at risk of gastrointestinal bleeding when using regular or even occasional non-steroidal anti-inflammatory drugs. Haemolysis is the correct answer here, since it is highly unlikely in the setting of a normal bilirubin concentration on liver function testing.

CASE 13

D: Given the low C4 and significantly elevated rheumatoid factor, a sample for cryoglobulins should be sent

Cyroglobulinaemia occurs in the presence of cryoglobulin-containing immune complexes. Depending on the type of cryoglobulin present, it can be classified into three different types. There is a recognised association between hepatitis C infection and the development of cryoglobulinaemia, particularly types II and III. The cutaneous manifestations of the condition are common and tend to occur in dependent areas. Skin biopsy is likely to show a leukocytoclastic vasculitis, and can occur either idiopathically or secondary to other systemic conditions. A skin biopsy is unlikely to confirm a diagnosis of a specific type of systemic vasculitis.

Patients can present to a number of different specialties, including rheumatology due to arthralgia. A significantly elevated rheumatoid factor (in types II and III) and low C3 are clues to the diagnosis, especially in a patient with hepatitis C. Low complement is found due to ongoing consumption by cryoglobulins or cryoglobulin-propagated immune complexes. Although rheumatoid arthritis and systemic lupus erythematosus are differential diagnoses, with the initial clinical picture the remaining blood results indicate that it is imperative to exclude cryoglobulinaemia associated with hepatitis C infection.

CASE 14

E: Helical CT scan of chest

The patient has Behçet's disease.

Pulmonary aneurysms are a life-threatening complication of the condition and carry a significant mortality rate. They may be suspected on chest X-rays with para- or peri-hilar opacities. However, pulmonary angiography is no longer recommended as the investigation of choice. Contrast studies of the arteries and veins carry risks in patients with Behçet's disease as catheter insertion can lead to venous thrombosis or aneurysm formation at the site of puncture. Helical CT scanning is now the investigation of choice as it does not carry these adverse risks. Ventilation perfusion scans can misdiagnose aneurysms as pulmonary emboli. Anticoagulation in this setting would lead to potentially fatal consequences. Anti-nuclear antibodies, lupus anticoagulant and anticardiolipin antibodies may be useful in excluding antiphospholipid syndrome in patients with pulmonary emboli, but will not identify the cause of haemoptysis in this patient.

CASE 15

D: Gadolinium enhanced cardiac MRI scan

This patient has adult onset Still's disease (AOSD) with myopericarditis.

Learning point

The Yamaguchi criteria for AOSD are listed below.[5]

Major criteria:

1. arthralgia greater than two weeks
2. fever greater than 39 °C
3. typical rash: maculopapular or salmon-pink rash
4. white cells greater than 10×10^9/litre with > 80% granulocytes.

Minor criteria:

1. sore throat
2. lymphadenopathy or splenomegaly
3. abnormal liver function tests
4. anti-nuclear antibody and rheumatoid factor negative.

There are many causes of myocarditis, and in the first instance a thorough screen for potential infective or viral agents should be completed. The clue to the diagnosis of AOSD is the significantly elevated ferritin. It is an important differential diagnosis in the investigation of patients with pyrexia of unknown origin, particularly in the setting of an elevated ferritin. Patients with AOSD can have serum ferritin levels exceeding 3000 µg/litre and levels of up to 10 000 have been reported. The classical AOSD rash is described as an evanescent salmon-coloured maculopapular rash that is more prominent during fever spikes. The fever is typically quotidian and temperature swings can be dramatic. Pharyngitis is also common, and findings of lymphadenopathy and splenomegaly are seen in roughly half of all patients.

Regardless of the underlying cause, the history points to a diagnosis of pericarditis and the raised troponin and wall motion abnormality suggest the possibility of myocarditis. Gadolinium enhanced cardiac MRI scanning would be the gold standard investigation for the assessment of myocarditis. It will also assess for muscle necrosis and scarring, global or regional wall abnormalities, pericardial effusions and cardiac function.

continued

Serial ECGs may assess the dynamic changes of pericarditis, but will give no information on the presence of myocarditis. Serial echocardiography can monitor cardiac function and wall motion abnormalities and indicate improvement, but it cannot confirm or exclude inflammation or necrosis within the wall of the myocardium. In a patient of this age, coronary angiography would not be the investigation of choice as the clinical scenario is not likely to represent a manifestation of coronary artery disease. Although a gated perfusion scan may detect hypertrophy or impairment of left ventricular function, these findings are not specific to myocarditis. The main purpose of a perfusion scan is to detect regional variations in epicardial blood supply. In myocarditis, epicardial blood flow is not normally affected.

CASE 16

E: Muscle biopsy

This patient has dermatomyositis, which is an idiopathic inflammatory myopathy. It typically presents with cutaneous findings or weakness due to muscle inflammation; however, the lungs, oesophagus and joints can be involved. The cutaneous findings described in this case include the 'shawl sign', which is an erythematous rash (also described as poikiloderma, which consists of erythema, hypopigmentation, hyperpigmentation and telangiectasia) over the anterior chest wall and/or upper back in the distribution of a shawl, and periungual telangiectasia. Gottron's papules on the knuckles, a periorbital heliotrope rash or even an erythematous rash on the lateral thighs (known as the 'holster sign') can also be seen in some cases.

The skin manifestations can precede, occur concurrently with or come on after the onset of muscle weakness. The weakness is proximal in distribution and can even result in respiratory difficulties. In patients with respiratory compromise, aspiration pneumonia due to dysphagia or interstitial fibrosis must also be considered. There is an association with underlying malignancy in 10–20% of patients, particularly in the elderly. Breast cancer, lung cancer, ovarian carcinoma and gastric carcinoma are usually implicated, and other investigations will be necessary in this case given that the patient smokes and has dysphagia. These tests would not, however, help in the diagnosis of dermatomyositis.

Although characteristic electromyography readings will support the diagnosis of polymyositis or dermatomyositis, this investigation cannot differentiate an inflammatory cause from other causes of myopathy. Early findings of increased insertional activity and spontaneous fibrillations, or decreased amplitude and duration of polyphasic motor unit potentials would certainly help differentiate from a neurogenic cause of weakness. Muscle imaging techniques such as magnetic resonance imaging have become more widely used to help define and localise the extent of muscle involvement in some patients. MRI scans may demonstrate signal intensity abnormalities of muscle due to inflammation, oedema or necrosis in an inflammatory myopathy, but cannot specify the underlying pathology.

Learning point

Dermatomyositis, polymyositis and inclusion body myositis can only be distinguished from each other and from other forms of myopathy by their histopathologic findings on muscle biopsy. In dermatomyositis this will show inflammation, vasculitis and perifascicular atrophy. A predominant B cell infiltration is seen around blood vessels, and vasculitis involving the perimysial capillaries and arterioles can be demonstrated. Fibres in varying stages of inflammation, necrosis and regeneration will also be seen. Muscle biopsy is the investigation of choice to confirm the correct diagnosis and guide appropriate treatment.

CASE 17

D: AA amyloidosis

Most cases of renal artery stenosis are asymptomatic and the condition is usually excluded during the investigation of a patient with difficult-to-control hypertension or those with declining renal function. A presentation with nephrotic syndrome would not be in keeping with this diagnosis.

Learning point

Patients with chronic systemic inflammatory disease are at risk of developing AA amyloidosis. In this condition, there is misfolding and irreversible transition of amyloid precursor proteins to insoluble fibrils which are deposited into various organs. Deposition occurs primarily in the kidneys, liver, spleen and gastrointestinal tract. Most patients present with proteinuria and renal failure. Hepatic and splenic deposits are rarely symptomatic.

Although gold and penicillamine treatment can cause proteinuria, the patient has probably not been treated with these drugs for many years since they have generally been replaced by other disease-modifying agents such as methotrexate.

There is no mention in this case of any stigmata of lupus, and although this diagnosis should be actively excluded, a far more likely diagnosis in someone with a chronic inflammatory condition that has been poorly controlled is systemic AA amyloidosis.

CASE 18

D: Drug-induced side effects

The patient most likely has anti-tumour necrosis factor (TNF) therapy-induced systemic lupus erythematosus. Constitutional symptoms of fatigue, weight loss and pyrexia are common, but patients can also present with new rashes, pleural or pericardial effusions, pneumonitis, or a deterioration in joint or muscle pain. Although anti-histone antibodies are not pathognomonic for drug-induced lupus and can be found in patients with idiopathic lupus, the previously normal anti-nuclear antibody screen, as well as the new onset of symptoms after treatment with anti-TNF therapy, make this the most likely diagnosis. Infection must be excluded in patients on immunosuppressive therapy, but all patients will undergo a thorough screen for tuberculosis before treatment.

CASE 19

D: Hughes syndrome

The clinical picture is in keeping with a pulmonary embolism. The patient is a smoker and on the oral contraceptive pill; however, the underlying cause is most likely Hughes syndrome which is another term for antiphospholipid syndrome.

Learning point

This is an autoimmune syndrome associated with vascular thrombosis (both arterial and venous), and pregnancy-related issues such as miscarriage and pre-eclampsia. Blood tests to confirm the diagnosis include anticardiolipin antibody, lupus anticoagulant and anti-β_2-glycoprotein. Clues in the history include the previous miscarriage, which in a patient with a diagnosis of lupus, should raise suspicions for the condition. Further clinical clues include the livedo rash, which is a purplish, net-like rash usually found in the extremities. It is due to stagnation of blood and dilation within capillaries. It has several associations, but patients with antiphospholipid syndrome can develop the rash attributable to obstruction of capillaries due to thrombi. The other clue to the diagnosis is the prolonged APTT which occurs due to interference from antibodies.

continued

CHAPTER 14 ANSWERS

Although there is a history of a previous fracture here, the patient has no prior history of steroid use and is currently premenopausal, which would put her in a low category for fracture risk. Serositis due to her lupus would indeed give pleuritic chest pain, but would be unlikely to cause significant dyspnoea. Tietze syndrome or costochondritis would be a diagnosis of exclusion, and other pathologies are more likely given the clinical scenario. Although patients with a community-acquired chest infection initially have a normal chest X-ray, the patient has a normal C-reactive protein concentration and no history of a productive cough. On balance, pulmonary embolism with the suspicion of underlying anti-phospholipid syndrome is the most likely diagnosis.

CASE 20

C: Plasmapheresis

The underlying diagnosis is thrombotic thrombocytopenic purpura (TTP).

> ### Learning point
>
> TTP is associated with the pentad of thrombocytopenia, fever, renal impairment, microangiopathic haemolytic anaemia and neurological symptoms. Lupus itself can present with all of the above features, but the finding of schistocytes on the blood film is strongly suggestive of TTP.

Aggregation of platelet thrombi with abundance of von Willebrand factor in the arterioles and capillaries of multiple organs is found in association with a disintegrin and metalloproteinase with a thrombospondin type 1 motif, member 13 (ADAMTS13) activity deficiency. The condition presents with haemolysis, thrombocytopenia and schistocytes on blood smears, often with neurological involvement. Mortality from the condition has improved in recent years due to the availability of plasmapheresis. Owing to the life-threatening severity of the condition, and the fact that drugs used to treat systemic lupus such as rituximab or cyclophosphamide take time to work, plasmapheresis is necessary here. The presence of schistocytes along with the remaining history is sufficient to diagnose TTP if the patient is too unwell for a bone marrow aspiration. Dialysis may be part of her supportive care but will not address the underlying pathology.

CASE 21

D: Eosinophilic granulomatosis with polyangiitis (EGPA)

Eosinophilic granulomatosis with polyangiitis is also known as Churg–Strauss vasculitis.

Learning point

The presence of four or more of these criteria has a sensitivity of 85% and a specificity of 99.7% for diagnosing this condition:

✦ asthma (a history of wheezing or the finding of diffuse high-pitched wheezes on expiration)

✦ greater than 10% eosinophils on the differential leukocyte count

✦ mononeuropathy (including multiplex) or polyneuropathy

✦ migratory or transient pulmonary opacities detected radiographically

✦ paranasal sinus abnormality

✦ biopsy containing a blood vessel showing the accumulation of eosinophils in extravascular areas.

Figure 14.5 represents a pericardial effusion, which was the cause of the cardiac arrest. EGPA can affect multiple systems. Asthma is the cardinal feature and is present in more than 95% of patients. It usually precedes the vasculitis phase by eight to ten years. Two thirds of patients have skin involvement, ranging from palpable purpura to subcutaneous nodules. Neurological involvement can present with a peripheral neuropathy, usually mononeuritis multiplex. Gastrointestinal involvement with abdominal pain, diarrhoea and bleeding has been reported, and renal involvement, although reported less commonly than in the other vasculitides, typically manifests as a focal segmental glomerulonephritis. This patient had predominantly nasal and cardiac involvement. Patients can have a history of allergic rhinitis or varying degrees of sinus polyposis with the maxillary sinus being the most frequently affected. Chronic serous otitis and sensorineural hearing loss are occasionally seen, and likely reflect the severity of rhinosinusitis. Although a positive anti-nuclear cytoplasmic antibody (ANCA) test is always reassuring in the setting of a possible vasculitis, only 40% of patients with EGPA are ANCA positive. Furthermore, patients with cardiac involvement are less likely to have a positive ANCA and are more likely to have higher peripheral blood eosinophil counts than other patients with this condition. Although each of the other diagnoses has potential merit, the clinical picture and pathology strongly support the diagnosis of a vasculitis and specifically EGPA.

**CHAPTER 14
ANSWERS**

CASE 22

A: 2–10 times the population prevalence of the disease

People with a first degree relative who is a patient with rheumatoid arthritis (RA) have 2–10 times the population prevalence of the disease. RA affects 0.5–1.5% of the population in industrialised countries.

CASE 23

E: Switch to subcutaneous methotrexate and consider the addition of a second disease-modifying anti-rheumatic drug (DMARD)

The management of RA has changed over the years, and the strategies used to gain rapid disease control and minimise joint destruction include 'treat to target' and 'TICORA' (tight control in RA) protocols. Ultimately, the aim is early diagnosis and remission, and patients diagnosed and treated within the first three months of symptoms have better outcomes.

Learning point

Clinical trials have shown that early combination of DMARDs to gain disease control with a subsequent 'step-down' strategy is more effective than serial monotherapy (ie answers C and D). Although switching to subcutaneous methotrexate may be necessary to try to improve her nausea, this patient has poor prognostic features with rheumatoid factor positivity and anti-CCP antibodies, and therefore early aggressive disease management and combination DMARDs are appropriate. In the UK, patients currently qualify for anti-TNF treatment once they have failed on two DMARDs, one of which should be methotrexate.

CASE 24

B: Sciatic nerve injury after gluteal injection

Mononeuritis multiplex is defined as nerve damage in two or more named nerves in separate parts of the body, eg foot drop due to damage to either the sciatic or peroneal nerve associated with wrist drop due to infarction of the radial nerve. This patient only has one area of nerve involvement. Compression or trauma to the sciatic nerve can occur in the sciatic notch or gluteal region. Trauma including hip fractures or dislocation, prolonged external compression or inaccurately placed injections can cause symptoms. Other compressive aetiologies include piriformis syndrome when the nerve is compressed in the sciatic notch by the piriformis muscle. This is more common in athletes when the piriformis muscle hypertrophies. Given the recent intramuscular injection in this case, the most likely answer is the first option.

Common peroneal nerve compression or injury will usually present with weakness on dorsiflexion and eversion, with sensory loss on the dorsum of the foot and preserved reflexes. Meralgia paraesthetica is frequently seen in people with recent weight gain due to compression of the lateral femoral cutaneous nerve at the inguinal ligament. It will cause paraesthesia and pain radiating down the lateral thigh to the knee, and sensory loss will be found on the lateral thigh. Sinus tarsi syndrome is characterised by anterolateral ankle pain secondary to trauma to the region that results in instability of the sub-talar joint, resulting in excessive supination and pronation.

References

1. Hunder G et al. 1990. The American College of Rheumatology 1990 criteria for the classification of giant cell arteritis. Arthritis and Rheumatism, 33, 1122–1128

2. Leavitt R et al. 1990. The American College of Rheumatology 1990 criteria for the classification of Wegener's granulomatosis. Arthritis and Rheumatism, 33, 1101–1107

3. Jennette J et al. 2012. 2012 Revised International Chapel Hill Consensus Conference Nomenclature of Vasculitides. Arthritis and Rheumatism, 65, 1–11

4. International Study Group for Behcet's Disease. 1990. Criteria for diagnosis of Behcet's disease. Lancet, 335, 1078–1080

5. Yamaguchi M et al. 1992. Preliminary criteria for classification of adult Still's disease. Journal of Rheumatology, 19, 424–430

CHAPTER 15

Therapeutics and Toxicology

Paul Hamilton

CASE 1

A 58-year-old man is reviewed at the medical clinic. He has been feeling unwell for several months, and his symptoms seem to be worsening. He describes abdominal cramps, intermittent vomiting, lethargy and some weakness of the fingers when working. Past medical history includes hypothyroidism and migraine. He takes levothyroxine 125 μg daily. There is no significant family history. He works in a scrap metal processing plant and uses an oxyacetylene cutter regularly.

Blood tests reveal the following: Haemoglobin 103 g/litre, MCV 92 fl, White cells 4.5×10^9/litre, Platelets 322×10^9/litre, Urinalysis: glucose +++, Sodium 136 mmol/litre, Potassium 3.7 mmol/litre, Urea 4.8 mmol/litre, Creatinine 68 μmol/litre, eGFR > 60 ml/min per 1.73 m².

Which of the following tests is most likely to lead to a diagnosis in this case?

- A. **Thyroid function tests**
- B. **Plasma protein electrophoresis**
- C. **IgA anti-transglutaminase antibody**
- D. **Oral glucose tolerance test**
- E. **Blood lead level**

CASE 2

A 78-year-old lady presents with pain in her left thigh. There is no history of trauma. Her medical history includes osteoporosis, diverticulitis and hypercholesterolaemia. On examination, her vital signs are stable. Her leg length is uniform and there is no abnormal rotation. An X-ray reveals an incomplete fracture of the mid-shaft of the femur. Which of these drugs for osteoporosis has been linked with this complication?

    A. **Calcitonin**
    B. **Strontium ranelate**
    C. **Teriparatide**
    D. **Denosumab**
    E. **Raloxifene**

CASE 3

A 44-year-old man with heterozygous familial hypercholesterolaemia is reviewed at clinic. He is being treated with combination lipid-lowering therapy comprising atorvastatin 40 mg daily, ezetimibe 10 mg daily and fenofibrate 200 mg daily. He is concerned regarding newspaper reports that he has read regarding the side effects of the drugs that he is taking. Which of the following is most unlikely to represent a potential adverse drug reaction in his case?

    A. **Rhabdomyolysis**
    B. **Diabetes mellitus**
    C. **Hyponatraemia**
    D. **Hepatitis**
    E. **Cholestasis**

CASE 4

A 62-year-old man with obesity, hypertension, gout and type 2 diabetes attends his GP for a general health check. He had been reviewed at a hospital diabetes clinic six weeks previously and was commenced on a new drug for diabetes since his glycaemic control was poor. He complains of penile discomfort that has been present in the last two weeks, with an occasional non-offensive urethral discharge. He has not had a sexual partner since the death of his wife five years previously. Which of the following agents is he most likely to have been commenced on?

A. **Acarbose**
B. **Sitagliptin**
C. **Exenatide**
D. **Dapagliflozin**
E. **Pioglitazone**

CASE 5

A 34-year-old lady with a history of schizophrenia presents to her GP complaining of intermittent discharge from the left nipple. On examination, no masses are detected in either breast, although the nipple is slightly indrawn on the left side. She is currently prescribed risperidone. A blood sample is sent for prolactin estimation and the following results are returned:

✦ Prolactin 1542 mU/litre

✦ Monomeric-prolactin 341 mU/litre

Which of the following management options is most appropriate?

A. **Arrange pituitary imaging, and commence cabergoline**
B. **Substitute risperidone for an alternative agent to be determined by her psychiatrist**
C. **Repeat prolactin testing after an interval of six to eight weeks**
D. **Arrange an urgent review at a breast clinic for triple assessment**
E. **Reassure her**

CASE 6

You review an 83-year-old man in the medical ward. He was admitted after a fall which is believed to have been due to him tripping over a mat at home. Medical history includes a previous stroke, atrial fibrillation, polymyalgia rheumatica, rheumatoid arthritis and osteoporosis. He is taking the following medication: prednisolone 5 mg daily, digoxin 125 µg daily, amiodarone 200 mg daily, hydroxychloroquine 200 mg daily and alendronic acid 70 mg daily. He mentions that he has been experiencing some unusual colour vision in recent months, and therefore undergoes a full visual assessment. Visual acuity is normal when wearing glasses, visual fields are full to confrontation, direct fundoscopy and slit lamp examination of the eyes are unremarkable. Which of his drugs should you consider changing on the basis of his visual symptoms?

A. **Prednisolone**
B. **Digoxin**
C. **Amiodarone**
D. **Hydroxychloroquine**
E. **Alendronic acid**

CASE 7

A 52-year-old man presents to the emergency department complaining of intermittent spasms of his hands that have been worsening over the last two weeks. His past medical history includes type 2 diabetes, gout, hypertension, gastritis and osteoarthritis of the knee. On examination you note a mild tremor of the outstretched hands and occasional twitching. Trousseau's sign is positive; Chvostek's sign is negative.

Blood testing reveals the following: Haemoglobin 142 g/litre, White cells 8.2 × 10⁹/litre, Platelets 352 × 10⁹/litre, Sodium 136 mmol/litre, Potassium 4.2 mmol/litre, Chloride 98 mmol/litre, Bicarbonate 23 mmol/litre, Urea 5.2 mmol/litre, Creatinine 62 µmol/litre, Albumin 35 g/litre, Calcium 2.03 mmol/litre.

Which of the following drugs that he is taking is most likely to be to blame for his presentation?

A. **Metformin**
B. **Allopurinol**
C. **Amiloride**
D. **Omeprazole**
E. **Diclofenac**

CASE 8

A 71-year-old lady is recovering in hospital following her third cycle of cisplatin and etoposide chemotherapy for extensive stage small cell lung cancer. She has had significant nausea and vomiting, and is now receiving a continuous infusion of levomepromazine subcutaneously. Her other medical history includes epilepsy and depression for which she takes carbamazepine and venlafaxine. Her vomiting settles after 48 hours and she is able to resume a normal diet. Over the course of an afternoon, she complains of an increasing headache and is felt by family members to have become a little confused. On assessment, she scores 6/10 on an abbreviated mental test. Her pulse rate is 94 bpm, and blood pressure is 96/48 mmHg lying and 72/50 mmHg standing. She feels dizzy on standing.

Laboratory tests show the following: Haemoglobin 102 g/litre, White cells 4.6×10^9/litre, Platelets 269×10^9/litre, Sodium 115 mmol/litre, Potassium 4.0 mmol/litre, Chloride 69 mmol/litre, Bicarbonate 21 mmol/litre, Urea 11.2 mmol/litre, Creatinine 70 μmol/litre, eGFR > 60 ml/min per 1.73 m², Serum osmolality 249 mOsmol/kg, Urine osmolality 352 mOsmol/kg, Urinary sodium 157 mmol/litre.

The last serum sodium concentration was checked five days previously when it was 133 mmol/litre. Which of the following is the most likely cause of her current situation?

    A. **Cisplatin**
    B. **Etoposide**
    C. **Levomepromazine**
    D. **Carbamazepine**
    E. **Venlafaxine**

CASE 9

A young woman is brought to the emergency department in a drowsy state. She was found in bed by her room-mate having left a suicide note. On your initial assessment, you note the following: airway patent; respiratory rate 12 breaths/min, oxygen saturations 94% breathing room air; pulse 124 bpm regular, blood pressure 74/52 mmHg; alert to pain only, pupils equally mid-sized and reactive to light; brief abdominal examination unremarkable, bilaterally upgoing plantar reactions. Her capillary blood glucose is 5.8 mmol/litre. An ECG is shown in Figure 15.1.

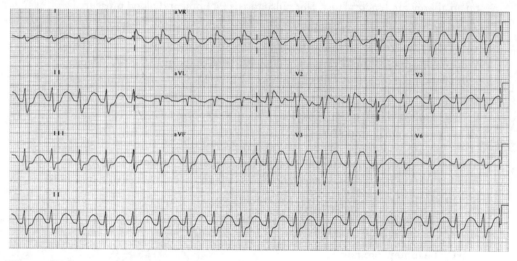

Figure 15.1

Which of the following is the most appropriate next stage in the patient's management?

A. **Arrange an urgent CT scan of head**
B. **Administer IV naloxone as a once-only dose**
C. **Administer IV naloxone by continuous infusion**
D. **Administer IV sodium bicarbonate**
E. **Administer IV flumazenil**

CASE 10

A 35-year-old man is admitted to the medical unit having taken a mixture of tablets from his mother's medicine cabinet while intoxicated about five hours previously. He utters expletives when you ask questions, and refuses to be properly examined. His clinical observations are as follows: temperature 36.7 °C, respiratory rate 14 breaths/min, pulse 72 bpm, blood pressure 124/82 mmHg, oxygen saturations 99% breathing room air. His ECG is shown in Figure 15.2.

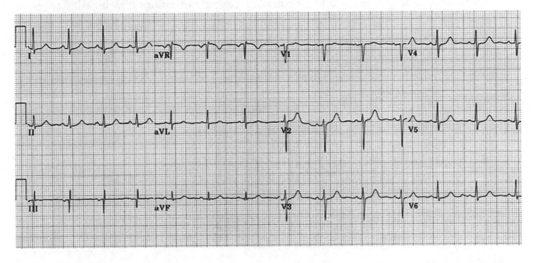

Figure 15.2

Which of the following is the most appropriate blood test to order for this patient?

A. **Digoxin level**
B. **Phenytoin level**
C. **Paracetamol level**
D. **Alcohol level**
E. **Coagulation screen**

CASE 11

A 74-year-old lady is admitted in a confused state. She has a history of hypertension, atrial fibrillation, chronic kidney disease (stage 3a) and gout. She takes the following medication: perindopril, amlodipine, warfarin, digoxin and allopurinol. She recently completed a course of clindamycin for cellulitis affecting her arm. She has had vomiting and diarrhoea for four days. Her clinical observations are as follows: temperature 38.2 °C, respiratory rate 20 breaths/min, pulse 52 bpm, blood pressure 132/88 mmHg, oxygen saturations 99% breathing room air.

Her biochemical blood tests show the following: Sodium 143 mmol/litre, Potassium 6.7 mmol/litre, Urea 17.2 mmol/litre, Creatinine 398 μmol/litre, eGFR 13 ml/min per 1.73 m^2, Digoxin 4.2 ng/ml.

Which of the following is the most important next stage in her management?

   A. Intravenous 0.9% sodium chloride infusion
   B. Intravenous 5% dextrose infusion
   C. Arrange for haemodialysis
   D. Administer digoxin-specific antibody fragments
   E. Commence metronidazole for likely *Clostridium difficile* infection

CASE 12

A middle-aged man is found unwell in the street by a passer-by and brought to the emergency department. He is drowsy, but rousable, and does not provide any sensible answers to your questions. On examination, his airway is patent, respiratory rate is 24 breaths/min, pulse rate 104 bpm, blood pressure 102/78 mmHg and temperature 36.4 °C. His cardiovascular, respiratory and gastrointestinal examinations are unremarkable. His Glasgow Coma Scale is 14/15 (E4 M6 V4). Pupils are equally mid-sized and react normally to light. There is no weakness and reflexes are normal. Capillary blood glucose is 5.2 mmol/litre.

His laboratory investigations reveal: Sodium 136 mmol/litre, Potassium 3.5 mmol/litre, Chloride 88 mmol/litre, Total CO_2 9 mmol/litre, Urea 6.4 mmol/litre, Creatinine 62 μmol/litre, eGFR > 60 ml/min per 1.73 m^2, Glucose 5.6 mmol/litre, Serum osmolality 321 mOsmol/kg.

Urinalysis: no evidence of blood, protein, glucose, nitrites or ketones.

Arterial blood gas analysis breathing room air: pH 7.22, PaO_2 13.2 kPa, $PaCO_2$ 2.3 kPa, Bicarbonate 8 mmol/litre.

Which of the following investigations would be most useful in planning his immediate treatment?

 A. **Salicylate level**
 B. **Urine screen for drugs of abuse**
 C. **Paraquat level**
 D. **Ethanol level**
 E. **Ethylene glycol level**

CASE 13

A 72-year-old man is reviewed at the respiratory clinic. He has been treated with a combination anti-tuberculous regimen for four months. He mentions that he has been feeling unwell for around three weeks. He describes mild fever, arthralgia and a facial rash which appears to flare when exposed to sunlight. Anti-nuclear and anti-histone antibodies are positive. His drug therapy is modified and, at next review four weeks later, his symptoms have largely resolved. Which of the following drugs are likely to be problematic for the patient if ever required in the future?

A. Suxamethonium
B. Hydralazine
C. Gliclazide
D. Ciprofloxacin
E. Nitrofurantoin

CASE 14

You attend a cardiac arrest in a medical ward. The initial rhythm is ventricular fibrillation, and the patient is successfully resuscitated following the delivery of a single shock from a defibrillator. He quickly regains consciousness and removes his laryngeal mask airway. Venous and arterial blood are drawn for analysis and his ECG is shown in Figure 15.3.

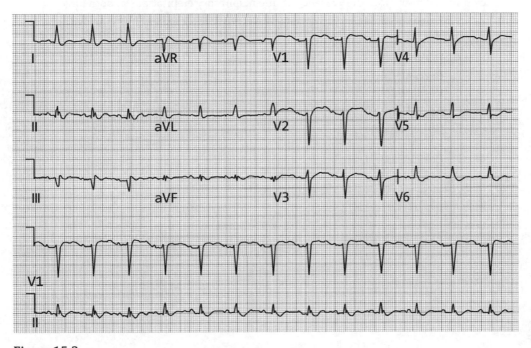

Figure 15.3

Which of the following drugs that the patient is taking is most likely to be responsible for the cardiac arrest?

    A. **Amitriptyline**
    B. **5-propylthiouracil**
    C. **Spironolactone**
    D. **Propafenone**
    E. **Amphotericin**

CASE 15

A 70-year-old lady with a history of heart failure is admitted after an episode of transient loss of consciousness. She has been feeling unwell for five days since commencing bisoprolol for blood pressure control. Her observations show a pulse rate of 36 bpm, respiratory rate 18 breaths/min, blood pressure 72/40 mmHg, oxygen saturation 94% breathing room air and temperature 36.4 °C. On examination you note the presence of fine inspiratory crepitations at both lung bases. Which one of these medications is she most likely to have been taking to account for this presentation?

A. **Ivabradine**
B. **Lercanidipine**
C. **Verapamil**
D. **Amiodarone**
E. **Chlortalidone**

CASE 16

A 35-year-old lady is admitted shortly after taking a deliberate drug overdose in an attempt at suicide. She is alert, but uncooperative, and refuses to tell you which drugs she has taken. On examination her pulse rate is 105 bpm, blood pressure 126/74 mmHg, respiratory rate 24 breaths/min, oxygen saturation 100% on room air and temperature 37.2 °C. Clinical examination is unremarkable. Her pupils are large, equal and reactive. An ECG shows sinus rhythm.

Blood tests reveal: Haemoglobin 132 g/litre, White cells 5.2×10^9/litre, Platelets 280×10^9/litre, Sodium 138 mmol/litre, Potassium 3.8 mmol/litre, Chloride 92 mmol/litre, Total CO_2 15 mmol/litre, Urea 6.2 mmol/litre, Creatinine 58 μmol/litre.

Arterial blood gas analysis (breathing room air): pH 7.36, PaO_2 12.2 kPa, $PaCO_2$ 2.8 kPa, bicarbonate 16 mmol/litre.

Lactate 0.8 mmol/litre.

Paracetamol 4 h after admission < 10 mg/litre.

Alcohol 65 mg/dl.

Coagulation screen normal.

Urinalysis – negative for blood, protein, leukocyte esterase, glucose and ketones.

Which of the following interventions is most likely to be beneficial?

    A. **N-acetylcysteine**
    B. **Fomepizole**
    C. **Enlist a family member's help to attempt to calm her down and reduce the respiratory rate**
    D. **Magnesium**
    E. **Sodium bicarbonate**

CASE 17

A 72-year-old man with end-stage renal failure is admitted with shortness of breath and fever. He is felt to have a combination of community-acquired pneumonia and pulmonary oedema, and receives emergency treatment. He improves over the next few hours. The next morning, he complains of increasing deafness and audiological testing that day reveals sensorineural hearing loss. Which drug that he has been given is most likely to be responsible for the deafness?

A. **Piperacillin-tazobactam**
B. **Gentamicin**
C. **Glyceryl trinitrate**
D. **Furosemide**
E. **Diamorphine**

CASE 18

A 52-year-old woman with resistant hypertension is being treated with perindopril 8 mg, bisoprolol 10 mg, amlodipine 10 mg, indapamide 2.5 mg, spironolactone 25 mg and doxazosin 16 mg daily. Her blood pressure remains elevated at review at the outpatient clinic, and this is confirmed on ambulatory measurement. What is the most appropriate next line of management?

A. **Admit for observation**
B. **Admit and commence intravenous labetalol**
C. **Commence methyldopa**
D. **Commence moxonidine**
E. **Arrange renal sympathetic denervation**

CASE 19

A 48-year-old man with type 1 diabetes is reviewed at a 6-monthly afternoon diabetes clinic. He is keeping well and his log of blood glucose readings shows good control. He is on a basal bolus insulin regimen with insulin glargine and insulin aspart, and also takes ramipril 10 mg daily and simvastatin 40 mg daily. You detect no retinopathy, and examination of the feet is unremarkable. Blood pressure is 148/94 mmHg.

Investigations reveal: HbA1c 43 mmol/mol, Sodium 136 mmol/litre, Potassium 4.2 mmol/litre, Chloride 88 mmol/litre, Total CO_2 25 mmol/litre, Urea 5.8 mmol/litre, Creatinine 58 μmol/litre, eGFR > 60 ml/min per 1.73 m^2, Total cholesterol 4.2 mmol/litre, HDL-cholesterol 1.6 mmol/litre, LDL-cholesterol 1.9 mmol/litre, Triglyceride 2.48 mmol/litre, Urinary albumin:creatinine ratio 96.

Which of the following changes to his treatment should most favourably affect long-term prognosis?

- A. **Add losartan 50 mg daily**
- B. **Add amlodipine 5 mg daily**
- C. **Add aliskiren 150 mg daily**
- D. **Switch from simvastatin to atorvastatin 40 mg daily**
- E. **Add fenofibrate 200 mg daily**

CASE 20

A 56-year-old lady presents to the emergency department with severe palpitations. Her medical history includes fibromyalgia, hypothyroidism, depression and a previous transient ischaemic attack. She normally takes gabapentin, levothyroxine, sertraline, dipyridamole, aspirin and atorvastatin. She is currently also being treated with nitrofurantoin for a urinary tract infection. Examination reveals: pulse rate 182 bpm, blood pressure 142/72 mmHg, respiratory rate 18 breaths/min, oxygen saturation 99% on room air and temperature 37.2 °C. The heart sounds are normal and the chest is clear. An ECG shows a regular narrow complex tachycardia.

Which of the following options would be the next most appropriate management step for this patient?

A. **Check thyroid function urgently**
B. **Give 2 g magnesium sulfate intravenously**
C. **Give amiodarone 300 mg intravenously**
D. **Give adenosine 1.5 mg by rapid intravenous injection**
E. **Sedate and deliver a synchronised DC shock**

CASE 21

A man who appears to be in his early twenties is brought into the emergency department having been found in a collapsed state in a nightclub toilet. No history is available. Examination reveals a patent airway, respiratory rate 14 breaths/min, a central trachea, symmetrical chest expansion, normal chest auscultation and oxygen saturation 99% on room air. The pulse rate is 94 bpm regular and blood pressure is 112/74 mmHg. His pupils are equally mid-sized and react to light. His Glasgow Coma score is 10/15 (E3 M4 V3). The capillary blood glucose is 5.2 mmol/litre. Abdominal and brief neurological examinations are non-contributory. He is given 400 µg of intravenous naloxone, which has no effect on his level of consciousness. A colleague then administers another intravenous antidote. Shortly after this, the patient has a generalised tonic-clonic seizure. Which of the following agents is your colleague most likely to have given?

A. **N-acetylcysteine**
B. **Dicobalt edetate**
C. **Dimercaprol**
D. **Flumazenil**
E. **Sodium bicarbonate**

CASE 22

A 42-year-old lady presents to the emergency department feeling very ill. She was last well one week ago. She developed a flu-like illness initially, dominated by coryzal symptoms and a sore throat. She took time off work on account of this. Over the last three days she has become increasingly tremulous and uncoordinated when using either hand. Her partner who returned from holiday today noted that her speech was slurred and is worried that she has had a stroke. She is unaware of the names of her medical problems, but her husband tells you that she is on a tablet to settle her nerves, and that she regularly attends for blood checks. Which of the following management options is most appropriate?

A. Call the stroke team and prepare for urgent thrombolysis
B. Monitor overnight and arrange a CT scan of brain for the next morning
C. Monitor overnight and arrange a MRI scan of brain for the next morning
D. Check full blood picture for neutropenia and administer a broad spectrum antibiotic with an antiviral agent
E. Check serum lithium level and commence intravenous hydration

CASE 1

E: Blood lead level

Occupational poisoning from lead and mercury produce very characteristic clinical features that are important to recognise. The use of high-temperature cutting equipment in the demolition industry can expose a worker to toxic lead fumes if the material being worked on contains lead paint.

Learning point

The characteristic features of lead poisoning include: abdominal colic, neuropathy, anaemia and nephropathy. The glycosuria is due to proximal renal tubular damage. Erythrocyte δ-aminolevulinic acid dehydratase (ALAD), urinary δ-aminolevulinic acid and blood zinc protoporphyrin levels can all point towards lead poisoning, as can the total blood lead level.

There are a number of distracters in this case. Abnormal thyroid function could account for the lethargy, gastrointestinal upset and anaemia, but not the other features. Multiple myeloma could cause lethargy and anaemia. Coeliac disease could explain the gastro-intestinal upset and anaemia. Diabetes could account for lethargy, neuropathy and glycosuria. Always look for an answer that can explain all of the abnormalities listed in the question. Occupational clues are often extremely relevant, as in this case.

CASE 2

D: Denosumab

This lady has sustained an atypical femoral fracture. This rare complication of osteoporosis treatment has recently been reported in the setting of patients taking long-term bisphosphonates or denosumab. It should be considered in any patient taking either of these medications who presents with pain in the groin, thigh or hip. No bisphosphonates are listed in the list of possible answers, making denosumab the correct choice here. Patients found to have this complication of treatment should always have the contralateral leg imaged also, since disease is often bilateral.

Calcitonin is no longer used in the treatment of osteoporosis, since its use is linked with the development of cancer. Strontium can cause gastrointestinal upset, but is also linked with venous thromboembolism and myocardial infarction. Teriparatide may cause gastro-intestinal upset, palpitations, shortness of breath and myalgia, among other effects. Raloxifene should be used with caution in patients at risk of venous thromboembolism or stroke, and it should not be used in patients who have breast cancer.

CASE 3

C: Hyponatraemia

Lipid-lowering therapy is commonly prescribed, and patients at high risk of cardiovascular complications often require combinations of lipid-lowering drugs to bring their lipid levels down to recommended targets.

Statins may cause muscle-related adverse effects ranging from myalgia to rhabdomyolysis. Deranged liver function tests (most commonly a hepatitis picture) may also be seen – hence patients should have their transaminases checked routinely after commencing treatment. Statins are largely very well tolerated, although many other side effects have been attributed to their use. A fairly recently reported side effect is the potential link between statin therapy and the development of hyperglycaemia or diabetes mellitus. Fibrates are also well tolerated in most individuals. When problems do occur, they are most commonly related to gastro-intestinal upset. These drugs are contraindicated in patients with gall bladder disease since they can cause cholestasis. They may also cause muscle disease, particularly when prescribed alongside a statin. Ezetimibe may cause gastrointestinal tract disturbance.

CASE 4

D: Dapagliflozin

There are now a vast array of drugs utilised in the treatment of patients with diabetes, and this question tests knowledge of the adverse effects of some of the newer agents.

Dapagliflozin is an inhibitor of the sodium-glucose co-transporter 2, and improves glycaemic control by increasing renal excretion of glucose. Adverse effects include dehydration, hypoglycaemia and infections of the genito-urinary tract. In this case, the patient has probably developed an infection with Candida.

Acarbose is not a new drug. It is an alpha-glucosidase inhibitor, and its use is greatly limited by the development of gastrointestinal side effects. Sitagliptin is a dipeptidyl peptidase-4 inhibitor. Adverse effects include gastrointestinal tract disturbance, oedema and upper respiratory tract symptoms. Pancreatitis has been reported. Exenatide is an agonist at the glucagon-like peptide-1 receptor. Side effects may include gastrointestinal upset, injection site reactions and pancreatitis. Pioglitazone is a thiazolidinedione. Although most patients take this drug without complication, liver dysfunction, heart failure, bone fractures and bladder cancer have been linked to its use.

CASE 5

D: Arrange an urgent review at a breast clinic for triple assessment

> ### Learning point
>
> There are a number of distracters here to try to lead you astray. This young lady has unilateral breast symptoms and an abnormal breast examination. She should be assumed to have breast cancer until proven otherwise.

Hyperprolactinaemia is commonly due to medications. In this case, however, the apparent hyperprolactinaemia is actually not grounds for concern. Some individuals, like the patient in this case, have unusually large forms of circulating prolactin. This 'macroprolactin' is not known to cause any clinical problems, but it does cause confusion when a doctor orders a prolactin blood test, since an extremely elevated prolactin concentration is 'falsely' reported. Most laboratories automatically go on to perform subsequent testing on prolactin when the level exceeds a predefined threshold (eg 700 mU/litre). In such circumstances, the 'monomeric-prolactin' concentration is reported, and this is the level to pay most attention to. In this case, the monomeric-prolactin level is normal, indicating that prolactin excess is not the cause for the presentation.

Commonly used drugs that can raise the prolactin level include: antipsychotics, antidepressants, antihistamines, anticonvulsants, antihypertensives, anti-dopamine agents, oestrogens and opioids.

CASE 6

B: Digoxin

This is a tricky question since all of the drugs listed can have adverse effects on the eye.

The list of adverse reactions of corticosteroids is an extensive one. It includes: hyperglycaemia, hypertension, osteoporosis, proximal myopathy, thinning of the skin and acne, peptic ulceration, immunosuppression and steroid-induced psychosis. In high doses, Cushing syndrome may result. In relation to the eye, steroids may cause the development of cataracts (typically posterior sub-capsular cataracts) as well as increasing intraocular pressure and causing papilloedema. One would expect these problems to have been picked up during the ophthalmic assessment of this patient.

Digoxin therapy can be linked with xanthopsia, a yellowish discoloration of the vision, and is the cause of the visual disturbance in this case. Other adverse effects associated with digoxin include nausea, vomiting and various types of cardiac arrhythmia.

Amiodarone is associated with a myriad of adverse effects. From an ocular perspective, the drug can cause corneal micro-deposits. These may cause glare at night, but should not affect colour perception. Rarely, optic neuritis or optic neuropathy can occur. Other adverse effects of this drug include: pulmonary fibrosis, abnormal thyroid function, skin discoloration, peripheral neuropathy, liver dysfunction and hypokalaemia.

Hydroxychloroquine is an uncommonly used drug that has a well-established link with ophthalmic complications. Screening for retinopathy is recommended and patients are encouraged to report any deterioration in eyesight. Other side effects include gastrointestinal upset, headache and rash. Hair and skin changes may occur, as may reductions in blood counts.

Bisphosphonates, like alendronic acid, are associated with gastrointestinal adverse effects, particularly irritation of the oesophagus. They can, however, cause uveitis and scleritis, although there was no evidence of either of these conditions in this patient. Other important potential adverse effects of this class of drugs include hypocalcaemia, osteonecrosis of the jaw and atypical femoral fractures.

CASE 7

D: Omeprazole

This man presents with neuromuscular irritability. This is commonly a feature of hypocalcaemia. Note that Trousseau's sign (spasm of the hands upon inflation of a cuff on the upper arm) may be abnormal despite a normal Chvostek's sign (spasm of the facial muscles after tapping on the facial nerve).

Learning point

Although this man's serum calcium concentration is low, when corrected for the hypoalbuminaemia, it is actually normal. Correction is performed by using the following formula: corrected calcium (mmol/litre) = calcium (mmol/litre) + [0.02 × (40 − albumin (g/litre)]. In this case the corrected calcium is 2.13 mmol/litre (2.03 + [0.02 × (40 − 35)]). Hypocalcaemia is therefore not to blame for his symptoms.

Hypomagnesaemia can also present in this way, and is the cause of the presentation here. The most common causes for hypomagnesaemia include: inadequate intake, alcohol excess, re-distribution (eg in re-feeding syndrome or during the treatment of diabetic ketoacidosis), disease of the gastrointestinal tract, renal disease or as an adverse effect of several drugs. Commonly implicated drugs include loop and thiazide diuretics, aminoglycosides, amphotericin B and calcineurin inhibitors (eg ciclosporin and tacrolimus). Recently, proton pump inhibitors such as omeprazole have been implicated in several cases of severe magnesium deficiency. The precise mechanism of action is unknown, but the phenomenon may relate to impaired magnesium absorption from the gut, possibly due to disruption of TRPM6 channel function. The problem tends to occur in patients who have been treated chronically. Other adverse effects of proton pump inhibitors include: gastrointestinal upset, headache and hyponatraemia.

Adverse effects of the other drugs listed that might be asked about include: metformin – gastrointestinal upset, lactic acidosis and risk of vitamin B12 deficiency; allopurinol – rash including Stevens–Johnson syndrome; amiloride – gastrointestinal bleeding and hyperkalaemia; diclofenac – gastrointestinal effects including ulceration, bronchospasm, acute kidney injury, hypertension and worsening of heart failure.

CASE 8

A: Cisplatin

This patient has symptomatic hyponatraemia and requires prompt treatment. She potentially has several reasons for developing hyponatraemia – lung cancer, nausea, vomiting and her medication.

Learning point

The key to answering this question correctly is to classify her hyponatraemia appropriately and to identify the most likely cause of this from the list of drugs given. Traditionally, the assessment of hyponatraemic patients is centred on an accurate assessment of volume status and categorisation of patients as either hypo-, normo- or hyper-volaemic.

This lady has symptomatic postural hypotension and is therefore likely to be hypovolaemic. Hypovolaemia is commonly due to fluid loss from either the gastrointestinal tract or the kidneys. She certainly has had excessive gastrointestinal fluid loss with her vomiting, but if this were the cause of the hyponatraemia in this instance, one would expect normally functioning kidneys to retain sodium, ie the urinary sodium would be expected to be < 15 mmol/litre. However, her urinary sodium excretion is very high indeed, so raising the possibility of renal salt wasting. Her eGFR is > 60 ml/min per 1.73 m^2 and she is not on diuretics. She has, however, been exposed to cisplatin, which in rare occasions can cause a renal salt wasting syndrome.

Levomepromazine is a first-generation phenothiazine antipsychotic drug that shares the side-effect profile of more familiar agents such as chlorpromazine, ie extrapyramidal effects (parkinsonism, acute dystonia, akathisia and tardive dyskinesia), cardiovascular effects, impaired temperature regulation, neuroleptic malignant syndrome and many others. Hyponatraemia can sometimes be seen with drugs in this class due to the syndrome of inappropriate antidiuresis (SIAD). Both carbamazepine and venlafaxine can also cause SIAD. This patient's volume status and laboratory results are not, however, compatible with this diagnosis. Other drug causes of SIAD include: selective serotonin reuptake inhibitors, tricyclic antidepressants, monoamine oxidase inhibitors, and various anticonvulsants.

CASE 9

D: Administer IV sodium bicarbonate

This is a case of tricyclic antidepressant (TCA) poisoning, and must not be missed either in the examination or in real-life medicine.

Learning point

The key to this diagnosis is appreciating the subtle ECG change shown. The most common ECG abnormality indicating severe TCA poisoning is QRS widening – beyond 100 ms is abnormal and indicates risk of arrhythmia and seizure. The more subtle change illustrated here is the presence of a dominant R wave in lead AVR. This is shown in more detail in Figure 15.4.

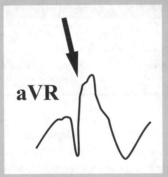

Figure 15.4

ECG changes and refractory hypotension are indications for bicarbonate treatment. Other pointers in poisoning cases that should make you suspect TCA overdose include urinary retention (due to anticholinergic actions of the drugs), cardiac arrhythmia and seizures.

Naloxone is an antagonist at opioid receptors and is indicated in opioid toxicity. Although drowsiness, slow respiratory rate and hypotension can be features of opioid poisoning, one would expect a slower respiratory rate and pinpoint pupils. Naloxone could be given if there was any concern of opioid toxicity, but a dramatic response would not be expected in this case based on the information given.

CASE 10

C: Paracetamol level

Do not be put off by normality. Recognising normal appearances in tests can be extremely difficult in examination settings, and their inclusion can distract many candidates who continue to search for minute abnormalities that are simply not present. The clinical observations and ECG are all normal here. This makes digoxin and phenytoin poisoning less likely. A blood alcohol level rarely influences treatment. In the setting of poisoning, a coagulation screen is most useful for picking up paracetamol-induced liver failure. This typically does not occur until at least 24 hours after ingestion, and so would be expected to be normal five hours post dosing, even if a significant quantity of paracetamol had been taken.

Learning point

A paracetamol level should be checked in all cases of poisoning, since the consequences of not picking up paracetamol toxicity could potentially be fatal for the patient. Levels must be taken at least four hours post ingestion, otherwise they cannot be interpreted with certainty.

You should be aware of the latest treatment guidelines concerning paracetamol toxicity. Points to note include: there is no longer a 'high-risk treatment line' on the nomogram (decision-to-treat graph) to assist in decisions regarding who to treat; you should not use the nomogram if the time of ingestion is unknown, slow-release preparations have been taken, drugs that delay gastric-emptying have been taken concomitantly or when the overdose has been staggered. Care should be taken in patients presenting late.

CASE 11

D: Administer digoxin-specific antibody fragments

The most important first stage in this patient's management would be the treatment of her life-threatening hyperkalaemia. This is taken as given, so none of the answers provided is of particular help in that regard. Administration of fluid would be helpful in replacing volume lost via the gastrointestinal tract. Haemodialysis might be necessary in due course – if the kidney function does not improve or if the potassium level does not settle with treatment, for example. *C. difficile* is a possible cause of the diarrhoea, but the presence of vomiting would perhaps make gastroenteritis more likely. Sending stool for analysis would seem reasonable before commencing metronidazole. In any case, this is not the pressing issue.

This lady has significant digoxin toxicity caused by accumulation of the drug secondary to reduced excretion due to the renal impairment. The key to answering this question correctly is appreciating the severity of the digoxin toxicity because of the hyperkalaemia. The combination of digoxin toxicity and hyperkalaemia confers a very poor prognosis. Digoxin toxicity in the context of hypokalaemia increases the risk of arrhythmia. Indications for the administration of the digoxin antidote are shown below.

Indications for digoxin-specific antibody fragments
Life-threatening arrhythmia
Potassium > 5 mmol/litre
Chronic poisoning with severe features
Digoxin level at least 10 ng/ml (at 6 h) or at least 15 ng/ml at any time
Ingestion of 10 mg or more
Non-digoxin cardiac glycoside poisoning

CASE 12

E: Ethylene glycol level

Poisoned patients are often not forthcoming with information that might assist you in planning their treatment. Careful examination of all the information at your disposal is essential. Performing two calculations in this case can help immensely in narrowing down the likely cause of the presentation.

First, you should appreciate that the patient has a metabolic acidosis. This should automatically trigger you to calculate the anion gap and decide whether this is raised or normal, since this will eliminate several possibilities as causes of the presentation. The anion gap (mmol/litre) = sodium + potassium – bicarbonate – chloride (where all concentrations are in mmol/litre). Commonly occurring causes of raised anion gap metabolic acidosis include lactic acidosis, renal failure, diabetic ketoacidosis, and poisoning with salicylates, paracetamol, tricyclic antidepressants or toxic alcohols (eg ethylene glycol, isopropyl alcohol, methanol). Normal anion gap metabolic acidosis is most commonly seen with excessive gastrointestinal tract losses and in renal tubular acidosis. The anion gap in this case is raised at 40 mmol/litre.

The second calculation to perform is the osmolal gap. You should consider calculating this when you are given the serum osmolality. The osmolal gap is the difference between the calculated and the measured osmolality. Calculated osmolality = (2 × sodium) + urea + glucose (all in mmol/litre). In this case, the osmolar gap is 30. A normal osmolal gap is around 2, so the gap here is clearly very high. This means that there is a significant quantity of an unmeasured osmotically active substance in the patient's blood. This abnormality is often due to the presence of ethanol or a toxic alcohol, most commonly ethylene glycol (antifreeze), in the patient's blood.

Bearing these results in mind, it would be imperative to order both an ethanol and an ethylene glycol level for the patient. More complex calculations can be performed to assess the contribution of the ethanol to the osmolar gap, but discussion of these issues is beyond the scope of this question.

CASE 13

B: Hydralazine

This case requires knowledge of two pharmacological phenomena to be answered correctly: drug-induced lupus erythematosus and slow acetylator status.

The patient's symptoms and immunological blood tests are in keeping with lupus. This could represent de novo systemic lupus erythematosus (SLE) or drug-induced lupus erythematosus (DILE). It would be relatively uncommon for a man in his seventies to present with SLE, and the additional presence of anti-histone antibodies make DILE more likely than SLE. The fact that the symptoms resolved quickly upon modification of his medication clinches this diagnosis. Drugs commonly implicated in DILE include isoniazid, minocycline (and various other antimicrobials), diltiazem, procainamide, carbamazepine, phenytoin, methyldopa and hydralazine. Given that this man was on treatment for tuberculosis, it is likely that this was a case of DILE related to isoniazid.

Learning point

Arriving at the correct answer in this question next requires appreciation of the fact that isoniazid-induced lupus is most likely in individuals who are genetically programmed to acetylate drugs slowly (so-called 'slow acetylators'). Problematic drugs in such people can be remembered using the mnemonic 'D-SHIP': dapsone, sulfonamides and sulfasalazine, hydralazine, isoniazid and procainamide. Hence, this patient is most likely to have problems if he is ever prescribed hydralazine.

The distractors in this case also deserve mention since they are all associated with other pharmacological problems. In patients with abnormal plasma pseudocholinesterase activity, the administration of suxamethonium may be associated with a markedly prolonged effect. This could cause problems if a general anaesthetic is ever required. In patients with mutations of the ryanodine receptor, administration of suxamethonium may also cause the rare condition malignant hyperthermia, necessitating treatment with dantrolene. This condition may also occur when other anaesthetic agents are administered.

Gliclazide, a sulfonylurea, is one in a long list of drugs that can trigger an attack of porphyria in susceptible individuals. The British National Formulary lists the following drug groups as the agents most likely to be associated with acute porphyria (although many more drugs have been implicated): alkylating drugs, amphetamines, anabolic steroids, antidepressants, antihistamines, barbiturates, calcium channel blockers, hormonal

continued

contraceptives, ergot derivatives, hormone replacement therapy, imidazole antifungals, non-nucleoside reverse transcriptase inhibitors, progestogens, protease inhibitors, sulfonamides, sulfonylureas, taxanes, thiazolidinediones and triazole antifungals.[1]

The other disorder affecting drug sensitivity that is commonly tested in examinations is that of glucose 6 phosphate dehydrogenase deficiency. Patients with this condition are prone to developing haemolysis if exposed to an implicated drug. Implicated drugs used in the UK include: dapsone, methylthionium chloride, nitrofurantoin, primaquine, quinolone antimicrobials (including ciprofloxacin), rasburicase and sulfonamides.[1] Drugs that may also be problematic include aspirin, chloroquine, menadione, quinine and sulfonylureas.

Adverse reactions of the commonly used anti-tuberculous drugs are frequently tested. They include: rifampicin – flu-like symptoms, haemolysis, thrombocytopenia, acute renal failure, hepatitis, red discoloration of bodily fluids; isoniazid – peripheral neuropathy, optic neuritis, hypersensitivity reactions, drug-induced lupus erythematosus, agranulocytosis, haemolysis, hepatitis and interstitial pneumonitis; pyrazinamide – hepatitis, sideroblastic anaemia, thrombocytopenia and rash; ethambutol – peripheral neuropathy, optic neuritis and colour blindness.

CASE 14

E: Amphotericin

The key to answering this question lies with correct interpretation of the ECG that shows features in keeping with severe hypokalaemia – flat T waves and the presence of U waves.

> **Learning point**
>
> Drugs linked with hypokalaemia include diuretics (except potassium-sparing agents), steroids, laxatives, insulin, phenothiazines, carbenoxalone and amphotericin. Drugs that commonly cause hyperkalaemia include ACE inhibitors, angiotensin receptor blockers, potassium-sparing diuretics and β blockers.

CASE 15

C: Verapamil

To answer this question correctly, you must correctly recognise that the presentation is likely to be related to her hypotension, and then appreciate which of the medications listed is most likely to interact with the recently commenced β blocker to account for this.

The non-dihydropyridine calcium channel blocker verapamil is the drug most likely to be responsible. Diltiazem is a similar agent.

Learning point

While verapamil and β blockers are sometimes combined for use in hypertension under expert supervision, this combination is not recommended in patients with impaired cardiac function (as in this case) or those with impaired cardiac conducting systems. A dangerous reduction in cardiac contractility, electrical conductivity (with ensuing heart block) or heart rate may occur when these drugs are used together. Other adverse effects of verapamil include gastrointestinal upset and nitrate-like vasodilator effects.

Lercanidipine is a dihydropyridine calcium channel blocker, like amlodipine and other similar-sounding drugs. This class of calcium channel blocker is less likely to result in deleterious cardiac interactions than verapamil or diltiazem, when used concomitantly with β blockers. Vasodilator effects are the most common complaint on these drugs.

Ivabradine is a relatively new anti-anginal agent that is commonly associated with visual adverse effects. It can also cause bradycardia and heart block. It could therefore account for the presentation in this case, but a verapamil/β blocker interaction is more likely. Dabigatran is a novel anticoagulant that has no significant interacting effects with β blockers. Its main adverse effect is bleeding, but gastrointestinal upset may also occur. Chlortalidone is a thiazide-like diuretic with no significant β blocker interaction. Its side effects are similar to those of thiazide diuretics and include metabolic abnormalities (hyponatraemia, hypokalaemia, hypomagnasaemia, hypercalcaemia, hyperglycaemia and hyperuricaemia).

CASE 16

E: Sodium bicarbonate

The diagnosis is not certain based on the limited information given. The patient is tachypnoeic, and the blood gas analysis reveals disturbances of both carbon dioxide and bicarbonate. She may therefore have an acute metabolic acidosis (with a raised anion gap) with complete respiratory compensation, a respiratory alkalosis with complete metabolic compensation or a mixed metabolic acidosis with respiratory alkalosis and an ensuing normal pH. The first and last of these options are realistic possibilities since the acid–base disturbance can be assumed to be relatively acute given the circumstances of a drug overdose. Option two (respiratory alkalosis with complete metabolic compensation) is less likely, since metabolic compensation typically takes time to develop. Based on the assumption that 'common presentations are common', it is likely that this patient has taken a salicylate overdose. This characteristically produces a mixed acid–base disturbance with a respiratory alkalosis (due to stimulation of the respiratory centre) and a metabolic acidosis. Mild salicylate overdoses may be managed with supportive care only. More serious overdoses require intervention. Urinary alkalinisation may be utilised to increase salicylate excretion. This is achieved by administering sodium bicarbonate. In more serious poisonings, dialysis may be required.

N-acetylcysteine is the antidote for paracetamol poisoning. There is no suggestion of a staggered overdose in this case or a late presentation, and a blood level taken more than four hours post ingestion is not elevated. Fomepizole is an inhibitor of alcohol dehydrogenase and may be utilised in poisoning with toxic alcohols. Further evidence of toxic alcohol ingestion would be necessary before administering this agent. Measurement of serum osmolality and comparison with the calculated osmolality would allow the calculation of the osmolal gap. The laboratory may also be able to measure toxic alcohol levels directly in the blood. It is possible that this patient has ingested a toxic alcohol (eg ethylene glycol or methanol), but it is more likely that they have taken salicylates. Calming measures may be helpful in patients with acute agitation in an attempt to slow the respiratory rate and settle the respiratory alkalosis. This is unlikely to be effective in this case.

CASE 17

D: Furosemide

Learning point

Commonly used drugs that are toxic to the ear include loop diuretics (eg furosemide), aminoglycoside antibiotics (eg gentamicin), macrolide antibiotics (eg erythromycin), vancomycin, platinum compounds (eg cisplatin) and isoniazid.

It is possible that the patient received all of the drugs listed in the management of his pneumonia and pulmonary oedema. The potentially ototoxic options are gentamicin and furosemide. Gentamicin ototoxicity is more common after a prolonged course of treatment than after a single dose. Furosemide ototoxicity is often linked with administration of a large quantity of the drug. In this case, since the patient has end-stage renal failure, it is most likely that he received a large dose of furosemide to stimulate a diuresis.

CASE 18

A: Admit for observation

This question is included for reasons of assessing principles of prescribing rather than testing complex knowledge of treatment options in hypertension.

Learning point

One should always be mindful of the possibility of poor patient concordance if a disease process proves to be extremely resistant to conventional treatment. This is particularly true for disease processes that are clinically silent (eg hypertension, dyslipidaemia) or where a patient lacks insight into their illness.

The vast majority of patients, even those with severely resistant hypertension, will achieve normalisation of blood pressure when taking six antihypertensive agents. Before further interventions are planned, it would be important to ascertain compliance with the treatment regimen.

Adverse effects of some of the less commonly used antihypertensive drugs are now listed: all centrally acting agents (methyldopa, clonidine and moxonidine) – sedation, dry mouth, oedema; methyldopa – haemolytic anaemia, gynaecomastia; clonidine – rebound hypertension on abrupt withdrawal; minoxidil – vasodilator effects, hypertrichosis; hydralazine – vasodilator effects, drug-induced lupus erythematosus, peripheral neuropathy, haemolytic anaemia and other haematological abnormalities.

CASE 19

B: Add amlodipine 5 mg daily

Relevant cardiovascular risk factors include smoking status, hypertension, dyslipidaemia, hyperglycaemia, renal dysfunction and microalbuminuria. The options given would modify either lipids or blood pressure +/– albumin excretion.

The patient's lipid profile shows a very well-controlled LDL-cholesterol with a relatively high HDL-cholesterol concentration. There would therefore be little point in switching his simvastatin to a more potent agent. His triglyceride concentration is higher than one might hope, but since this was an afternoon clinic, the level may simply reflect the recent intake of food. Even if this was a fasting lipid profile, the merits of lowering a triglyceride concentration of 2.48 mmol/litre would be questionable.

The patient's blood pressure is suboptimal, as is their urinary albumin excretion. The addition of another antihypertensive should hopefully address both of these factors. There is evidence that treatment with drugs active against the effects of the renin–angiotensin system are particularly helpful in such patients, but of note, this patient is already being treated with ramipril. Until relatively recently, it would have been common practice to combine an ACE inhibitor with either an angiotensin receptor blocker (like losartan) or, less commonly, a direct renin inhibitor (aliskiren). It is now known that the combination of more than one such agent increases the likelihood of hyperkalaemia and poor renal outcomes. Combination treatment is therefore no longer advocated. The correct answer in this scenario therefore relates to lowering blood pressure using a drug from a different class – a calcium channel blocker in this case.

CASE 20

D: Give adenosine 1.5 mg by rapid intravenous injection

This lady's palpitations are due to a regular, narrow, complex tachycardia. The Resuscitation Council provides a useful treatment algorithm for treating patients with tachyarrhythmias.[2] Following this algorithm, a synchronised DC shock should only be considered if a patient is in shock, has had syncope, shows features of myocardial ischaemia or is in heart failure. None of these features applies in this case. Magnesium should be considered in polymorphic ventricular tachycardia, or in other arrhythmias when the serum magnesium is known to be low. Amiodarone is useful in the treatment of several tachyarrhythmias; however, it should not be used first line in a regular, narrow, complex rhythm such as in this case. It would be useful to check thyroid function in this case, since an excessive daily dose of thyroxine might exacerbate tachycardia. The results of this test would not be immediately available, however, so other measures must be taken immediately.

Learning point

Standard treatment of a regular, narrow, complex tachycardia involves using vagal manoeuvres to slow the heart rate. In the absence of a sustained response, it would be routine to administer adenosine by rapid intravenous injection. The usual starting dose of 6 mg is normally followed by up to two 12 mg boluses if it is ineffective. Adenosine has an established interaction with dipyridamole. Administration of the standard dose of adenosine to patients taking dipyridamole can result in a significantly exaggerated effect of the adenosine. If required for such patients, a much lower dose of adenosine than normal should be used. Patients with a heart transplant should also receive very cautious dosing of adenosine if it is required.

CASE 21

D: Flumazenil

Flumazenil is a benzodiazepine antagonist, which can be extremely useful for reversing the effects of benzodiazepines given for sedation, for example at the time of a short procedure such as DC cardioversion. The drug is not licensed for use in the treatment of patients who have overdosed themselves on benzodiazepines. Unlike naloxone, which can be used relatively safely in a sedated patient as a test for opioid effects, flumazenil should not be administered to unconscious patients in the hope that their presentation is due to benzodiazepine overdose, unless the administration is supervised by an expert with full resuscitation equipment at hand. The danger of using naloxone in this way is that administration in such a manner has been linked with seizures and adverse outcomes for patients. Seizures are particularly likely in patients who have taken tricyclic antidepressants in overdose and in those with epilepsy.

Antidotes that you should be familiar with are listed below.

Poison	Therapy/antidote
Beta blockers	Atropine, glucagon, isoprenaline
Carbon monoxide	Oxygen
Cyanide	Oxygen, dicobalt edetate, hydroxocobalamin, sodium nitrite with sodium thiosulfate
Digoxin	Digoxin-specific antibodies
Ethylene glycol	Ethanol or fomepizole
Heavy metals	Dimercaprol, penicillamine
Iron salts	Desferrioxamine
Lead	Penicillamine, calcium sodium edetate
Methanol	Ethanol or fomepizole
Opioids	Naloxone
Organophosphate insecticides	Atropine, pralidoxime
Paracetamol	N-acetylcysteine
Tricyclic antidepressants	Sodium bicarbonate
Warfarin	Vitamin K

CASE 22

E: Check serum lithium level and commence intravenous hydration

There are two medications that should immediately come to mind from the description given – being used 'to settle nerves' and requiring regular blood monitoring. These are clozapine, an atypical antipsychotic, and lithium, used in the treatment of mania and other psychiatric conditions. Clozapine can cause agranulocytosis leaving affected patients susceptible to infections. While an intracranial infection might account for some of this patient's symptoms, this would certainly not be a typical presentation for meningitis or encephalitis.

This patient has lithium toxicity, most likely brought on by the self-administration of non-steroidal anti-inflammatory drugs at the time of her flu-like illness. Several drugs interact with lithium, making toxicity more likely. These include: ACE inhibitors, angiotensin receptor blockers, diuretics and non-steroidal anti-inflammatory drugs. Checking a lithium level, witholding the drug and providing adequate hydration is generally effective in the management of mild lithium toxicity. In more serious cases, dialysis may be required.

The fact that her symptoms have developed gradually and are not unilateral would point away from stroke as the cause. Disease of the cerebellum (best visualised using MRI), could account for some of the features described, but lithium toxicity is a more satisfactory provisional diagnosis based on the evidence given.

References

1. Joint Formulary Committee. 2015. British National Formulary (BNF) 69. Pharmaceutical Press, London, UK

2. Resuscitation Council (UK). 2011. Peri-arrest arrhythmias. www.resus.org.uk/resuscitation-guidelines/updates-to-guidelines-2010

Practice Examination

All authors

QUESTIONS

Question 1

A 79-year-old woman has been admitted to hospital with confusion. You are working through a delirium screen and review her drug chart.

Which of the following drugs would be least likely to contribute to her confusion?

A. **Oxybutynin**
B. **Ramipril**
C. **Co-codamol**
D. **Digoxin**
E. **Amitriptyline**

Question 2

You are called by a colleague who informs you that she has accidentally pierced her finger while withdrawing blood from a patient known to have a past history of heroin use. Which of the following is true for risks of transmission of blood-borne infections following a needle stick injury?

A. **3% if donor is hepatitis B e antigen positive**
B. **0.3% if donor is hepatitis B e antibody positive**
C. **30% if donor is hepatitis C antibody positive**
D. **3% if donor is HIV positive**
E. **There is a rare risk of transmission of emerging or unknown agents**

Question 3

A 46-year-old lady complains of neck pain and a pulling sensation to the right which has worsened since its onset nine months ago. There is no past medical history and no family history of neurological disease. On examination, there is torticollis to the right and hypertrophy of the neck muscles on the left. The remainder of the neurological examination is normal. Which of the following treatments is most likely to be effective in this case?

A. **Botulinum toxin injection**
B. **Baclofen**
C. **Trihexyphenidyl**
D. **Tetrabenazine**
E. **Levodopa**

Question 4

A 65-year-old lady is seen at clinic with a several-month history of lethargy. She also complains of the new onset of loose motions associated with abdominal cramps and bloating. She thinks she may have lost some weight. She has also been referred to a dermatologist for the assessment of a pruritic blistering rash on her elbows.

Blood tests reveal: Haemoglobin 90 g/litre, MCV 75 fl, MCH 26 pg,
White cells 4.0×10^9/litre, Platelets 164×10^9/litre, Ferritin 8 ug/litre.

What is the diagnostic investigation of choice for this lady's clinical presentation?

A. **Flexible sigmoidoscopy and serial colonic biopsies**
B. **Colonoscopy**
C. **OGD and duodenal biopsies**
D. **CT scanning of abdomen and pelvis**
E. **Capsule endoscopy**

Question 5

You are asked to see a 46-year-old man as an emergency. He gives a 1-week history of a progressive skin rash and difficulty eating. On examination, he has a widespread rash consisting of numerous 'atypical target' lesions and blisters affecting 8% of his body surface area with a marked conjunctivitis and haemorrhagic mucositis. Which of the following is the most likely trigger?

A. **Bisoprolol**
B. **Ciclosporin**
C. **Paracetamol**
D. **Ramipril**
E. **Sulfamethoxazole-trimethoprim**

Question 6

An 84-year-old man is under investigation for a small unilateral pleural effusion of unknown cause. He is an ex-smoker and has multiple co-morbidities. Previously he complained of reduced exercise tolerance and dry cough. Previous pleural aspiration showed an exudative effusion with no organisms and cytology was negative. A CT scan was carried out which showed a slightly nodular and thickened appearance of the pleura. No definite mass. He was reluctant for further investigation at that time. At review he complains of increasing chest pain, dyspnoea with minimal exertion and weight loss. His history is reviewed – he had some asbestos exposure at work more than 30 years ago. On X-ray, the effusion has increased in size and a chest drain is inserted. Fluid analysis showed: pH 7.21, glucose low, cytology negative. A CT scan is repeated showing increased pleural thickening with some chest wall invasion. Ultrasound guided biopsy confirms mesothelioma.

What is the likely prognosis?

A. **Curative with surgery**
B. **< 6 months' survival**
C. **Median survival is 8–14 months**
D. **Survival of > 3 years is typical**
E. **Radical/curative radiotherapy possible depending on size**

Question 7

A 42-year-old man from sub-Saharan Africa presents with weight loss and malaise. On examination he is cachexic and dehydrated; he is also noted to have multiple pigmented lesions affecting his skin and oral mucosae. Blood tests demonstrate CD4 count < 200ul/mm^3. CT scanning demonstrates multiple lesions affecting the liver, gastrointestinal tract and lungs. What is the most appropriate management?

A. HAART
B. Systemic chemotherapy
C. HAART and intravenous aciclovir
D. HAART and systemic chemotherapy
E. Palliative care and symptom control only

Question 8

Which of the following is not associated with scleroderma?

A. Aspiration pneumonia
B. Macrocytosis and vitamin B12 deficiency
C. Gastric antral vascular ectasia
D. Photosensitive facial rash
E. Malignant hypertension

Question 9

A 45-year-old woman presents to hospital following a deliberate overdose of paracetamol. She was diagnosed with HIV infection one year ago and has been drinking heavily over the past six months. She has recently split from her partner of ten years. Which of the following is not a recognised risk factor for completed suicide?

A. Being single (rather than married etc)
B. Alcohol dependence
C. Female sex
D. History of previous suicide attempts
E. Physical illness

Question 10

A 22-year-old lady is admitted following an episode of transient loss of consciousness. As part of her investigations, she is noted to have a prolonged QT interval on her ECG. In a woman, what corrected QT interval is considered abnormal?

    A. > 450 ms
    B. > 460 ms
    C. > 470 ms
    D. > 480 ms
    E. > 490 ms

Question 11

A 22-year-old woman with a body mass index of 32 kg/m², but no significant past medical history, presents to the ophthalmology department with a 2-week history of headaches and bilateral blurred vision. She has horizontal diplopia which is more marked on left gaze. Her visual field test results are shown in Figure 16.1.

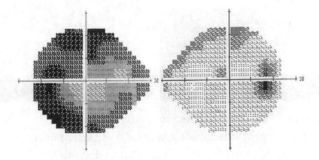

Figure 16.1

An MRI scan of brain and orbits was reported as normal. Which investigation should be done next?

    A. **MRI scan of brain with MR venogram**
    B. **Lumbar puncture**
    C. **Optical coherence tomography**
    D. **Ocular ultrasound scan**
    E. **CT-angiogram**

Question 12

A 62-year-old lady is admitted with abdominal pain and is found to have marked constipation. She has a history of a severe peanut allergy. Ten minutes after administering treatment for constipation, she becomes acutely unwell with hypotension, wheeze, an urticarial rash and lip swelling. Which of the following agents is she most likely to have been prescribed?

A. Lactulose
B. Glycerol suppository
C. Arachis oil enema
D. Phosphate enema
E. Senna

Question 13

Which of the following drugs does not prolong the QT interval?

A. Risperidone
B. Lithium
C. Citalopram
D. Digoxin
E. Fluconazole

Question 14

A 65-year-old retired accountant presents with joint pain, fatigue and 5 kg weight loss. His past medical history includes hypertension and the recent onset of Raynaud's phenomenon. On systemic questioning he admits to decreased exercise tolerance over six months and shortness of breath on climbing stairs. On examination he has thickened and cracked skin on the radial side of his fingers and multiple tender small joints in the hands. On auscultation he has fine bilateral basal crepitations in the lungs, and he is unable to hold his arms at shoulder height for more than a few minutes. He is also unable to stand from a seated position with his arms folded. Which of the following antibodies is most likely to be associated with this condition?

A. Anti-Jo-1
B. Anti-Mi-2
C. Anti-Scl 70
D. Anti-centromere
E. Anti-cyclic citrullinated peptide

Question 15

You are asked to check the lipid profile of a man with type 2 diabetes with a previous myocardial infarction. His low-density lipoprotein cholesterol (LDL-C) level is 2.4 mmol/litre. Which statement is false?

A. **He is classed as very high risk for the development of a cardiovascular event and his LDL-C level should therefore be < 1.8 mmol/litre**

B. **He is classed as very high risk for the development of a cardiovascular event and his LDL-C level should therefore be < 2.5 mmol/litre**

C. **LDL-C is the recommended target for treatment in current European guidelines**

D. **He is at high risk of a cardiovascular event and his target LDL-C is < 2.5 mmol/litre**

E. **A statin should be prescribed to the highest recommended/tolerated dose to reach target lipid levels**

Question 16

A 45-year-old farmer presents with intermittent facial flushing associated with a recurrent papulopustular eruption on the cheeks, chin and forehead. On examination he has erythema, telangiectasia and papulopustular lesions on the cheeks and chin with swelling and prominent sebaceous glands on the nose. What is the most appropriate first-line management?

A. **A 3-month course of doxycycline**

B. **Pulsed-dye laser therapy**

C. **Nasal shave**

D. **Topical retinoids**

E. **Topical mild potency steroids**

Question 17

You are asked to see a 60-year-old man in the coronary care unit who is unwell after having been treated for an ST elevation MI. His heart rate has risen suddenly to 180 bpm and his blood pressure has fallen to 90/60 mmHg. He is clammy and describing chest discomfort. You review his 12-lead ECG, which shows a broad complex tachycardia (shown in Figure 16.2), and decide to electrically cardiovert him. His rate returns to 80 bpm, his blood pressure rises to over 100 mmHg systolic. Which statement is false?

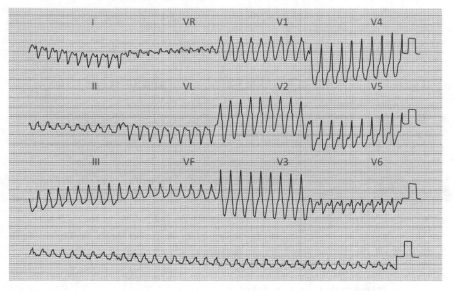

Figure 16.2

A. A previous history of myocardial infarction makes ventricular tachycardia (VT) the most likely diagnosis

B. A positive QRS complex in lead AVR makes VT the most likely diagnosis

C. Negative concordance across the chest leads makes VT the most likely diagnosis

D. A history of severe LV systolic dysfunction makes VT the most likely diagnosis

E. Right bundle branch block morphology indicates the VT originates in the right ventricle

Question 18

You are asked to see a 54-year-old man with a new rash. On examination a widespread rash consisting of scaly plaques and patches with overlying silver scale consistent with psoriasis is noted. What medication is not likely to have precipitated his psoriasis?

A. **Bisoprolol**
B. **Atenolol**
C. **Hydroxychloroquine**
D. **Warfarin**
E. **Lithium**

Question 19

A 52-year-old man with type 2 diabetes attends for clinic review. He has had diabetes for 13 years and is on metformin 1 g twice daily and gliclazide 160 mg twice daily, with simvastatin 40 mg and losartan 50 mg daily. He feels well and blood pressure at clinic was 135/78 mmHg.

Blood results reveal: Sodium 136 mmol/litre, Potassium 4.6 mmol/litre, Urea 5.6 mmol/litre, Cr 178 µmol/litre, eGFR 46 ml/min per 1.73 m^2, Albumin:creatinine ratio (ACR) 12 (previously 7).

Which of the following would suggest renal disease other than diabetic nephropathy as a cause of the declining renal function?

A. **Presence of retinopathy**
B. **ACR rising despite the addition of angiotensin receptor blocker therapy**
C. **Gradual trend downwards in eGFR**
D. **Finding the patient to be systemically unwell**
E. **Presence of microscopic haematuria**

Question 20

A 75-year-old man presents with a two-year history of a non-healing lesion on his nose. On examination, you observe the lesion seen in Figure 16.3.

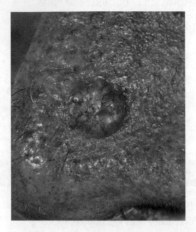

Figure 16.3

What is the diagnosis?

    A. **Basal cell carcinoma**
    B. **Bowen's disease**
    C. **Actinic keratosis**
    D. **Pyogenic granuloma**
    E. **Haemangioma**

Question 21

A 22-year-old lady attends as an unscheduled review. She has had type 1 diabetes for over 15 years. She had poor control throughout her adolescent years and early adulthood but improved as she was keen to get pregnant. Her HbA1c one year ago was 89 mmol/litre and it is now 53 mmol/litre. She informs you that she woke up this morning with the sensation of a 'curtain' over her left visual field. Visual acuity in that eye is reduced to hand movements. In which of the following conditions is an urgent/emergency review not required by an ophthalmologist?

    A. **Retinal detachment**
    B. **Rubeosis iridis**
    C. **Vitreous haemorrhage**
    D. **Sudden loss of vision**
    E. **Circinate exudates within the macula**

Question 22

A 21-year-old woman is seen at the gastrointestinal clinic with a several-month history of dysphagia mainly to solids, regurgitation and weight loss. She has not responded to a trial of acid suppression prescribed by her GP. Her OGD shows mild oesophagitis and her barium swallow shows only a minimally dilated oesophagus. What is the next most appropriate diagnostic test for this woman?

A. **Oesophageal manometry**
B. **CT scan of her chest and abdomen**
C. **24-hour ambulatory oesophageal pH studies**
D. **Videofluoroscopy**
E. **Repeat OGD**

Question 23

A 40-year-old lady presents with severe hirsutism. This appears to have developed over the last three months. She has not had a menstrual period in the last three months, but before this had been well with regular periods. Menarche was at age 13 years. Although her appetite is poor, she feels she has gained weight, particularly around her abdomen. On examination, she has coarse, thick hair on her face, chest and abdomen. She has mainly abdominal obesity. She does not have any abdominal tenderness but does describe a dull ache in her lower back.

Investigations are as follows: Urinary cortisol: elevated, Urinary catecholamine levels: normal, CT scan of abdomen: 6cm irregular mass in the right adrenal gland.

What is the approximate overall 5-year survival of a patient with an adrenocortical carcinoma?

A. **1%**
B. **10%**
C. **30%**
D. **80%**
E. **100%**

Question 24

A 50-year-old lady presents with a two-month history of lethargy, right upper quadrant discomfort and anorexia. The only significant past medical history is of recurrent urinary tract infections for which she has been prescribed a prophylactic antibiotic for the past six months.

Blood tests reveal: Bilirubin 20 μmol/litre, ALP 88 U/litre, ALT 480 U/litre, AST 400 U/litre, Albumin 43 g/litre, INR 1.3 s, Hepatitis virus A, B and C serology: negative, Ferritin 8 μg/litre, Anti-smooth muscle antibody titre: 1 in 320, IgG 22.8 g/litre

Which is the most likely antibiotic to have caused this presentation?

A. **Amoxicillin**
B. **Ciprofloxacin**
C. **Trimethoprim**
D. **Co-amoxiclav**
E. **Nitrofurantoin**

Question 25

A 76-year-old man presents with falls and difficulty walking. His gait is slow and shuffling, and he has difficulty turning in bed. Examination reveals increased tone bilaterally in the lower limbs. There is no tremor. His Folstein mini-mental test score is 20/30. A ^{123}I-ioflupane SPECT scan (DaT scan) is negative. Medications: aspirin 75 mg, perindopril 4 mg, simvastatin 40 mg, ranolazine 375 mg.

What is the most likely diagnosis?

A. **Idiopathic Parkinson's disease**
B. **Progressive supranuclear palsy**
C. **Vascular parkinsonism**
D. **Dementia with Lewy bodies**
E. **Drug-induced parkinsonism**

Question 26

A 19-year-old female clerical worker presents with a 6-month history of fatigue and daytime sleepiness. She has been researching narcolepsy on the internet and wishes to undergo assessment for this condition. Which of the following features is not suggestive of narcolepsy?

    A. **Low cerebrospinal fluid hypocretin level**

    B. **Cataplexy**

    C. **Mean sleep latency of less than 20 minutes**

    D. **Sleep paralysis**

    E. **HLA-DR2 haplotype**

Question 27

A 42-year-old lady is admitted with a several-hour history of acute epigastric pain radiating to her back, associated with nausea and vomiting. She has had a previous laparoscopic cholecystectomy for gallstones, but is otherwise fit and healthy. On examination, she was tender in the epigastrium.

Blood tests reveal: Bilirubin 10 μmol/litre, ALP 90 U/litre, ALT 35 U/litre, Albumin 43 g/litre, Amylase 1500 U/litre, C-reactive protein 125 mg/litre, White cells 15×10^9/litre.

Which of the following tests is the most appropriate in diagnosing and assessing the severity of this lady's illness?

    A. **CT scan of the abdomen**

    B. **Ultrasound scan of the abdomen**

    C. **Plain abdominal X-ray**

    D. **MR cholangiopancreatography**

    E. **ERCP**

Question 28

An 84-year-old man with a past history of ischaemic heart disease, porcine aortic valve replacement, atrial fibrillation, previous transient ischaemic attack and severe chronic obstructive pulmonary disease is admitted following a fall down a flight of stairs. There is nothing to suggest a stroke. X-ray confirms a displaced intracapsular fractured neck of femur. His INR is 4.2 and haemoglobin concentration 92 g/dl. Which of the following statements is correct?

A. Bone cement must be used intraoperatively
B. A sliding hip screw is the preferred surgical option
C. Carotid Doppler ultrasound should be performed preoperatively
D. Dalteparin 5000 units should be given
E. Attempt to stand the patient on the day after surgery

Question 29

Signs and symptoms in patients with urethritis may include which of the following?

A. Urethral discharge which may be yellow, green, brown, or tinged with blood. The production is related to sexual activity
B. In men, dysuria is usually localised to the meatus or distal penis, worst during the first morning void, and relieved by alcohol consumption
C. In men, typical symptoms include urinary frequency and urgency
D. In women, symptoms may occasionally worsen during the menstrual cycle
E. Systemic symptoms, eg fever, chills, sweats, nausea, are invariably absent

Question 30

A 60-year-old lady, with a background history of scleroderma, presents with recurrent abdominal pain, bloating and diarrhoea. Stool cultures are negative, duodenal biopsies normal and a colonoscopy shows normal colonic mucosa. What is the most likely cause for this lady's presentation?

- A. **Small intestinal bacterial overgrowth**
- B. **Irritable bowel syndrome**
- C. **Non-coeliac gluten intolerance**
- D. **Microscopic colitis**
- E. **Lactose intolerance**

Question 31

A 74-year-old man with multiple sclerosis was admitted with urinary retention and was treated for an uncomplicated urinary tract infection. The residual urine volume after urinary catheter insertion in the emergency department was 695 ml. A trial removal of catheter was successful before discharge. He has a structurally normal urinary tract on departmental ultrasound. He represents with urinary incontinence. A post-void bladder scan reveals a residual volume of 500 ml.

What is the most appropriate management of this man's incontinence?

- A. **Long-term indwelling urinary catheter**
- B. **Intermittent self-catheterisation**
- C. **Adhesive continence pads**
- D. **Urine sheath**
- E. **Solifenacin 5mg OD**

Question 32

An 81-year-old man is 12 days post right hip hemiarthroplasty following a fractured neck of femur. He developed pneumonia four days post surgery, and was empirically commenced on IV piperacillin-tazobactam (as per the hospital's protocol) and a sputum specimen was sent for culture. This specimen cultured MRSA and the patient was therefore changed to IV vancomycin two days after commencing piperacillin-tazobactam, and he seemed to be improving.

You are asked to review him because routine bloods tests now show several abnormal values:

- ✦ White cells 24×10^9/litre (predominantly neutrophils) – rising
- ✦ Urea 14 mmol/litre (previously normal)
- ✦ Creatinine 142 µmol/litre (previously normal)

Findings from your initial assessment include the following: the patient is alert and orientated, pulse 85 bpm, blood pressure 115/70 mmHg, oxygen saturation 97% breathing room air. You note good air entry bilaterally with a few crepitations at the right lung base. The surgical wound is healing well and there is no evidence of any other skin infection. Nursing staff report he is eating and drinking satisfactorily, although there have been several episodes of loose stools (type 7 on Bristol stool chart) over the past 48 hours. The physiotherapists are happy with his progress in mobilising. The patient reports no significant pain nor does he complain of any urinary symptoms.

Which of the following actions is likely to be the most appropriate?

A. **Discussion with the orthopaedic team to exclude prosthetic joint infection**
B. **CT scan of chest to exclude complications of MRSA pneumonia**
C. **Stool sample for culture and testing for *Clostridium difficile* toxin**
D. **Trial of ciprofloxacin with improved coverage for gram-negative bacteria**
E. **Testing of the MRSA sputum isolate for the presence of Panton–Valentine leukocidin toxin**

Question 33

A 25-year-old lady attends with a 4-month history of headache. It occurs on a daily basis and is worse in the mornings on wakening. She describes two episodes of visual loss lasting less than a minute in the previous week when putting on her shoes. On assessment, blood pressure is 142/80 mmHg, weight 72 kg and height 156 cm. Findings on neurological examination include reduced abduction of the right eye. Her optic discs appear swollen on fundoscopy. A CT scan of brain and CT venogram (shown in Figure 16.4) are reported as normal. Lumbar puncture was performed. CSF opening pressure 27 cm CSF, protein 0.4 g/litre, 3 leucocytes per mm^3 and glucose 3 mmol/litre (plasma glucose 4.5 mmol/litre).

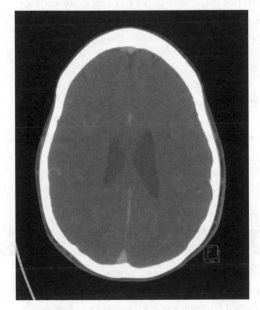

Figure 16.4

Which is the most likely diagnosis in this case?

    A. **Chiari malformation**
    B. **Dural venous sinus thrombosis**
    C. **Malignant hypertension**
    D. **Malignant meningitis**
    E. **Idiopathic intracranial hypertension**

Question 34

A 60-year-old lady is receiving chemotherapy as an outpatient. She has a past medical history of hypertension, congestive cardiac failure and type 2 diabetes. She presents to the emergency department in the early evening with an acute history of feeling unwell. Findings from initial assessment include: temperature 38.5 °C, respiratory rate 20 breaths/min, oxygen saturation 94% breathing 2 litre/min oxygen via nasal cannulae, pulse rate 108 bpm and blood pressure 88/56 mmHg. She has a peripherally inserted central catheter (PICC) in situ and there are widespread crepitations bilaterally. On questioning, the symptoms began shortly after the community nurse had attended to dress and flush her PICC. Her white cell count had been in normal range three days ago, but today's results show a total count of 3.1×10^9/litre (neutrophils 0.8×10^9/litre). If an infective process underlies her acute problems, which of the following is likely to be the most helpful in making a diagnosis?

A. **CT scan of chest**
B. **Bronchoalveolar lavage for microscopy and culture**
C. **Blood cultures**
D. **Urinary antigens to test for evidence of pneumococcal and legionella infection**
E. **Bronchoalveolar lavage for PCR (polymerase chain reaction) to detect viruses and atypical agents of infection**

Question 35

A 62-year-old man complains of right ankle weakness and a tendency to trip. This has worsened since beginning four months previously. On examination, muscle wasting is evident over the dorsal aspect of the right ankle. There is moderate weakness of ankle dorsiflexion and mild weakness of ankle plantar flexion, inversion and eversion. Knee jerks are brisk, the right ankle jerk is reduced and plantar responses are flexor. There is no sensory loss. Upper limb and cranial nerve examination are normal. EMG is performed and shows active denervation in muscles innervated by the peroneal and tibial nerves. What is the most likely diagnosis?

A. **Lumbar canal stenosis**
B. **Motor neurone disease**
C. **Multifocal motor neuropathy with conduction block**
D. **Common peroneal nerve palsy**
E. **Spinal muscular atrophy**

Question 36

A 39-year-old man is referred to the renal team having been admitted on the medical take. He is well known to the department due to frequent admissions with alcohol and heroin-related issues. This evening, his friends summoned an ambulance as he was found unresponsive in his room at a local hostel. He was last seen two days earlier when he had been drinking heavily. He required an IV naloxone infusion before his Glasgow Coma Scale rose to 14/15. He had become quite agitated in the emergency department and complained of painful legs, which were noted to be moderately swollen. His legs are uncomfortable to touch but distal pulses are maintained with a capillary refill time of two seconds. He is transferred to the medical assessment unit and catheterised, with 45 ml residual dark urine being obtained. Chest and abdominal examination is unremarkable. The pulse is 120 bpm, blood pressure 110/60 mmHg, temperature 37.8 °C, respiratory rate 28 breaths/min, oxygen saturation 99% breathing 3 litre/min oxygen.

Investigations are shown below. Haemoglobin 178 g/litre, MCV 92 fl, White cells 19.1×10^9/litre (neutrophils 17.5), Platelets 490×10^9/litre, Sodium 131 mmol/litre, Potassium 6.4 mmol/litre, Chloride 103 mmol/litre, Bicarbonate 12 mmol/litre, Urea 20.5 mmol/litre, Creatinine 370 μmol/litre, C-reactive protein 28 mg/litre, Corrected calcium 1.7 mmol/litre, Phosphate 2.9 mmol/litre, Bilirubin 11 μmol/litre, ALP 40 U/litre, AST 3480 U/litre, GGT 50 U/litre, Albumin 45 g/litre.

Arterial blood gas analysis: pH 7.24, PaO_2 18.5 kPa, $PaCO_2$ 2.9 kPa, bicarbonate 12 mmol/litre.

Lactate 3.2 mmol/litre.

Urinalysis: blood +++.

Ultrasound scan of legs: oedema in soft tissues; no evidence of venous thrombosis.

Ultrasound scan of renal tracts: normal-sized kidneys, no hydronephrosis, empty bladder with catheter tip in situ.

Chest X-ray: normal.

ECG: sinus tachycardia, rate 112 bpm. Normal QRS and T-wave morphologies.

What treatment is best advised at this stage?

A. **0.9% Saline infusion**
B. **8.4% Sodium bicarbonate infusion**
C. **Bilateral fasciotomies**
D. **Broad spectrum antibiotic cover**
E. **Haemodialysis**

Question 37

A 40-year-old lady presents with a progressive history of weakness in her limbs and numbness and paresthesiae in her hands and feet over two weeks. Two months previously she had been diagnosed with severe, bilateral optic neuritis which was treated with a 3-day course of intravenous steroids. There is no recent history of infection, vaccination or travel outside the UK. On examination, bilateral disc pallor is noted and corrected visual acuity is 6/18 in both eyes. There is moderate quadriparesis with reduced proprioception and fine touch to the elbows and knees. Blood tests including herpes, HIV, hepatitis serology and anti-double-stranded DNA antibody were all negative. Cerebrospinal fluid was negative for oligoclonal bands and had 60 lymphocytes per mm^3. MRI brain was normal. MRI spine showed a high signal lesion in the cervical cord on T2-weighted imaging, extending over 4 vertebral segments..

Which of the following serum antibody tests is likely to be diagnostic in this case?

A. **Aquaporin-4 antibody**
B. **C-ANCA**
C. **JC virus antibody**
D. **Anti-myelin oligodendrocyte glycoprotein antibody**
E. **Anti-La antibody**

Question 38

A 39-year-old man with previously mild and very well-controlled asthma presents to his GP with worsening asthma control. Despite titrating up his therapy with the addition of inhaled steroids and long-acting β agonists, he does not feel as well as he had two months previously. He has had to rehome his cat as he began to sneeze uncontrollably when she was near him. He has also noticed in the past two days that his left ankle is weak and that he is getting a 'pins and needles' feeling in his hands. His GP refers him urgently and a battery of blood tests is performed.

Haemoglobin 135 g/litre, MCV 88 fl, White cells 17×10^9/litre (neutrophils 48%, eosinophils 24%, lymphocytes 18%, monocytes 7%), Platelets 145×10^9/litre, Sodium 137 mmol/litre, Potassium 5.1 mmol/litre, Chloride 99 mmol/litre, Bicarbonate 25 mmol/litre, Urea 14 mmol/litre, Creatinine 155 µmol/litre, Corrected calcium 2.45 mmol/litre, Phosphate 1.8 mmol/litre, Total bilirubin 18 µmol/litre, ALP 80 U/litre, ALT 24 U/litre, AST 34 U/litre, GGT 40 U/litre, Albumin 36 g/litre, C-reactive protein 58 mg/litre, Erythrocyte sedimentation rate 74 mm/1st hour, Glucose 6.8 mmol/litre.

Given this presentation, which antibody is most likely to be detected in elevated titres in his serum?

A. **Anti-double-stranded DNA (anti-dsDNA)**
B. **Anti-glomerular basement membrane (anti-GBM)**
C. **Anti-topoisomerase (anti-SCL70)**
D. **C-ANCA**
E. **P-ANCA**

Question 39

A 38-year-old woman presents during the second trimester of pregnancy with a breast lump. Biopsy confirms invasive ductal carcinoma and staging imaging suggests early stage (I/II) disease with no radiological evidence of metastatic disease. What is the optimal management in this case?

A. **Modified systemic chemotherapy using a taxane-based regimen**
B. **Targeted radiotherapy only with uterine shielding**
C. **Surgery now, with consideration of adjuvant radiotherapy deferred until post-partum**
D. **Surgery with adjuvant chemotherapy using a taxane-based regimen**
E. **Termination of pregnancy followed by surgery and adjuvant chemotherapy**

Question 40

A 38-year-old man with a history of deliberate self-harm and personality disorder is found confused and disoriented outside his home by his neighbour. An empty 500 ml bottle of antifreeze is brought in with him. On arrival in the emergency department, the Glasgow Coma Scale is 13/15, respiratory rate 38 breaths/min, pulse rate 125 bpm, blood pressure 120/70 mmHg and temperature 36.7 °C. Oxygen saturations on room air are 99%.

Bloods results show: Sodium 134 mmol/litre, Potassium 4 mmol/litre, Chloride 97 mmol/litre, Bicarbonate 3 mmol/litre, Urea 7 mmol/litre, Creatinine 115 μmol/litre, Glucose 6 mmol/litre, Corrected calcium 1.85 mmol/litre, Venous pH 7.01, Serum osmolality 296 mOsmol/kg, Lactate 4 mmol/litre, Serum ketones < 0.1 mmol/litre, Serum ethanol < 20 mg/dl, Urinalysis: bland.

What is the best treatment to be instituted now?

A. **Continuous veno-venous haemofiltration**
B. **Ethanol**
C. **Fomepizole**
D. **Haemodialysis**
E. **Sodium bicarbonate infusion**

Question 41

A 35-year-old gentleman presents with a several-month history of epigastric pain radiating to the back, associated with weight loss and diarrhoea. He admits to drinking excess alcohol in the past, although he has reduced his consumption of late.

His blood test results show: Haemoglobin 13.7 g/litre, White cells 11×10^9/litre, Platelets 400×10^9/litre, Sodium 135 mmol/litre, Potassium 4.5 mmol/litre, Urea 1.9 mmol/litre, Creatinine 27 μmol/litre.

CT scan of abdomen: chronic calcification in the pancreas and some peripancreatic fat stranding.

What would be the most appropriate next management step for this gentleman?

A. **Advise him to abstain from alcohol completely**
B. **Start him on empirical proton pump inhibitor**
C. **Start him on nutritional supplements**
D. **Start him on pancreatic enzyme replacement therapy**
E. **Refer him to the pain team for analgesia advice**

Question 42

A 56-year-old woman who has been receiving adjuvant docetaxel chemotherapy for breast cancer has been admitted with febrile neutropaenia. She was initiated on broad spectrum intravenous antibiotics and fluids. Three days after admission you are asked to review her on the ward. She complains of malaise and rigors, and you note that she is continuing to have temperatures of up to 39 °C. Physical examination reveals that she looks unwell, skin is clammy, heart rate is 120 bpm and blood pressure is 110/60 mmHg. There is a 'Hickman' line in situ, but no localising features of infection. Her latest blood counts demonstrate a neutrophil count of 0.0×10^9/litre, and C-reactive protein of 245 mg/litre (rising).What is the most appropriate management?

A. Contact microbiology and if no growth on any cultures, continue current antibiotics

B. Contact microbiology and if no growth on any cultures, stop all antibiotics and initiate antifungal therapy

C. Contact microbiology, change to alternative broad spectrum antibiotics, add a glycopeptide to cover line infection

D. Repeat blood and urine cultures, and perform lumbar puncture to send CSF for urgent analysis

E. Remove the 'Hickman' line and continue current antibiotic therapy through peripheral venous access

Question 43

An 86-year-old lady is referred to the general medical team by the orthopaedic house officer who notices that she has a persistently low serum bicarbonate. She was admitted nine days earlier with a fractured neck of femur that is so far being managed conservatively. She fell at night when trying to go to the toilet. She has a history of hypertension, paroxysmal atrial fibrillation, osteoarthritis, type 2 diabetes, glaucoma and hysterectomy. Two days after her admission she developed loose bowel movements up to three times each day. On examination she is euvolaemic, early warning scores have been consistently zero and blood pressure stable at 145/80 mmHg. She is alert and oriented and, apart from some ongoing hip discomfort, has no new complaints. Her medications include amlodipine, warfarin, co-codamol, metformin, sodium docusate, senna, ranitidine and brinzolamide eye drops. She states that she never misses taking her medications as she feels they give her good relief from her symptoms.

Investigations show: Sodium 137 mmol/litre, Potassium 3.9 mmol/litre, Chloride 115 mmol/litre, Bicarbonate 16 mmol/litre, Urea 6.5 mmol/litre, Creatinine 110 μmol/litre, Urinalysis: bland, Urinary sodium 35 mmol/litre, Urinary potassium 40 mmol/litre, Urinary chloride 20 mmol/litre.

What is the cause of her acidosis?

A. **Brinzolamide**
B. **Diarrhoea**
C. **Metformin**
D. **Ranitidine**
E. **Renal impairment**

Question 44

A 25-year-old man has a family history of colorectal cancer. Genetic testing is performed and he is diagnosed with hereditary non-polyposis colorectal cancer syndrome (HNPCC, or Lynch syndrome). What is his lifetime risk of developing colorectal cancer?

A. **100%**
B. **70–80%**
C. **40–50%**
D. **20–30%**
E. **<10%**

Question 45

A 72-year-old woman with type 2 diabetes is recorded as having a Snellen visual acuity of 6/24. She has been receiving intravitreal ranibizumab injections to her left eye as treatment for a choroidal neovascular membrane secondary to wet age-related macular degeneration. Two days following her most recent injection, she presents to the emergency department with a painful red eye and hand movements vision. What is the most likely diagnosis?

A. Trauma to the crystalline lens
B. Infective endophthalmitis
C. Rhegmatogenous retinal detachment
D. Central retinal artery occlusion
E. Uveitis

Question 46

You review a 62-year-old man who has liver cirrhosis due to excessive consumption of alcohol. He has been on an alcohol binge for ten days and has come to hospital because he has become jaundiced. He normally has ascites, but this appears to have increased in volume markedly. You diagnose decompensated alcoholic liver disease. He is alert and not confused in any way.

His blood tests show: Bilirubin 132 µmol/litre, AST 121 U/litre, ALT 114 U/litre, ALP 98 U/litre, GGT 201 U/litre, Albumin 27 g/litre, PT 20 s.

Later that night he becomes aggressive and a junior doctor prescribes a dose of clomethiazole to settle him. Shortly afterwards, he is unrousable. What characteristic of clomethiazole has resulted in the profound effect seen with this patient?

A. It is a hydrophilic drug
B. It exhibits a low degree of protein binding
C. It has high hepatic extraction
D. It has a tendency to cause salt retention
E. It is toxic to the kidney

Question 47

A 17-year-old girl is admitted to the medical ward with an electrolyte imbalance. Doctors suspect she has an eating disorder. Which of the following is a feature of atypical anorexia nervosa?

A. Absence of amenorrhoea
B. Body mass index 15% below the normal/expected weight for age and height
C. Self-perception of being too fat, despite being underweight
D. Fear of fatness
E. Self-set low weight threshold

Question 48

A 30-year-old lady is admitted with acute dyspnoea and left-sided chest pain. She has a history of a non-productive cough and has had some recent minor haemoptysis. A chest X-ray shows a significant left-sided pneumothorax and a chest drain is inserted (20 G). The drain continues to bubble, with some improvement in X-ray appearances. After 48 hours, the situation has remained unchanged. A CT is requested, and a representative image is shown in Figure 16.5.

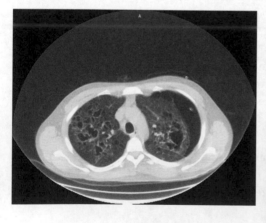 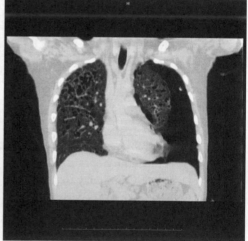

Figure 16.5

The CT report also mentions small cystic areas throughout both lungs, which are thin walled, with no particular distribution. Suction is applied and slowly things begin to improve.

What prognosis is expected for this lady in regards to her underlying condition?
- A. **Full recovery with no residual effects**
- B. **Full recovery from this event but at high risk of further pneumothoraces**
- C. **Relapsing and remitting symptoms**
- D. **Gradual progression to respiratory failure**
- E. **Will need surgical correction**

Question 49

A 16-year-old boy is reviewed by an adolescent psychiatrist on account of severe depressive symptoms. It is decided that he warrants pharmacological therapy in relation to his illness. Which of the following drugs would be most likely to lead to a favourable long-term outcome, assuming that adequate monitoring and follow-up is provided?

- A. **Fluoxetine**
- B. **Citalopram**
- C. **Mirtazepine**
- D. **Venlafaxine**
- E. **Sertraline**

Question 50

Rheumatoid arthritis is not associated with which of the following?
- A. **Shared epitope**
- B. **Anti-cyclic citrullinated peptide antibodies**
- C. **HLA-B27**
- D. **The same cardiovascular risk as type 2 diabetes**
- E. **Smoking**

Question 51

The GP of an 81-year-old lady who attends the clinic with normally stable bronchiectasis has been in contact asking for an earlier than planned review as the lady has been increasingly unwell with cough, spit and weight loss. When assessed she is not distressed, respiratory rate is 20 breaths/min, oxygen saturation 93% on room air (usually > 94%) with other observations normal. There were crackles heard at the right base and a few in the right upper zone. A chest X-ray was organised, which showed chronic changes at the bases in keeping with bronchiectasis and some new infiltrates in the right upper lobe. There were no soft tissue densities and no cavities. She is a life long non-smoker. Sputum has been sent for culture and testing for tuberculosis.

What organism is this least likely to be?

- A. *Mycobacterium tuberculosis*
- B. *Mycobacterium kansasii*
- C. *Staphylococcus aureus*
- D. *Chlamydia burnetti*
- E. *Klebsiella pneumonia*

Question 52

A 50-year-old lady presents to her GP with increasing wheeze. She has had troublesome asthma all her life, but it has deteriorated in recent months. Her co-morbidities include a hyperprolactinoma and glaucoma. She was treated for breast cancer three years ago, and is currently actively trying to stop smoking. She is currently taking cabergoline, tamoxifen, timolol eye drops and varenicline. She buys St John's wort over the counter. Which of her drugs is most likely to be exacerbating the wheeze?

- A. **Cabergoline**
- B. **Tamoxifen**
- C. **Timolol**
- D. **Varenicline**
- E. **St John's wort**

Question 53

A 19-year-old girl is admitted via the emergency department following a collapse at home. She gives a three to four month history of malaise, intermittent pyrexia and weight loss of approximately 6 kg. Clinically she looks pale and unwell. There is no evidence of rash. Cardiovascular examination reveals a bruit in the left carotid territory. The left radial pulse is faint. The blood pressure (BP) is 110/72 mmHg in the right arm and 96/63 mmHg in the left arm with no postural drop evident.

Baseline blood tests reveal: Haemoglobin 10.1 g/litre, MCV 86 fl, ESR 114 mm/1st hour, C-reactive protein 83 mg/litre.

Which of the following tests is the most appropriate next investigation to confirm the diagnosis?

    A. **Tissue biopsy**
    B. **Ultrasound scan**
    C. **MRI or CT scan**
    D. **Transthoracic echocardiogram**
    E. **CT-PET scan**

Question 54

A 53-year-old lady initially presents with foot pain. She had a fracture in her right foot 30 years ago and had been doing a lot of walking recently with the subsequent onset of pain. Her GP had arranged an X-ray, which did not show any new fracture but it did reveal possible osteopenia. She had an early menopause at the age of 44 years, but never started hormone replacement therapy due to a family history of breast carcinoma. She does not take any regular medications. Her mother had osteoporosis, and two of her sisters were diagnosed with breast cancer. She informs you that she is awaiting genetic testing for a breast cancer gene.

A DEXA scan shows T-score: vertebra –2.8; left hip –2.5.

Which of the following is the most appropriate therapy?

    A. **Hormone replacement therapy**
    B. **Raloxifene**
    C. **Strontium ranelate**
    D. **Calcitonin**
    E. **Risedronate**

Question 55

For pregnant patients, which one of the following factors would mandate screening for congenital heart block in the fetus?

A. **A maternal history of systemic lupus erythematosus**
B. **A maternal history of Sjögren syndrome**
C. **A maternal history of anti-Ro/SSa antibodies or anti-La/SSB antibodies**
D. **A maternal history of high anti-double-stranded DNA antibody levels**
E. **A maternal history of thromboembolic disease**

Question 56

A 52-year-old man with a history of hypertension, angina, depression and hypoadrenalism is prescribed sildenafil for erectile dysfunction. After using the drug for the first time, he is admitted following a collapse episode. On initial assessment in the emergency department, he is found to have a respiratory rate of 16 breaths/min, pulse rate of 112 bpm, blood pressure 78/42 mmHg, oxygen saturations 99% on room air and a temperature of 36.2 °C. Which of his other drugs is most likely to have interacted with the sildenafil to have caused this presentation?

A. **Nicorandil**
B. **Sertraline**
C. **Isosorbide mononitrate**
D. **Doxazosin**
E. **Fludrocortisone**

Question 57

A 45-year-old woman presents with a 2-year history of gradually enlarging asymptomatic skin lesions on her lower legs. On examination there are bilateral, yellow–brown, waxy plaques with telangiectasia consistent with necrobiosis lipoidica.

Which of the following investigations would you perform next?

A. **Autoantibody screen**
B. **Fasting serum glucose**
C. **Fasting lipid profile**
D. **Thyroid function tests**
E. **Thyroid autoantibodies**

Question 58

A 22-year-old lady is referred to clinic. She is currently pregnant at 16 weeks' gestation. She has a history of hypothyroidism following a complete thyroidectomy for medullary thyroid carcinoma when aged nine years. She continues on levothyroxine 250 µg daily. She is feeling tired but otherwise well, with no cold or heat intolerance and no skin dryness. She has occasional palpitations that she has been putting down to pregnancy. She has no other medical history but her sister also has a history of medullary thyroid carcinoma. She informs you that genetic tests confirmed multiple endocrine neoplasia syndrome type two (MEN 2 syndrome). On examination she is well, blood pressure is 128/78 mmHg and heart rate is 90 bpm.

Biochemical tests reveal: Sodium 135 mmol/litre, Potassium 4.8 mmol/litre, Urea 5.0 mmol/litre, Creatinine 58 µmol/litre, Glucose 5 mmol/litre, Corrected calcium 2.4 mmol/litre, Free thyroxine 14 pmol/litre, TSH 1.2 mU/litre, Calcitonin 9 ng/litre.

Which additional test should be carried out?

A. **Prolactin**
B. **Chromogranin A**
C. **Fasting gut hormones**
D. **24-hour urinary catecholamines**
E. **Free triiodothyronine**

CHAPTER 16
QUESTIONS

609

Question 59

A 75-year-old lady is admitted following the successful resuscitation of a cardiorespiratory arrest she suffered at home. She has no significant past medical history.

The next day blood results show: Bilirubin 24 µmol/litre, ALP 100 U/litre, ALT 8500 U/litre, AST 10 100 U/litre, Albumin 43 g/litre, INR 3.5 s.

What is the most appropriate treatment?

A. **Start anticoagulation therapy**
B. **Provision of supportive care and treatment of underlying condition**
C. **Start lamivudine**
D. **Start N-acetylcysteine**
E. **Start a course of steroids**

Question 60

A 44-year-old woman who gives no past medical history is admitted on the medical take. She is complaining of worsening headache and lethargy over the past three days. This is on a background of 12 weeks of severe heartburn and dysphagia, as well as painful lesions on her fingers. She states that she has to wear gloves all the time as even cool weather can worsen the pain in her fingers. Other than this she denies nausea, vomiting, diarrhoea, changes in vision, weakness or weight disturbance. On examination she is pale and somewhat jaundiced. Chest auscultation reveals a systolic murmur, and the second heart sound is heard louder at the second intercostal space on the left compared to the right. The chest is clear, and an abdominal examination is unremarkable. There is mild pitting oedema at the ankles and distal pulses are readily palpable. There are no vascular bruits detected. On examination of the hands there are some exquisitely tender nodules on the finger tips and the skin is smooth and shiny. Fundoscopy reveals bilateral papilloedema and no other retinal changes. The pulse rate is 110 bpm, blood pressure 230/135 mmHg, temperature 37.4°C, oxygen saturation 98% breathing room air and the respiratory rate is 24 breaths/min.

Bloods tests reveal the following: Haemoglobin 87 g/litre, White cells 9.5 × 10⁹/litre, Platelets 52 × 10⁹/litre, Sodium 136 mmol/litre, Potassium 5.2 mmol/litre, Chloride 99 mmol/litre, Bicarbonate 20 mmol/litre, Urea 21 mmol/litre, Creatinine 380 µmol/litre, Glucose 6.2 mmol/litre, Total bilirubin 87 µmol/litre, Conjugated bilirubin 11 µmol/litre, ALP 86 U/litre, ALT 210 U/litre, AST 650 U/litre, GGT 40 U/litre, Albumin 38 g/litre, LDH 1310 U/litre, PT 14 s, APTT 37 s, Fibrinogen 2.74 g/litre, C-reactive protein 16 mg/litre.

Blood film: schistocytes +++.

Urinary β-HCG is normal, and urinalysis demonstrates protein +++ and blood ++.

An urgent bedside ultrasound scan shows two normal kidneys.

Based on the above information, which of the following treatments is most strongly indicated?

- A. **Enalapril orally**
- B. **Immunoglobulins intravenously**
- C. **Labetalol IV infusion**
- D. **Methylprednisolone intravenously**
- E. **Plasma exchange**

Question 61

A 75-year-old previously fit and healthy man complains of bright red rectal bleeding, tenesmus and weight loss. Physical examination including digital rectal examination is unremarkable. What is the most appropriate investigation?

- A. **CT scan of chest, abdomen and pelvis**
- B. **MRI scan of pelvis**
- C. **Flexible sigmoidoscopy**
- D. **Barium enema**
- E. **Colonoscopy**

Question 62

A 35-year-old woman who has been diagnosed with chronic hepatitis C virus infection is referred to the liver clinic for assessment for antiviral treatment with pegylated interferon and ribavirin. Which of the following tests is not required before the initiation of pegylated interferon and ribavirin?

- A. **Full blood picture**
- B. **Serum bilirubin**
- C. **Thyroid function tests**
- D. **Hepatitis C virus genotype**
- E. **Pregnancy test**

Question 63

A 67-year-old woman presents with an ischaemic stroke. Her brother also had an ischaemic stroke and his admission was complicated by seizures. She is concerned about her risk of seizures over the next five years.

What proportion of stroke survivors go on to develop seizures?

    A. **0–4%**
    B. **5–20%**
    C. **20–40%**
    D. **50–60%**
    E. **75–85%**

Question 64

A young man gets bitten by a bat while exploring a Scottish castle. A bat watcher witnesses this and identifies the bat as a Daubenton's bat. What is the best course of action?

    A. **Do nothing**
    B. **Try to catch the bat to see if it becomes unwell**
    C. **Give normal human immunoglobulin**
    D. **Give a rabies vaccination and rabies immunoglobulin**
    E. **Give rabies vaccination only**

Question 65

A patient with an inherited neuromuscular disorder is admitted with an abnormal ECG (see Figure 16.6).

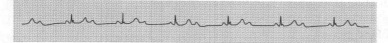

Figure 16.6

Genetic testing reveals a defect in the *DMPK* gene. What is the likely underlying diagnosis?

    A. **Myotonic dystrophy type 1**
    B. **Emery–Dreifuss muscular dystrophy (EDMD)**
    C. **Laminopathy**
    D. **Desminopathy**
    E. **Myotonic dystrophy type 2**

ANSWERS

Answer 1

B. Ramipril

Older people are more susceptible to drug–drug interactions, adverse drug reactions and drug–disease interactions, and these can result in morbidity, mortality and increased cost/length of hospital stays. This susceptibility is on the basis of age-related changes in pharmacodynamics and pharmacokinetics. Older people are often not routinely included in drug trials, leading to an absence of hard data on how it can be expected they will react in the real prescribing world.

In the absence of an acute kidney injury, ramipril is the least likely drug to have resulted in delirium. There is an anticholinergic burden scale to guide you. Anticholinergic stimulation predisposes to delirium. Amitriptyline and oxybutynin carry the highest activity, while digoxin and codeine both carry anticholinergic activity as well.

Answer 2

E. There is a rare risk of transmission of emerging or unknown agents

Following a needle stick injury, there is 30% risk of acquiring hepatitis B if the donor is hepatitis B e antigen positive, and 3% if the donor hepatitis B e antibody positive. There is a 3% risk of hepatitis C if the donor is hepatitis C antibody positive and a 0.3% risk of HIV if donor is HIV positive. There is also the unknown rare chance of acquiring emerging or unknown infectious agents.

Answer 3

A. Botulinum toxin injection

This is cervical dystonia (spasmodic torticollis), most likely idiopathic in nature given the lack of evidence for generalised dystonia or a genetic predisposition. Focal dystonia usually responds to botulinum toxin type A injection, which may need to be repeated at 3- to 6-month intervals.

Answer 4

C. OGD and duodenal biopsies

The diagnosis here is coeliac disease, and the rash described is dermatitis herpetiformis. The gold standard diagnostic test is duodenal biopsy while the patient is still taking a gluten-containing diet.

Answer 5

E. Sulfamethoxazole-trimethoprim

The patient is suffering from Stevens–Johnson syndrome (SJS). This is an idiosyncratic reaction involving the skin and mucous membranes most commonly due to medications. The incidence per year is 1–2 per million, compared with toxic epidermal necrolysis (TEN), which has an incidence of 0.4–1.2 per million per year.

Learning point

The main difference between the two conditions is the degree of skin detachment: < 10% SJS, 10–30% SJS/TEN overlap, > 30% TEN.

The most commonly implicated medications are similar to those causing TEN and include: anticonvulsants, sulfonamides, non-steroidal anti-inflammatory drugs, beta-lactam antibiotics and allopurinol.

Treatment includes stopping the culprit medication with supportive management including analgesia, mouth care and wound dressings. Mortality is determined by the degree of skin detachment. In SJS where the detachment is < 10%, the mortality rate is 1–5%, which increases to 30–40% for patients with > 30% detachment with TEN. Bacteraemia and sepsis appear to play a major role in increased mortality. The other medications listed can rarely cause SJS, but the most obvious answer in this question is sulfamethoxazole-trimethoprim.

Answer 6

C. Median survival is 8–14 months

Patients with mesothelioma have a median survival of 8–14 months. Surgery is rarely possible and is unlikely to be curative. Clinical trials are ongoing. Radiotherapy can be used in the management of mesothelioma; however, it will not be curative. It can be used to manage pain (especially where chest wall invasion occurs), or prophylactically at drain and aspiration sites to prevent tumour tracking. Prognosis may be worse if male, of poor performance status and advanced age. Few patients will survive more than three years. Effusions should be managed with a chest drain and pleurodesis if possible.

If the performance status is good, entry into clinical trials is possible and referral should be made to an oncologist involved in these.

Compensation is available for asbestos-related disease. A consensus diagnosis at a lung multidisciplinary meeting or a tissue biopsy is required. Claims can be made through government schemes and through the courts. Exposure history should be clear. There are increasing amounts available with increasing severity of disease burden.

All deaths associated with asbestos should be discussed with the coroner. If a definitive diagnosis has not been achieved, a post-mortem may be required, especially if compensation is being pursued. It is important to discuss this with the patient if possible, and with the family to make them aware.

Asbestos has many other effects in the lungs. Due to a long latency period of 20–40 years, the peak forecast for asbestos-related disease is 2020. Many have a clear exposure history, for others it is not clear. Other family members of those affected can present with asbestos-related disease possibly due to exposure from the fibres on the clothes of the patient.

Pleural plaques can be seen on chest X-ray. They are often calcified, bilateral and symmetrical on the posterior and lateral walls, mediastinal pleura and on the dome of the diaphragm. They are usually asymptomatic. There is no evidence that they are pre-malignant.

Benign asbestos-related pleural effusions are an early manifestation, usually presenting after around ten years post exposure. They are often small, unilateral and asymptomatic. They are usually exudative and often blood-stained. Other causes should be excluded. This manifestation can precede diffuse pleural thickening and there is no association with mesothelioma. Patients should be treated symptomatically.

Diffuse pleural thickening can present with exertional dyspnoea, pain, restrictive pulmonary function tests and hypercapnic respiratory failure. Chest X-rays may show

continued

smooth, uninterrupted pleural opacities over at least one quarter of the chest. CT scans will show more detail – typical findings are > 8 cm cranio-caudally, 5 cm laterally and > 3 mm deep. A biopsy may be needed to exclude mesothelioma. Treatment is difficult – decortication fails to give functional benefit in many.

Rounded atelectasis or folded lung can also be seen, when visceral fibrosis twists underlying lung. On CT, it is typically 2.5–5 cm with a comet tail of vessel and bronchi, usually adjacent to thickened pleura. Reduced lung volume is common. It is usually asymptomatic and no specific treatment is required. Surgery should be avoided.

Asbestosis is pulmonary fibrosis secondary to asbestos and it presents with dyspnoea, dry cough and bibasal late inspiratory crepitations. 40% will have finger clubbing. It can progress to cor pulmonale and respiratory failure. Spirometry is restrictive and transfer factor is reduced. Chest X-rays often show bilateral symmetrical reticulo-nodular shadowing from lower lobe up to the mid-zones in some cases. High-resolution CT scanning is most sensitive. In early disease there is ground glass change with parenchymal bands, subpleural lines and intralobular septal thickening. In more advanced disease, a more fibrotic picture is seen with traction bronchiectasis, loss of lobular architecture and honeycombing. A tissue biopsy is the gold standard for diagnosis. There are no specific treatments and management is supportive. There is a risk of developing lung cancer, especially in smokers.

Answer 7

D. HAART and systemic chemotherapy

This patient has HIV with an AIDS-defining disease: Kaposi's sarcoma (KS). The most appropriate management is immediate initiation of HAART (highly active antiretroviral therapy) to control the HIV infection, and concurrent systemic chemotherapy which is indicated due to the diffuse nature of his KS, which involves multiple viscera. First-line chemotherapy would be liposomal doxorubicin, which is well tolerated and has a similar response rate to multi-agent regimens. Intravenous aciclovir might be considered a rational choice due to the underlying pathogenesis of KS being due to human herpesvirus 9; however, it is not routinely utilised. Palliative care may well be appropriate for symptom control in conjunction with definitive therapy.

Answer 8

D. Photosensitive facial rash

Patients with scleroderma can develop involvement of the gastrointestinal tract at any level. The oesophagus is the most commonly affected site, with reflux and oesophagitis reported frequently. Subsequent strictures or recurrent aspiration pneumonia can occur in more severe cases. Due to dysmotility of the gastrointestinal tract caused by fibrosis, the small bowel is at risk of bacterial overgrowth and malabsorption, which can lead to vitamin B12 and other deficiencies. Gastric antral vascular ectasia (GAVE) is also known as 'watermelon stomach', and can cause bleeding and anaemia. Malignant hypertension is seen in a scleroderma renal crisis. It is characterised by the acute onset of renal failure, with hypertension and hyper-reninaemia, and a relatively normal urinary sediment. Other features can include a microangiopathic haemolytic anaemia, heart failure and pulmonary oedema, and in severe cases hypertensive encephalopathy. Ultraviolet light exposure can cause or exacerbate the cutaneous involvement in lupus but not scleroderma.

Answer 9

C. Female sex

Known risk factors for completed suicide include male sex, marital status (increased risk in single, divorced and widowed people), alcohol/drug dependence, social isolation, unemployment, diagnosed mental illness and previous suicide/self-harm attempts. Concurrent physical illness is also a recognised risk factor. Decisions about referral, discharge and admission to hospital for patients who have self-harmed, should be based on a comprehensive assessment, including a risk assessment.

Answer 10

B. > 460 ms

In women a corrected QT (QTc) interval > 460 ms is considered abnormal, in men a QTc > 450 ms is the cut-off. Long QT syndrome (LQTS) is not necessarily the diagnosis. Patients must be questioned regarding medication use, as many drugs can prolong the QTc interval without necessarily indicating the presence of an underlying channelopathy. A QTc of > 500 ms identifies those patients at highest risk of becoming symptomatic by the age of 40 years. There are over ten subtypes of LQTS, but types 1–3 are the most common in descending order of prevalence.

continued

Type 1 involves a defect of the *KCNQ1* gene, type 2 is a *KCNH2* defect (both result in potassium channelopathies), while type 3 is a sodium channelopathy involving the *SCN5A* gene. Jervell and Lange-Nielsen syndrome is an autosomal recessive form of LQTS which is associated with congenital deafness. It is caused by a mutation of the *KCNE1* and *KCNQ1* genes and has a particularly high risk of ventricular arrhythmia.

The ESC recommends that those with LQTS 1 avoid swimming unsupervised, while LQTS 2 patients minimise acoustic stimuli. All LQTS patients must avoid drugs known to prolong the QT interval. Beta blockers are the mainstay of treatment with an ICD only recommended in those who have survived a cardiac arrest (level Ia evidence) or in those who have experienced syncope and have documented ventricular tachycardia despite β blockade (level IIa).

Answer 11

A. MRI scan of brain with MR venogram

The most likely diagnosis is idiopathic intracranial hypertension (IIH), although it must be remembered that this is a diagnosis of exclusion. The visual fields reveal enlarged blind spots in both eyes, with superior and inferior arcuate scotomas in the left eye (left image); such defects are associated with papilloedema. The papilloedema is the result of raised pressure in the cerebrospinal fluid and subarachnoid space causing an interruption to the axoplasmic flow in the optic nerve.

Learning point

As this change can be caused by an intracranial lesion or venous sinus thrombosis, these differential diagnoses must be promptly investigated. An MRI scan and MR venogram would be ideal due to the increased sensitivity of imaging and lack of radiation. If an MRI scanner is not available, a CT scan with CT venography would be appropriate.

Cerebral angiography is not beneficial in the investigation of IIH.

Optical coherence tomography scanning of the optic nerve head is helpful in confirming that papilloedema is present and can help to differentiate between optic nerve head drusen (calcium deposits) and true optic nerve head swelling. Ocular ultrasound can help confirm the presence of papilloedema, as an echolucent area within the optic nerve sheath (known as the crescent sign) may be seen. This is due to separation of the nerve sheath from the nerve due to increased subarachnoid fluid. Although these investigations are useful adjuncts, the priority must be the ruling out of serious intracranial pathology.

Answer 12

C. Arachis oil enema

Arachis oil is derived from peanuts, and may be used as a faecal softener. It may trigger an allergic or anaphylactic reaction in patients with a peanut allergy, and should be avoided in patients with a known allergy. It is generally believed that refined arachis oil should not contain allergenic peanut proteins, and hence administration to a person with allergy may be safe. Manufacturers of these agents do, however, advise against their use in patients known to be allergic to peanuts.

Other laxatives are generally well tolerated. They may be associated with cramps or abdominal discomfort, and can on occasion cause electrolyte disturbance.

Answer 13

D. Digoxin

There is an extensive list of drugs which can prolong the QT interval and which should be avoided in those with long QT syndrome. Digoxin has no meaningful effect on the QT. Antipsychotic agents and tricyclic antidepressants are among the commonest causes of drug-induced long QT syndrome. Prolongation of the QT interval can lead to an 'R on T' phenomenon resulting in Torsades de Pointes ventricular tachycardia, which can deteriorate to ventricular fibrillation.

Answer 14

A. Anti-Jo-1

This gentleman has anti-synthase syndrome which can present with any of the triad of interstitial lung disease, polymyositis and/or a small joint polyarthropathy. 'Mechanic's hands' as described above, and the presence of Raynaud's phenomenon, support the diagnosis. The most common antibody is Jo-1 and this can indicate a higher risk of pulmonary involvement. Anti-Mi-2 is also a myositis-associated antibody. Anti-centromere and anti-Scl 70 antibodies are seen in scleroderma, and anti-cyclic citrullinated peptide antibodies are associated with rheumatoid arthritis.

Answer 15

D. He is at high risk of a cardiovascular event and his target LDL-C is < 2.5 mmol/litre

Current ESC guidelines recommend the risk stratification of patients to decide upon target lipid levels most appropriate for individuals.[1] LDL-C is now the preferred target over total cholesterol with levels to be achieved dependent on the individual's assigned risk as shown in Table 16.1. The European guidelines favour the SCORE risk estimator which has been validated in a European cohort.

Risk group	LDL-C target (mmol/litre)	Class of evidence
Very high risk (established CVD, type 2 diabetes (aged over 40 with ≥ 1 other risk factor), type 1 diabetes with target organ damage, moderate–severe CKD, SCORE risk ≥ 10%)	< 1.8	Ia
High risk (type 2 diabetes aged (< 40 with no other risk factors), markedly elevated single risk factors, SCORE level ≥ 5–< 10%)	< 2.5	IIa
Moderate risk (SCORE level > 1–< 5%)	< 3.0	IIa

CVD, cardiovascular disease; SCORE, systemic coronary risk evaluation.

Table 16.1: European Society of Cardiology guidelines on the management of dyslipidaemia[1]

Current NICE guidance is to institute statin therapy when an individual has a 10-year risk of a cardiovascular event of > 10% calculated using an appropriate risk estimator.[2] Atorvastatin is the recommended starting agent.

Answer 16

A. A 3-month course of doxycycline

Rosacea is an inflammatory skin disease most often affecting middle-aged men (but it may occur in younger patients).

> **Learning point**
>
> It can be subdivided into various types including:
>
> + erythrotelangiectatic
> + ocular
> + rhinophymatous
> + papulopustular.
>
> In reality, however, there are often overlapping subtypes as in this case.

Trigger factors include sunlight, alcohol, exercise, extremes of temperature and spicy food. Ocular rosacea can cause blepharitis, conjunctivitis or keratitis. Treatment includes topical therapy for mild to moderate disease, eg metronidazole or azelaic acid. For more severe or resistant cases, systemic therapy is used, most often erythromycin or tetracycline antibiotics for two to three months. However, many patients require long-term treatment. In severe recalcitrant cases, isotretinoin may be used.

Recently the α-adrenergic agonist brimonidine in a gel formulation has been shown to be efficacious in the treatment of the persistent facial erythema of rosacea. Other therapies include β blockers or clonidine for the flushing. Although pulsed-dye laser is an appropriate therapy for the telangiectasia in rosacea and nasal shave for the rhinophyma, first-line therapy in this case should aim to treat the papulopustular element, following which adjuvant therapy may be added. Topical steroids should not be used due to the risk of exacerbating rosacea. Topical retinoids, although useful in acne vulgaris (particularly comedomal acne), are unhelpful in rosacea, as patients with rosacea do not have comedomes. This is one of the distinguishing features between the two conditions.

Answer 17

E. Right bundle branch block morphology indicates the VT originates in the right ventricle

The diagnosis is VT in this case. The history of a STEMI means that there is likely to be scarring in either ventricle which is acting as a focus for VT. Infarction impairs the function of sodium channels, which ordinarily have a major role in the heart's conducting network. The loss of cells through scarring leads to abnormal rhythm origin and re-entry around the scar.

Learning point

As VT originates in the ventricles, it can lead to negative concordance (all the QRS complexes pointing downwards) in the chest leads, as the rhythm can originate at the apex and move upward through the ventricles, therefore away from the chest leads. A right bundle branch block morphology means that the rhythm is originating in the left ventricle and vice versa as the ECG reflects the delay in depolarisation of the ventricle which is depolarised last.

Lead AVR essentially 'looks down' at the heart from the right shoulder. Therefore, any positive QRS complexes in this lead reflect electrical activity coming towards the right shoulder and therefore originating at the bottom of the heart (ventricles) and travelling upwards. This is different to the usual atrial starting point with electrical activity travelling downwards and leading to a negative complex in AVR. Fascicular VT arises from the fascicles of the left bundle and usually has a narrower QRS with a RBBB morphology. See Figure 16.7.

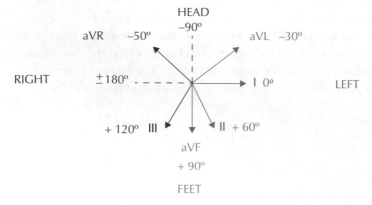

Figure 16.7: Cardiac axis

Answer 18

D. Warfarin

The patient has developed latent psoriasis triggered by medication. Psoriasis is a common condition affecting approximately 2% of the population. It is polygenic, and may be triggered by medications, among other factors.

Learning point

The most commonly known drug triggers for psoriasis include lithium, β blockers, antimalarials, ACE inhibitors and interferon. Other triggering events that may precipitate latent psoriasis include infections (both viral and bacterial, with streptococcal infection particularly associated with guttate psoriasis), psychogenic stress, endocrine factors (eg pregnancy) and cutaneous injury (ie the Koebner phenomenon).

In this question, all medications except warfarin (which is not known to precipitate psoriasis) may have triggered the onset.

Answer 19

D. Finding the patient to be systemically unwell

Diabetic nephropathy is a common complication of diabetes. It generally has an onset of about ten years from diagnosis. In the UKPDS trial, 30% of patients had developed nephropathy at 15 years.[3]

Learning point

Renal disease other than nephropathy should be considered if:

+ there is no significant or progressive retinopathy
+ the blood pressure is particularly high or resistant to treatment
+ heavy proteinuria (ACR > 100 mg/mmol) develops in a patient with a previously normal ACR
+ there is significant haematuria
+ eGFR has worsened rapidly
+ the patient is systemically unwell.

CHAPTER 16 ANSWERS

Answer 20

A. Basal cell carcinoma

This patient presents with a history of a slow-growing, non-healing lesion on the nose with typical appearances of a basal cell carcinoma (BCC), ie telangiectatic, rolled pearly edges with central ulceration. There are various types of BCC including: pigmented, morphoeic, superficial and nodular (as in this case). Risk factors for BCC include: chronic sun exposure, genetic syndromes such as Gorlin syndrome, arsenic ingestion, radiotherapy and immunosuppression.

The treatment of choice for nodular BCC would be surgical excision with appropriate clinical margins. Pyogenic granuloma is a benign growth, which usually presents in children and young adults as a rapidly growing shiny red papule/nodule with a raspberry surface that bleeds easily. The aetiology is unknown but may be due to trauma or infection. The majority occur on the head, neck, hands and feet. The treatment of choice is removal with curettage and cautery or excision to gain an histological diagnosis. Haemangioma are also benign growths of endothelial cells (cells lining blood vessels), which usually result in a red or blue/purple compressible swelling. Diagnosis is on clinical grounds, and if the patient is asymptomatic and there are no clinical concerns, the treatment is reassurance. Actinic keratoses usually present as rough, skin-coloured or erythematous scaly spots on sun-exposed areas. Bowen's disease (intraepithelial carcinoma in situ) usually presents with irregular, flat, erythematous, scaly lesions on chronically sun-exposed skin. Neither of these lesions presents with pearly well-defined lesions.

Answer 21

E. Circinate exudates within the macula

Retinal detachment is likely here. This can occur if rapid glycaemic control is achieved on a background of poor control. This would warrant urgent review by an ophthalmologist. Emergency review by an ophthalmologist would be recommended for: sudden loss of vision, rubeosis iridis, pre-retinal or vitreous haemorrhage, and retinal detachment. Non-urgent review by an ophthalmologist would be required with maculopathy (circinate or group of exudates within the macula; or exudative or retinal thickening within one disc diameter of the centre of the fovea), or an unexplained drop in visual acuity.

Answer 22

A. Oesophageal manometry

Achalasia should be suspected in this case despite a non-specific barium swallow finding. Oesophagitis is not uncommon in achalasia due to the food stasis in the oesophagus.

Learning point

Patients with achalasia can have a fairly normal OGD and barium swallow, therefore a high index of suspicion is required, especially in young patients who present with dysphagia, regurgitation, vomiting and weight loss. The diagnostic test of choice is oesophageal manometry.

The manometric criteria for the diagnosis of achalasia include: absence of peristalsis in the oesophagus with swallow; incomplete relaxation of the lower oesophageal sphincter (LES); and elevated resting LES pressure.

Answer 23

C. 30%

This is a case of adrenocortical carcinoma. This is an aggressive carcinoma originating from the adrenal gland. It usually presents at 30–40 years of age in adults with virilisation. At the time of diagnosis it has often invaded local tissues or metastasised. Cushing syndrome is often associated with adrenal cortical carcinoma. Surgery offers the only chance of cure, although palliation may be the only approach for some patients. Chemotherapy including using mitotane (an inhibitor of steroid synthesis) may be used. A rapid development or progression of hirsutism increases the likelihood that a patient has an androgen-secreting neoplasm. The overall survival is approximately 20–35%.

CHAPTER 16 ANSWERS

Answer 24

E. Nitrofurantoin

Nitrofurantoin-induced autoimmune hepatitis is commonly associated with hypergammaglobulinaemia and elevated anti-nuclear and anti-smooth muscle antibodies. The liver histology resembles that of idiopathic autoimmune hepatitis. Treatment is withdrawal of nitrofurantoin if the causal relationship is identified. The hepatitis is usually reversible if nitrofurantoin is withdrawn early. However, if abnormal liver enzymes persist despite drug discontinuation, immunosuppression with steroids is required.

Answer 25

C. Vascular parkinsonism

His medications suggest that he has a history of atherosclerosis. None of the drugs listed causes parkinsonism. Examples would include metoclopramide and betahistine. ^{123}I-ioflupane is a radiopharmaceutical imaging agent that works by binding to presynaptic dopamine transporters in the brain to form a visual interpretable image using single photon emission CT.

Parkinsonian variants are in practice predominantly distinguished by clinical history and examination, with the passage of time often providing enlightenment. The diagnosis should always be revisited at follow-up appointments. Non-nigrostriatal, non-dopamine-dependent neurodegenerative processes, such as vascular parkinsonism, do not show binding in the 'comma-shaped' putamen and circular caudate bilaterally. In idiopathic Parkinson's disease, the putamen tends to be involved initially and the caudate latterly.

The UK Parkinson's Disease Society's 'brain bank criteria' are sensitive but there is a risk of jeopardising specificity. A DaT scan can be useful to discriminate the diagnosis in patients with an incomplete/atypical parkinsonian syndrome, those with mild symptoms and if a supportive diagnosis of non-nigrostriatal system disease is being considered (eg drug-induced, psychogenic, vascular, post-traumatic, juvenile onset dystonia).

Answer 26

C. Mean sleep latency of less than 20 minutes

The features of narcolepsy include excessive daytime somnolence, cataplexy and parasomnias (eg sleep paralysis or hypnagogic hallucinations). Confirmatory findings on polysomnography include a mean sleep latency of less than five minutes and at least two sleep onset rapid eye movement periods. Additional supportive tests may include CSF with a low hypocretin-1 level and HLA typing (demonstrating DQB1*0602 or DR2 positivity).

Answer 27

A. CT scan of the abdomen

A CT scan of abdomen, specifically using a CT pancreas protocol with intravenous contrast, is the modality of choice for assessing the severity of the acute pancreatitis and for determining the presence of pancreatic necrosis. An ultrasound scan of the abdomen is usually of limited value due to the poor transmission of ultrasound waves through the bowel gas that normally obscures the pancreas. A plain abdominal X-ray is of no use in this case. MR cholangiopancreatography is not superior to CT scanning in assessing the pancreas. ERCP is generally contraindicated in acute pancreatitis unless there is concurrent cholangitis, or when therapeutic ERCP is indicated.

Answer 28

E. Attempt to stand the patient on the day after surgery

Patients should be sitting out and standing the day after surgery. The British Geriatrics Society and British Orthopaedic Association have issued joint guidance on hip fracture patient management called 'The Blue Book'. 10% of patients are dead within one month of hip fracture and around one third are dead at one year. 10–20% admitted from home are discharged to institutional care with all the incumbent costs. In the UK, around 310 000 people present to hospital with fracture each year; approximately one quarter of these cases are hip fractures. The incidence of fracture is expected to rise as the population ages.

Learning point

One per cent of patients will have a normal X-ray. 10–15% patients will not have limb shortening or external rotation as the fracture can be undisplaced.

continued

CHAPTER 16
ANSWERS

For undisplaced intracapsular fractures, internal fixation with sliding hip screws or three parallel screws are the preferred options. Arthroplasty is preferred for displaced intracapsular fractures. However, if the patient is 65–70 years old, their life expectancy may exceed that of the arthroplasty, in which case internal fixation is the preference.

Cementless versus cemented arthroplasties is a matter of debate in the literature. Dalteparin is not appropriate given the current INR.

Answer 29

D. In women, symptoms may occasionally worsen during the menstrual cycle

Signs and symptoms in patients with urethritis may include the following:

+ urethral discharge; this could be yellow, green, brown, or tinged with blood; production is unrelated to sexual activity
+ dysuria (in men) is usually localised to the meatus or distal penis, is worst during the first morning void, and is made worse by alcohol consumption
+ urinary frequency and urgency are typically not present
+ sensation of urethral itching or irritation between voids
+ orchalgia (heaviness in the male genitals)
+ in women, symptoms may worsen during the menstrual cycle (occasionally)
+ systemic symptoms (eg fever, chills, sweats, nausea) may be present.

Answer 30

A. Small intestinal bacterial overgrowth

Small intestinal bacterial overgrowth is common in patients with scleroderma. This is due to the loss of or abnormal migrating motor complex, which functions to clear secretions and bacteria from the small intestines. Stasis and pooling of secretions promotes bacterial overgrowth. Atrophy and wall-thinning of the small intestine can result in diverticulae, which predispose to bacterial overgrowth as well. In severe cases, patients can present with symptoms of malabsorption.

Answer 31

B. Intermittent self-catheterisation

Providing he has normal visual acuity and is physically able to undertake clean intermittent self-catheterisation, this is the preferred option. The Center for Disease Control and Prevention has identified urinary tract infection (UTI) as the second most common type of infection in a hospital setting. Catheter-associated UTI can lead to cystitis, pyelonephritis, bacteraemia, prostatitis, epididymitis, orchitis and, less commonly, endocarditis, vertebral osteomyelitis, septic arthritis, endophthalmitis and meningitis. Complications of such infections include discomfort, prolonged hospitalisation and increased cost and mortality.

Absorptives are always a last resort or a 'holding' option. Condom or sheath-based urinary collection devices rely on the ability to void the bladder. There is nothing to suggest over-active bladder here, and for that reason solifenacin is not a valid option.

Answer 32

C. Stool sample for culture and testing for *Clostridium difficile* toxin

Where there is a significantly high white cell count that is attributable to infection, it is prudent to think about abscesses, septic collections and *C. difficile* infection. A collection of infected fluid at the site of the hip prosthesis is unlikely in this patient on the grounds that both his surgical wound is satisfactory and, importantly, he seems to be mobilising at an appropriate rate and without reports of significant pain. *Staphylococcus aureus* pneumonia can become complicated by the formation of lung abscesses. These are, however, likely to show some clinical signs and all of the respiratory findings in this patient point towards a resolving pneumonia.

Panton–Valentine leukocidin is a toxin produced by some strains of *S. aureus* (both sensitive species (MSSA) and MRSA species) that has been associated with transmissibility and virulence. However, it is not known whether the pathogenicity of PVL–*S. aureus* is the direct result of the PVL toxin or, indeed, what role is played by any of the wide variety of other virulence factors known to exist in *S. aureus* species.

C. difficile disease can manifest anywhere on a spectrum from very mild gastrointestinal upset to life-threatening toxic megacolon. Accordingly, it is crucial that a doctor makes regular assessments of a patient with *C. difficile* infection to ensure that they are receiving optimal management. The latest UK guidance on *C. difficile* recommends a thorough assessment of the patient's clinical status in helping to determine disease severity.[4]

continued

CHAPTER 16 ANSWERS

> ## Learning point
>
> Some of the markers that may be suggestive of severe illness include any of the following: total white cell count > 15×10^9/litre, blood creatinine > 50% above normal, temperature > 38.5 °C and evidence of severe colitis.

Some 'ribotypes' of *C. difficile* bacteria have an association with more severe disease, such as ribotype 027. While very mild disease may not require medical intervention, successful treatment for *C. difficile* disease usually requires:

- ✦ diligent supportive care (with particular attention to fluid and electrolyte balance)
- ✦ antimicrobial therapy targeted at the *C. difficile* bacteria (metronidazole is generally used for mild/moderate disease and oral vancomycin is generally used for severe disease)
- ✦ avoidance of unnecessary antimicrobials
- ✦ strict attention to good hygiene practices to prevent re-infection as well as to prevent transmission to other patients.

Review of gastric acid-suppressing medications has also been suggested and surgical intervention may be indicated in some severe cases.

Note: Vancomycin is a very large molecule and only negligible amounts of intravenously administered drug penetrate the gut. Likewise, only negligible amounts of the drug orally administered is absorbed systemically. It follows that enteral vancomycin is the only route that can be used to treat *C. difficile* infection.

Answer 33

E. Idiopathic intracranial hypertension

A syndrome of raised intracranial pressure (ICP) is suggested by the features of postural headache, transient visual obscurations, optic disc swelling, abducens nerve palsy and elevated CSF opening pressure (above 25 cm H_2O). In this case, the most likely diagnosis is idiopathic intracranial hypertension, given that the patient is an overweight woman (body mass index over 29 kg/m^2) with no other explanation for raised ICP (normal cerebral venography and CSF constituents).

Answer 34

C. Blood cultures

The history is suggestive of a PICC-related bloodstream infection. There is a temporal relationship between the nurse accessing the line and the patient developing symptoms. Organisms (bacteria or fungi) can colonise any vascular access device, entering the bloodstream when the device is used. The nature of a subsequent bloodstream infection is a function of the specific organism, its biological load and the host's immune status. Common organisms include: staphylococci (both coagulase-positive (*Staphylococcus aureus*) and coagulase-negative) species, candida species and coliforms (eg *Escherichia coli*).

Learning point

If the same organism is cultured more quickly in the central line blood specimen than from blood simultaneously sampled via venepuncture (also referred to as a 'peripheral' sample), a central line-associated infection of the patient's bloodstream is suggested. This is because infected lines normally accommodate a greater concentration of organisms than are present in the rest of the circulation. A bloodstream infection involving the central line can also be suggested by the culture of the same organism from a removed central line tip and a venepuncture blood sample.

The respiratory findings in this patient are a secondary phenomenon to the PICC-related bloodstream infection. The host's immune response to sepsis can produce pulmonary oedema through mechanisms such as decreased systemic vascular resistance and capillary leakage. These effects can be further exaggerated in the setting of a patient with impaired baseline cardiac function. Nonetheless, it would be important to consider respiratory infection and its differentials in a real patient scenario. Bacterial pneumonia, viral infection, infection with 'atypical' organisms and infection with more opportunistic agents such as aspergillus species, *Pneumocystis jiroveci* and cytomegalovirus should be considered. Factors influencing the aetiology of respiratory infection include: whether there is underlying lung disease, colonisation with resistant organisms (eg MRSA, ESBL-producing *E. coli*, *Pseudomonas aeruginosa*), prior antimicrobial exposure, and the length and depth of immunosuppression.

CHAPTER 16
ANSWERS

Answer 35

B. Motor neurone disease

There is progressive distal lower limb weakness without sensory involvement. The presence of mixed upper and lower motor neurone signs suggests that the cause is motor neurone disease. The EMG findings of denervation are non-specific but indicate a neurogenic process such as anterior horn cell disease or peripheral neuropathy.

Answer 36

A. 0.9% Saline infusion

This gentleman has a clinical diagnosis of rhabdomyolysis causing renal injury associated with acidosis and hyperkalaemia. Additionally, he has a systemic inflammatory response syndrome (SIRS) (tachycardic, elevated white cells and a raised lactate) and a grossly elevated AST with decreased calcium and increased phosphate. The suggestion is that he has taken alcohol and opiates and has had a prolonged lie, leading to muscle breakdown.

Learning point

Patients with rhabdomyolysis get renal injury through a variety of mechanisms. First, myoglobin, released from muscles, is toxic to renal tubular cells. Myoglobin also precipitates intraluminally, causing cast obstruction. An inflammatory cytokine cascade occurs, leading to a rise in white cells and often C-reactive protein – this causes renal vasoconstriction. Additionally, fluid is sequestered in muscles that are being broken down and several litres can quite rapidly move out of the circulating volume causing haemodynamic compromise and further renal injury. Phosphate released from dying muscles can precipitate with calcium and dangerous hypocalcaemia can follow.

The treatment initially, given the scenario, is vigorous fluid resuscitation with 0.9% saline to expand the intravascular volume as well as to allow the kidneys a chance to excrete myoglobin (detected here as 'blood' on the dipstick). Several litres in the first 24 hours may be required, with careful attention to fluid balance, especially if the patient remains oligo/anuric due to the development of acute tubular necrosis.

Sodium bicarbonate is a useful strategy in both addressing systemic acidosis and alkalanising the urine, which aids in excretion of myoglobin and other haem pigments. Although he is acidotic, he is not severely so and does not yet require aggressive alkali therapy. If he did warrant it, a lower strength solution such as 1.4% should be used rather than 8.4%, which is reserved for the treatment of tricyclic antidepressant poisoning with cerebral or cardiac dysfunction. Bilateral fasciotomies may well be required in the next 24 to 48 hours if fluid sequestration continues, but are not indicated at this stage. Broad spectrum antibiotic cover should be considered early; however, although he has a SIRS, he has little objective evidence of sepsis. Bilateral cellulitis would be unlikely and chest and urinary examinations do not suggest presence of infection. At this stage, if occult infection (endocarditis/discitis/skin abscess from injection sites etc) was suspected, it would be more rational to take blood cultures and continue fluid resuscitative efforts. Finally, haemodialysis may well be avoided if his urine output improves with fluids. His potassium is elevated due to a combination of renal dysfunction and acidosis. This can be managed medically at this stage, although there is no definite indication for treatment at this time given his ECG findings.

Answer 37

A. Aquaporin-4 antibody

This is a case of neuromyelitis optica (NMO), an inflammatory syndrome of the central nervous system characterised by severe optic neuritis and longitudinally extensive transverse myelitis (a cord lesion extending over at least three vertebral segments). Serum aquaporin-4 antibody testing is highly specific for NMO. Although phenotypically similar in some cases, it is important to distinguish NMO from multiple sclerosis as NMO requires immunosuppressant therapy to prevent NMO relapses.

Answer 38

E. P-ANCA

This man's presentation with worsening asthma, the new onset of allergies with a mononeuritis multiplex as evidenced by paresthesiae in his hands and foot drop, very high eosinophil count and mild renal dysfunction is highly suggestive of eosinophilic granulomatosis with polyangiitis (Churg–Strauss syndrome). This is a multisystem vasculitic disorder in which P-ANCA antibodies (with MPO staining) are seen in up to 50% of cases. Renal dysfunction tends to be mild initially and patients can have symptoms for several years before involvement of the kidneys, lungs and gastrointestinal tract results in destructive necrotising lesions.

In Goodpasture's disease, anti-GBM antibodies against the alpha-3 chain of type four collagen arise and incite an inflammatory response against this protein which is mainly

continued

CHAPTER 16
ANSWERS

located in the basement membranes of the lungs and nephrons. The clinical features are usually those of frank haemoptysis and acute renal failure. In some cases presentation with isolated lung or kidney damage is seen. Granulomatosis with polyangiitis (Wegener's granulomatosis) tends to present like Goodpasture's disease, but also with upper airway, eye and ear pathology such as epistaxis, nasal stuffiness, perforation of the nasal septum, hearing loss and uveitis, in addition to arthritis and peripheral neuropathies. Elevated titres of C-ANCA (with PR3 staining) antibodies are typically associated with this condition. Anti-double-stranded DNA antibodies are found in association with lupus nephritis and patients will tend to have other features such as a malar rash, mouth ulcers, positive anti-nuclear antibodies, arthritis, hair loss, serositis (pleural/pericardial effusions) and photosensitivity.

Anti-topoisomerase antibodies are seen in generalised systemic sclerosis, a multisystem connective tissue disorder in which fibrosis causing hardening of the skin is seen. It can involve other organs such as the lungs, gastrointestinal tract and kidneys. Arthritis and Raynaud's phenomenon leading to digital colour changes, pain and, in some cases, infarction can be seen.

Answer 39

C. Surgery now, with consideration of adjuvant radiotherapy deferred until post-partum

The incidence of cancer during pregnancy is increasing and now affects up to 1 in 1000 pregnancies. Breast and cervical cancers are the most commonly detected in this population. Investigation of a breast lump during pregnancy should be performed with ultrasound, or shielded mammography, and biopsy since the sensitivity of mammography in pregnancy is reduced.

Learning point

Surgery may be performed as clinically indicated during pregnancy (for example modified radical mastectomy and axillary node dissection); however, if possible, adjuvant radiotherapy should be deferred until post-partum. Data on the safety of cytotoxic agents is limited and all chemotherapy should be avoided in the first trimester. Some agents may be considered in the second and third trimesters including cyclophosphamide, methotrexate and 5-fluorouracil (CMF) which are associated with a 1.3% risk of fetal malformation. Data on taxanes are limited and they are not currently recommended. Termination of pregnancy is not recommended except in unusual circumstances.

Answer 40

D. Haemodialysis

This gentleman presents with a profound metabolic acidosis, hypocalcaemia and mild renal impairment. His lactate is elevated above the normal range but is not sufficient to account for the severity of acidosis.

Learning point

When faced with any acidotic patient (in life as in exams), it is important to calculate the anion gap. This separates 'normal' gap acidoses (caused by renal or gastrointestinal losses of bicarbonate) from 'raised' gap acidoses (where an extra, unmeasured anion is present). This gentleman has an anion gap of 34 mmol/litre ($Na-Cl-HCO_3$). Causes of a raised anion gap are most commonly diabetic ketoacidosis, starvation ketoacidosis, alcoholic ketoacidosis, lactic acidosis, renal failure, ingestion of an organic alcohol (methanol or ethylene glycol in antifreeze and windscreen wiper wash), and some drugs and chemicals (isoniazid, toluene, salicylates). A lesser-known cause of a raised gap acidosis is the accumulation of pyroglutamic acid (also known as 5-oxoproline), which can be seen in malnourished or otherwise sick individuals who are chronically treated with paracetamol, especially if given intravenously – this is worth bearing in mind when the cause of the acidosis is not clear. It will resolve on stopping the paracetamol.

There is a suggestion in the question that the patient has ingested antifreeze (ethylene glycol) and this would be very consistent with the severe acidosis and confusion. One extra step when encountering a raised gap acidosis is to see if the fall in bicarbonate is proportionate to the 'extra' acids present. There is a 1:1 ratio of increase in the anion gap above normal to fall in bicarbonate. So for every extra anionic acid present (reflected in the anion gap), the bicarbonate should decrease by 1 mmol/litre. For example, in this question the normal anion gap is taken as 12. The anion gap measured is 34, therefore there are 34 – 12 = 22 'extra' anions present. These would be expected to decrease the bicarbonate by 22 from its normal value, conventionally taken as 25. In this case we would expect to see a bicarbonate of 25 – 22 = 3 mmol/litre, which is what is seen. Therefore, this patient has a pure gap acidosis. If the serum bicarbonate in this case was 15 mmol/litre and the anion gap was still 32, then the patient would not be as acidotic as expected. This usually occurs because the patient has started out with a higher baseline bicarbonate as the result of a previously existing metabolic alkalosis, as in the case of patients with chronic, compensated type two respiratory failure, or if the patient has been dehydrated as a result of vomiting or diuretics and developed a hypochloraemic contraction alkalosis.

continued

Conversely, if the measured bicarbonate is substantially (> 3 mmol/litre) lower than expected, it suggests there is a 'normal' gap acidosis also present (remember it is possible to have **both** an acidosis caused by extra anions **as well as** an acidosis due to renal or gastrointestinal bicarbonate losses). This situation could occur in the above scenario if the patient, for example, had also had several days of profuse diarrhoea and suffered gastrointestinal losses of bicarbonate.

Treatment of organic acid poisoning is dependent on time of presentation. A subset of patients, presenting early, with no renal dysfunction and no acidosis can often be treated on a medical ward with intravenous fomepizole, a competitive inhibitor of alcohol dehydrogenase. Alcohol dehydrogenase is the enzyme that converts methanol and ethylene glycol, themselves not particularly toxic apart from their inebriating effects, into toxic acid metabolites that are responsible for renal and neurological damage and metabolic acidosis. Apart from taking a reliable history, a clue to very early ingestion is that the osmolar gap (the gap between the measured and calculated osmolarity) will be raised (substantially > 10 mOsmol/kg). As the parent alcohol is metabolised to its toxic metabolites, the osmolar gap will steadily decrease.

In the question stem the calculated osmolarity (2(Na + K) + urea + glucose) = 289 mOsmol/kg and the measured osmolarity is close to this at 296 mOsmol/kg. This suggests poisoning has happened at least several hours, if not one to two days, before, as almost all the parent alcohol (ethylene glycol in this case) has been metabolised to toxic metabolites. The half-life of ethylene glycol is three to nine hours, and fomepizole permits the parent alcohol to be renally cleared before it is metabolised by alcohol dehydrogenase. Giving ethanol, which competes with alcohol dehydrogenase for metabolism, has a similar effect to fomepizole but the required volumes to be administered lead to the patient becoming inebriated. This is at best a minor inconvenience on the ward. At worst, it can mask or complicate some of the neurological and cardiorespiratory complications of organic alcohol toxicity.

Intravenous sodium bicarbonate can be helpful in replenishing the diminished stores of bicarbonate, but will do little to ameliorate the injurious effects of the toxic metabolites. Given that the patient has a severe acidosis, and a raised creatinine (as a result of calcium oxalate deposition in the kidney – reflected in the low serum calcium levels), then some form of dialysis is required. Continuous veno-venous haemofiltration is commonly available in the intensive care unit, but is not effective in clearing ethylene glycol and its metabolites. Instead, haemodialysis, because of its additional methods of solute removal, is more efficient.

Answer 41

D. Start him on pancreatic enzyme replacement therapy

This gentleman has malabsorption (weight loss and diarrhoea, typically steatorrhoea) due to pancreatic insufficiency caused by alcohol-induced chronic pancreatitis. As the pancreatic insufficiency progresses, lipid digestion and malabsorption become the overriding problems, which ultimately lead to clinical symptoms, nutrient and fat-soluble vitamins deficiencies. Pancreatic enzyme replacement therapy remains the mainstay of treatment for pancreatic insufficiency. Dosages vary from patient to patient, but the general advice is to give 25 000–50 000 units of lipase with each main meal and 5000–25 000 units of lipase with snacks. Alcohol abstinence, nutritional support and optimising analgesia are all appropriate management, but pancreatic enzyme replacement to improve his weight and diarrhoea is the key treatment.

Answer 42

C. Contact microbiology, change to alternative broad spectrum antibiotics, add a glycopeptide to cover line infection

This is a patient who was appropriately treated initially for febrile neutropaenia but has unfortunately not responded. This is a common scenario in oncological medicine. Guidelines vary from hospital to hospital, but if a patient is deteriorating after 72 hours of antibiotics, it is generally recommended to switch to second-line cover (eg from tazocin/gentamicin to meropenem), and add a glycopeptide such as vancomycin to treat infected indwelling venous catheters (even when there is no clinical evidence of such). If an indwelling catheter has multiple lumens, antibiotics should be administered through each lumen in rotation. If a patient continues to deteriorate despite the above measures, an antifungal agent should be added and it may be appropriate to remove any indwelling lines. If the patient was improving clinically and inflammatory markers were dropping, it may be appropriate to continue current antibiotic therapy despite ongoing fever, but careful clinical monitoring would be required. Antibiotics should never be stopped in the context of febrile neutropaenia until the patient has recovered. Finally, lumbar puncture is contraindicated in the absence of neutrophils due to risk of introducing infection or causing bleeding due to concurrent thrombocytopaenia.

Answer 43

A. Brinzolamide

This lady has an acidosis. The first question is to see whether this is a normal gap or raised gap acidosis. In this case her anion gap is 137 – 115 – 16 = 6 mmol/litre. This is a normal gap acidosis. In view of this, causes of a raised gap acidosis can be excluded – renal failure and lactic acidosis secondary to metformin.

> ### Learning point
>
> Causes of a normal gap acidosis can easily be divided into those in which bicarbonate is lost from the gut (eg from diarrhoea, pancreatic fistulae, high-output stomas) or from the kidneys (either due to losses, lack of reabsorptive capacity or failure of manufacture). Renal causes can include drugs such as carbonic anhydrase inhibitors (acetazolamide, brinzolamide), some chemotherapeutic drugs such as ifosfamide, autoimmune and metabolic causes of renal tubular acidosis, eg Sjögren syndrome, systemic lupus erythematosus, Wilson's disease and inherited metabolic disorders.

Distinguishing between causes of a normal gap acidosis can be straightforward in cases where there is, for example, an obvious loss of bicarbonate-rich fluid from the gastrointestinal tract. In this present case, however, things are less clear. One way to determine the difference is to see whether, in the face of systemic acidosis, the kidneys are able to appropriately excrete an acid load. This can be determined by looking at the urinary anion gap.

The urinary anion gap is determined by summing the positive ions (Na + K) and subtracting the negative ion (– Cl⁻). If the value is overall strongly positive, then the acidosis is due to a renal cause. If the value is negative, it is due to a gastrointestinal cause. Remember, 'NeGUTive urinary anion gap is due to GUT causes'.

The major unmeasured anion in urine (accounting for any 'gaps') is the ammonium ion, which is secreted by the kidney. These ions complex with chloride to form ammonium chloride and this is the major way in which the kidneys excrete acid. Overall electroneutrality needs to be maintained and so if there is an excess of chloride ions over the measured positive Na and K ions, this suggests that there is excretion also of ammonium ions, ie the kidney is able to generate ammonium ions in the face of systemic acidosis and therefore renal issues are not the cause of the acidosis. If the positive ions are greater numerically than chloride ions during a systemic acidosis, this suggests that there is a relative lack of ammonium ion generation and therefore the kidneys are not able to excrete an appropriate acid load. In such cases, renal issues are therefore the cause of the acidosis.

The easiest way to remember this is to remember that GUT losses cause a 'neGUTive' urinary anion gap, ie Cl⁻ ions numerically outweigh the sum of Na and K. In the present scenario the urinary anion gap is $35 + 40 - 20 = 55$. Despite the acidosis, there is a positive gap. There is therefore a lack of ammonium ions being excreted (complexed with the measured chloride ions), and so the problem lies with the kidneys. Diarrhoea is therefore **not** the cause.

The last two answers then are brinzolamide or ranitidine. Ranitidine is an H_2 receptor antagonist which reduces acid secretion into the gut, but does not have an effect on renal acid handling. Brinzolamide is a carbonic anhydrase inhibitor used to treat glaucoma. Although it is given topically via the eye, there have been case reports of significant systemic absorption leading to symptoms and, in some cases, a normal gap acidosis. Carbonic anhydrase is found in the proximal tubular cells and its inhibition leads to reduced sodium chloride and bicarbonate reabsorption in the proximal tubule, causing a modest diuresis and also metabolic acidosis (due to the alkali lost in urine). The present question writer encountered a very similar situation where it was believed that there was systemic absorption of brinzolamide as this was the only explanation for the normal gap acidosis seen.

Answer 44

B. 70–80%

There are two important hereditary colorectal cancer syndromes to be aware of: familial adenomatous polyposis (FAP), which is associated with a 100% lifetime risk of colorectal cancer, and HNPCC, which is associated with approximately a 70% lifetime risk. HNPCC is also associated with an increased incidence of endometrial cancer (up to 40% lifetime risk) and ovarian cancer (up to 20%). For affected patients, screening should be performed from age 25 years upwards, and should include annual colonoscopy, annual pelvic/transvaginal ultrasound and annual CA125 measurement.

Answer 45

B. Infective endophthalmitis

An acute post-operative endophthalmitis is the most serious ophthalmic complication associated with intravitreal injections. It occurs in < 1/1000 post-injection eyes, but its occurrence should be presumed until ruled out by an ophthalmologist, as it can rapidly lead to complete loss of vision. Patients present with a red, painful eye and reduced vision. If suspected, patients should have urgent anterior chamber and vitreous samples taken for microscopy, culture and sensitivity, followed by the administration of intravitreal antibiotics and subsequent close follow-up.

continued

In the case of intraocular lens trauma, the area of damage may be visible on dilated ocular examination. Ocular inflammation would be noted due to leakage of lens proteins into the anterior chamber and there may be an associated intraocular pressure rise and discomfort. This would, however, be unlikely to cause hand movements vision. A retinal detachment could cause hand movements vision if there is involvement of the macula, but this would not be associated with pain and would be visible on dilated fundoscopy. An arterial occlusion could cause hand movements vision, but again would be unlikely to be painful. In the minority of patients experiencing this complication, it tends to occur immediately following the injection due to the associated intraocular pressure rise experienced with administrating an intravitreal substance and would therefore be unlikely to present two days post procedure. Uveitis can cause a red painful eye but hand movements vision is unusual unless there is severe inflammation or macular involvement. Having said that, this does occur in some cases and should be considered once endophthalmitis has been ruled out.

Answer 46

C. It has high hepatic extraction

Clomethiazole is a drug with high hepatic extraction. Normally, when clomethiazole is administered orally, around 90% of the dose is extracted by the liver. In patients with liver impairment, this effect is diminished since there is a reduction in hepatic blood flow. Less drug is therefore extracted, meaning that a much higher quantity of drug is delivered to the systemic circulation. Exaggerated drug effects can therefore result. Other drugs with high hepatic extraction include chlorpromazine, levodopa, midazolam, morphine, nitrates, some antidepressants, some β blockers, some calcium channel blockers and some statins.

Answer 47

A. Absence of amenorrhoea

Anorexia nervosa is a condition commonly affecting young women (1 : 10 men : women ratio). It is characterised by deliberate/self-induced weight loss (body mass index 15% below normal or less), a marked distortion of body image (patients commonly perceive themselves as 'fat') and a pathological desire for thinness. There is usually evidence of a widespread endocrine disorder involving the hypothalamic–pituitary–gonadal axis. Typically, serum LH, FSH, progestogens and oestrogens are reduced, with resulting amenorrhoea. Growth hormone and cortisol are elevated. In atypical anorexia nervosa, some of the expected features of anorexia nervosa (eg amenorrhoea) are absent.

Answer 48

D. Gradual progression to respiratory failure

This lady has lymphangioleiomyomatosis (LAM), a rare condition affecting women of childbearing age.

Learning point

LAM is hormone-dependent and associated with abnormal smooth muscle cell proliferation. It affects lungs and potentially other organs. In two thirds of cases, it presents with pneumothorax, dyspnoea (42%), cough (20%), haemoptysis (14%) and chylothorax (12%). Examination is non-specific. Spirometry is normal or obstructive and transfer factor is often reduced. Chest X-ray is normal or hyperinflated. High-resolution CT scan images are characteristic with multiple cysts of mostly uniform size, usually small and thin walled, that are scattered and not in a zonal pattern. A biopsy is often needed for diagnosis. Pneumothoraces should be managed as secondary pneumothoraces. Other elements of treatment include recommending a low-fat diet, avoidance of pregnancy (as symptoms often worsen), hormone manipulation, avoidance of oestrogens, smoking cessation, avoidance of air travel, and use of bronchodilators. If these patients are transplanted, the disease can recur.

There is a national centre for LAM in Nottingham and patients can be referred for assessment and for involvement in clinical trials. LAM has a poor prognosis with a slow progression to respiratory failure. At ten years, 70% are alive, 23% are on long-term oxygen therapy and 10% are housebound.

Another rare lung condition that may cause pneumothorax is histiocytosis X or pulmonary Langerhans' histiocytosis X. This affects younger male adult smokers. The lungs are infiltrated with histiocytes that cause nodules, which progress into pulmonary cysts. It is a systemic condition. 25% are asymptomatic; others can have cough, dyspnoea, fever and weight loss. 20% present with pneumothorax. Chest X-rays can show diffuse reticulo-nodular shadowing with cystic change. High-resolution CT scan images can show bizarre-shaped cysts with thick walls in a mid- and upper-zone predominance; associated emphysema can also be seen. Spirometry measurements are variable, with reduced transfer factor and often hypoxia on exertion. The disease is associated with severe pulmonary hypertension, lymphoma and lung cancer. Management includes smoking cessation and steroids, although there is no evidence for a benefit. The disease can recur in transplanted lungs. Prognosis is variable; it can progress to respiratory failure and can shorten life expectancy.

Answer 49

A. Fluoxetine

Fluoxetine is currently the only antidepressant recommended for use in children and adolescents. There is concern about the incidence of self-harm, including suicide, when all antidepressants are used in young people. Fluoxetine is not free from this problem, hence appropriate follow-up should be in place before the drug is used and it should only be used under specialist supervision.

Antidepressants are commonly prescribed drugs, and a knowledge of their common adverse reactions is important. Some of the most important effects are detailed here.

Tricyclic antidepressants (eg amitriptyline): postural hypotension, effects on cardiac conduction, anxiety, confusion, dry mouth, blurred vision, constipation, urinary retention, gynaecomastia, galactorrhoea and hyponatraemia.

Selective serotonin reuptake inhibitors (eg sertraline): gastrointestinal upset, hypersensitivity reactions, dry mouth, anxiety, galactorrhoea, hyponatraemia. A 'serotonin syndrome' is occasionally seen in overdose. This comprises features of serotonin excess including autonomic instability, neuropsychiatric effects, hyperthermia and rhabdomyolysis.

Monoamine oxidase inhibitors (eg isocarboxazid): postural hypotension and jaundice. It is important to remember the 'cheese reaction' for patients taking these drugs. Owing to enzyme inhibition, consumption of tyramine-containing food (eg mature cheese, meat/yeast extracts, red wine, beer, 'out-of-date' meat/fish) can cause severe hypertension, as can co-prescription with tricyclic antidepressants, amphetamines and some other agents.

Answer 50

C. HLA-B27

All of the others are associated with rheumatoid arthritis (RA). One of the strongest genetic risk factors for RA is the shared epitope. In patients with the disease, several HLA-DRB1 molecules share a common amino acid sequence at position 70–74 in the third hyper-variable region of the DRB1 chain. This sequence has been named the 'shared epitope' and contributes around 30% of the total genetic effect. Citrullination is a physiological process, which is believed to be important for degradation of intracellular proteins during apoptosis. The modified (citrullinated) protein is assumed to be foreign to the body, and auto-reactive antibodies are formed. In RA they have a sensitivity of 72% and specificity of 99.7%. HLA-B27 is typically associated with ankylosing spondylitis and not RA. RA is a chronic inflammatory disease and is associated with increased cardiovascular risk. This risk is comparable to that in patients with type 2 diabetes. Cigarette smoking is the most important environmental risk factor for RA. This risk is increased further in the presence of the shared epitope.

Answer 51

D. *Chlamydia burnetti*

This lady could have any of the above organisms in the options list; however, *C. burnetti* is least likely as it is generally seen in epidemics related to animal sources and it is very uncommon. The others could all cause upper lobe pneumonia. However, in this lady, non-tuberculous mycobacteria would be suspected with this clinical picture if *M. tuberculosis* was ruled out.

Learning point

Non-tuberculous mycobacteria are a group of bacteria commonly found in the environment. There are many different species. They are low-grade pathogens in humans. They cause pulmonary infections in the older population and in those with pre-existing lung disease such as bronchiectasis or in those who are immunocompromised. Clinically they present with a subacute illness or with atypical features of their underlying disease. Chest X-ray findings can be non-specific. In some cases, upper lobe infiltrates are similar to those of *M. tuberculosis*. Sputum (or washings from bronchoscopy) may yield a Ziehl–Neelsen stain positive culture (*M. tuberculosis* PCR is negative). Multiple positive cultures are required for significance. Pulmonary disease is likely if the chest X-ray is suggestive and if there are three or more positive cultures, more than a week apart. Alternatively, one culture from a sterile site or two cultures from lavage, on different days, would be in keeping. The clinical significance is also important to bear in mind, as treatment is intensive and difficult, especially if the patient is very elderly or if they have multiple co-morbidities.

Examples include *M. kansasii*, which needs treatment as it will progress without. Treatment is with rifampicin and ethambutol for at least nine months. There is generally a 100% response rate and < 10% relapse with full compliance.

M. avium complex can be asymptomatic and does not always require treatment, which would be rifampicin, ethambutol and isoniazid for two years. It has a 50% response rate and 20% relapse rate. Maximising the treatment of any underlying lung disease may be effective alone. Other culprit organisms include *M. malmoense* and *M. xenopi*.

continued

**CHAPTER 16
ANSWERS**

Non-tuberculous mycobacteria disease does not need to be notified; those cases that are notified and subsequently found not to be due to *M. tuberculosis* can be de-notified and treatments can be adjusted.

Pneumocystis jiroveci infection, previously known as *Pneumocystis carinii*, can be present without causing active pneumonia. Exposure in susceptible hosts can cause *P. jiroveci* pneumonia. Those at risk include patients with HIV who have CD4 counts < 200/mm^3, as well as patients receiving chemotherapy, other immunosuppressants or long-term steroids. The incidence has reduced since patients have been given prophylactic co-trimoxazole. Infected patients generally present with a dry cough, dyspnoea on exertion, chest tightness, fever, increased respiratory rate and pneumothoraces. They can be profoundly hypoxic. Diagnosis can be confirmed on culture from sputum, bronchoscopy or transbronchial biopsy. First-line treatment is with high doses of IV co-trimoxazole. The treatment can then be changed to the oral route and continued for two to three weeks. If suspected, treatment should not be delayed, since results can take some time to come through. If patients are hypoxic, steroids should be given. The prognosis is dependent on the underlying condition: in HIV, mortality is < 10%, in cancer it is around 30%, and if the patient is intubated and ventilated, mortality is around 60%.

Answer 52

C. Timolol

Timolol is a β blocker, which may be given topically to the eyes in the treatment of glaucoma. Systemic absorption may cause toxicity, such as the bronchospasm detailed in this case.

Cabergoline is an ergot derivative dopamine agonist, most commonly used in the treatment of hyperprolactinaemia. It, and related drugs, may cause troublesome fibrosis that can affect the heart, lung and retroperitoneal regions. Regular echocardiography and spirometry is recommended for patients using these drugs in the long term. Tamoxifen is an anti-oestrogen agent. Serious adverse effects include an increased risk of thrombo-embolic disease and endometrial cancer. Varenicline may be used to assist patients with stopping smoking. Its use has been linked with seizures, depression and suicidal ideation, and it may cause a wide range of adverse effects. St John's wort is a herbal remedy that may be purchased over the counter. It is a hepatic enzyme inducer, and hence can have significant interacting effects when used alongside other drugs also metabolised by the same enzymes.

Answer 53

C. MRI or CT scan

The diagnosis is Takayasu's arteritis. The patient is young (< 40 years) and presents with systemic upset and an episode of collapse. Clinically she has a > 10 mmHg difference in systolic BP between each upper limb and there is an audible bruit in the carotid region. She therefore fulfils three out of six of the 1990 American College of Rheumatology diagnostic criteria for the condition. In addition she has markedly elevated inflammatory markers and prodromal systemic upset.

Tissue biopsy is rarely attempted on a routine basis due to the major risks associated with the procedure. The features seen on biopsy are similar to those seen in classical temporal arteritis with multinucleated giant cells and granulomatous inflammation. An ultrasound examination of the aorta may detect alteration in aortic calibre but is rarely used to confirm diagnosis as it is technically challenging to achieve a detailed picture of the entire aorta and its branches. MRI and CT scanning are the gold standard investigations. These can be performed with or without angiography. Either modality can be used with similar features seen in both modalities. Imaging demonstrates smooth tapering of the lumen and focal areas of vessel wall thickening due to occlusive lesions more proximally. Transthoracic echocardiography has no place in the diagnostic work-up for Takayasu's arteritis. CT-PET scanning is occasionally used in this clinical setting, although currently there is limited access to this form of CT imaging, which uses fluorodeoxyglucose (FDG) uptake, and there have been no validated studies in Takayasu's arteritis. The modality does, however, sound promising with a possible association between FDG uptake and the activity of inflammation within the vessel wall.

Answer 54

B. Raloxifene

This lady has osteoporosis. This results from reduced bone mass and disruption of the microarchitecture of bone with subsequent decreased bone strength. It is defined by a T-score of −2.5 standard deviations or below, as measured by dual-energy X-ray absorptiometry. Risk factors in this case include early menopause, lack of oestrogen replacement and a positive family history.

Raloxifene is an oral selective oestrogen receptor modulator (SERM) that has oestrogenic actions on bone and anti-oestrogenic actions on the uterus and breast. Therefore, in a case like the one presented where treatment of osteoporosis is required in a lady at risk of breast carcinoma, SERM therapy may be the preferred option. This would need to be balanced against the increased risk of venous thromboembolism resulting from this treatment.

continued

Raloxifene reduces risk of vertebral fractures by 30–50% but evidence in the prevention of other fractures is not as convincing.

Otherwise, bisphosphonates are generally regarded as the first-line treatment in post-menopausal women with osteoporosis. The use of hormone replacement therapy is controversial but would definitely be contraindicated here with the history of breast carcinoma. Strontium ranelate is recommended as an alternate option for primary prevention in women who are intolerant or unable to comply with instructions for administration of a bisphosphonate. Its use has been linked with arterial and venous complications.

Answer 55

C. A maternal history of anti-Ro/SSa antibodies or anti-La/SSB antibodies

The development of congenital heart block is not dependent on a mother's diagnosis, but rather the presence of anti-Ro/SSa antibodies or anti-La/SSB antibodies. Congenital heart block is the most severe manifestation of neonatal lupus syndrome when placental transfer of antibodies to the fetus causes irreversible damage to the developing conducting system.

Learning point

Women with lupus and Sjögren syndrome should be screened for the presence of antibodies, and referred for careful monitoring if they are present. High anti-double-stranded DNA antibody levels in isolation have not been associated with fetal heart block.

Answer 56

C. Isosorbide mononitrate

Sildenafil is a phosphodiesterase type five inhibitor, which may be used for erectile dysfunction or pulmonary hypertension. This group of drugs should not be used alongside nitrates, such as isosorbide mononitrate, due to potentiation of their antihypertensive effects. Side effects include gastrointestinal upset, headache, dizziness, nasal congestion and visual disturbances.

Answer 57

B. Fasting serum glucose

The history of gradually expanding, waxy, atrophic, yellow–brown patches on the shin is consistent with necrobiosis lipoidica (although necrobiosis may appear elsewhere on the body). The investigation of choice in this scenario would be fasting glucose test because the condition is strongly associated with diabetes.

Learning point

Necrobiosis can precede the diagnosis of diabetes mellitus in approximately 15% of cases, occur following the diagnosis in 60% and appear concurrently in 25% of patients.

The aetiology is uncertain, and the presence of the condition in patients with diabetes is not associated with poor diabetic control. The condition is more common in women than men, and usually presents in early middle-aged patients.

Answer 58

D. 24-hour urinary catecholamines

MEN 2 syndrome is an autosomal dominant syndrome with a high penetrance for medullary thyroid carcinoma. It consists of two main forms: MEN 2A consists of medullary thyroid carcinoma, phaeochromocytoma and parathyroid adenomas; MEN 2B comprises medullary thyroid carcinoma, phaeochromocytoma and a characteristic marfanoid appearance. The association of phaeochromocytoma with MEN 2 is important to consider. This lady is also pregnant and a phaeochromocytoma must be ruled out.

Prolactin levels increase in pregnancy and are often not useful for monitoring. MEN 1 is associated with prolactinomas. Chromogranin A would be non-diagnostic and therefore not recommended on its own. Although thyroxine levels are in the lower range of normal, the TSH level is satisfactory. In pregnancy, the target TSH level is < 2.5 mU/litre. Testing free triiodothyronine is unlikely to be helpful.

Answer 59

B. Provision of supportive care and treatment of underlying condition

The cause for the acute transaminitis in this case is ischaemic hepatitis. It is universally caused by tissue hypoxia, either from hypoperfusion from cardiac failure, systemic hypoxaemia from respiratory failure or increased oxygen demand from sepsis. The elevated transaminases are usually in the thousands range. In most cases, ischaemic hepatitis is transient and self-limiting. The overall prognosis depends on the severity of the underlying cause. Treatment for ischaemic hepatitis is supportive and directed at improving tissue perfusion and oxygenation.

Answer 60

A. Enalapril orally

To decide the best treatment for this sick patient it is important to broadly establish the correct diagnosis. She is severely hypertensive with anaemia, thrombocytopaenia and renal dysfunction. It is as yet undetermined whether this is acute, chronic or acute on chronic – the working hypothesis is that this has to be acute. Her fundoscopy would suggest she has not been severely hypertensive for very long – there is papilloedema only. LDH and unconjugated bilirubin are substantially elevated along with liver transaminases. The blood film demonstrates schistocytes or fragmented red cells. This lady is suffering from a microangiopathic haemolytic anaemia (MAHA), also known as thrombotic microangiopathy (TMA) when associated with end-organ damage due to microthrombi.

There are a number of different types and mechanisms of this condition, but commonly endothelial dysfunction permits the activation of platelets on capillary surfaces and the development of fibrin strands which mechanically 'cheese-wire' red cells causing haemolysis. Some of these platelet–fibrin clots can embolise to organs such as brain, kidney, heart and liver.

Learning point

Clues in the clinical history include her symptoms of an upper GI disorder, clinical signs of pulmonary hypertension (loud pulmonary component of the second heart sound), skin changes and painful lesions on her fingers. The skin on her hands is shiny and smooth. These clinical findings would be consistent with a diagnosis of systemic sclerosis. In this setting, the diagnosis of scleroderma renal crisis (SRC) has to be the top differential.

Other conditions such as thrombotic thrombocytopenic purpura (TTP), haemolytic uraemic syndrome (both diarrhoea-associated and non-diarrhoea-associated) and malignant hypertension per se could cause the biochemical abnormalities, but would not explain the skin findings. Additionally, TTP is often associated with neurological involvement due to microthrombi lodging in the brain.

So the treatment indicated now, even despite her advanced renal dysfunction, is oral enalapril, which is the best treatment aimed at reversing the pathological process in SRC. Immunoglobulins are of use if TTP is suspected. Plasma exchange is also indicated in the setting of TTP and, especially, 'atypical' haemolytic uraemic syndrome, which can be associated with a range of genetic and acquired disorders of complement regulation. A titrated IV labetalol infusion would be a sensible idea, but will not directly target the underlying SRC pathology. Steroids are indicated for adjunctive treatment of both TTP and atypical haemolytic uraemic syndrome but are absolutely contraindicated in SRC. They can actually precipitate renal crisis in patients with scleroderma and are therefore best totally avoided.

Answer 61

E. Colonoscopy

In this case, left-sided colorectal cancer is suggested by the history of bright-red fresh blood and tenesmus. It is important to visualise the full extent of the colon where possible to exclude synchronous tumours. If colonoscopy was contraindicated, barium enema may be utilised to identify areas of stricturing. CT and MRI scanning would be performed after a tumour has been identified to fully stage the patient and to plan definitive management.

CHAPTER 16 ANSWERS

Answer 62

B. Serum bilirubin

It is important to determine the hepatitis C virus (HCV) genotype, as this will guide the duration of treatment. HCV genotype one patients receive a maximum treatment of 48 weeks, whereas patients with genotypes two and three are treated for 24 weeks. Side effects of the combination treatment include anaemia, neutropaenia, thrombocytopaenia and thyroid function abnormalities. It is therefore prudent to obtain baseline blood tests before treatment and these should be monitored during treatment. Ribavirin is teratogenic, hence pregnancy has to be excluded first in female patients of reproductive age.

Answer 63

B. 5–20%

Approximately 4–22% of patients develop seizures within five years of an ischaemic stroke. In the over 65-years age group, up to 40% of seizures are as a result of cerebrovascular ischaemia. Early onset seizure prevalence in subarachnoid haemorrhage is around 6.5%, compared to 6.5–8.5% with ischaemic stroke, and up to 15.4% with intra-cerebral haemorrhage. Early onset seizures occur within two weeks, with 45% of those occurring within the first 24 hours. Late onset seizures peak within 6–12 months, with an up to 90% recurrence rate in this group versus 35% in the early onset group.

Mortality is higher in patients who have post-stroke seizures of any kind. It is very difficult to predict who will have seizures, but stroke-damaged areas act as a focus for localisation epilepsy. For example partial onset motor seizures can occur in an affected limb.

For the treatment of partial onset seizures, the International League Against Epilepsy suggest that lamotrigine and gabapentin are as effective as carbamazepine and are better tolerated in older patients.[5] The Scottish Intercollegiate Guidelines Network (SIGN) and the National Institute for Health and Care Excellence (NICE) suggest that carbamazepine, valproate, lamotrigine or oxcarbazepine can all be used as monotherapies for partial onset seizures with secondary generalisation.[6, 7]

Answer 64

D. Give a rabies vaccination and rabies immunoglobulin

The UK is free of terrestrial rabies, and rabies post-exposure prophylaxis (PEP) is not required for exposures apart from bats. Risk assessment for rabies should be undertaken as soon as possible following exposure so that PEP can be started promptly. The incubation period for rabies is typically one to three months, but may vary from < 1 week to > 1 year. Owing to the potentially long incubation period for rabies, there is no time limit for giving PEP and all potential exposures should be risk assessed. If the exposure was more than one year ago, rabies immunoglobulin is not indicated.

Answer 65

A. Myotonic dystrophy type 1

This patient has the defect for myotonic dystrophy type 1 and now has developed a high degree of AV block. Myotonic dystrophy is an autosomal dominant disorder manifesting with myotonia and dystrophy. The development of AV conduction disturbances is well described in this condition. The CTG trinucleotide repeat on chromosome 19q13 is transcribed in mRNA that is expressed in tissues affected by myotonic dystrophy. The normal population has between 5 and 27 copies, while those with myotonic dystrophy have anything from 50 to over 2000 copies, with more copies correlating with increased disease severity. Cardiac conduction problems are common and may relate to the extent of the CTG expansion. The atrioventricular block seen in myotonic dystrophy is usually infra-Hisian and due to fibrosis, fatty infiltration and atrophy of the conduction system.[8]

Emery–Dreifuss muscular dystrophy is an X-linked trait, caused by emerin mutations or as an autosomal dominant disorder resulting from mutations in the gene encoding lamins A and C. Like emerin, lamins A and C are components of the nuclear coat, but are located in the lamina. Conduction system disease is caused by defects in the head or tail domain of the lamin gene or by emerin mutations (see Table 16.2).

continued

CHAPTER 16 ANSWERS

Inherited primary arrhythmias	Gene and gene symbol or proteins	Cardiac phenotype
Familial long QT syndrome	KCNQ1, KCNH2, SCN5A	Brady-dependent VA
Progressive familiar AV block, autosomal dominant sick sinus syndrome	HCN4, SCN5A, TRPM5, GJA5 genes	Bradycardia, nodal rhythm, PAF, AV block
Neuromuscular disorders		
Myotonic dystrophy type 1 (Steinert's disease)	Myotonin kinase DMPK	AV block, fascicular block, bundle branch block, atrial flutter and fibrillation, VA, DCM
Myotonic dystrophy type 2 (proximal myotonic myopathy: PROMM)	Zinc finger protein 9 ZNF9	PAF, AV block, VA
X-linked Emery–Dreifuss muscular dystrophy (EDMD)	Emerin EMD or STA	AV block, atrial paralysis, VA, atrial flutter and fibrillation, DCM
Laminopathies (including automomal EDMD, limb girdle muscular dystrophy type IB (LGMDIB) and lamin-associated protein defects)	Lamin AC (LMNA) FHLI	AV block, atrial arrhythmia, VA, DCM, ARVC, SCD
Desminopathies	Mutated desmin (DES)	Conduction defects, arrhythmias, sudden death
Metabolic disorders		
Anderson–Fabry disease (alpha-galactosidase A deficiency)	Alpha-galactosidase A GLA	Progressive AV block, sinus node dysfunction, HCM
Familial amyloidosis	Transthyretin TTR	Varies with mutation: AV block, cardiomyopathy
Mutations in AMP kinase	PRKAG2	HCM, AV block, WPW
Mitochondrial cytopathies (including Kearns–Sayre disease)	Mitochondrial DNA (mtDNA) deletions	AV block, atrial and ventricular arrhythmia, ventricular pre-excitation, cardiomyopathy (HCM, DCM)
Danon disease	LAMP2	

continued

Inherited primary arrhythmias	Gene and gene symbol or proteins	Cardiac phenotype
Developmental disorders		
ASD with conduction disease, tetralogy of Fallot	NK2 homeobox 5 gene NKX2.5	ASD, VSD, tetralogy of Fallot, AV conduction
Holt–Oram syndrome	TBX5	Congenital heart defects, AV block, sinoatrial disease, WPW

Table 16.2: Diagnoses recognised to be associated with conduction system disease. Inherited primary arrhythmias

References

1. Reiner et al. 2011. ESC/EAS Guidelines for the management of dyslipidaemias. European Heart Journal, 32, 1769–1818

2. NICE. 2014. Lipid modification: cardiovascular risk assessment and the modification of blood lipids for the primary and secondary prevention of cardiovascular disease. NICE clinical guideline 181. www.nice.org.uk/guidance/cg181

3. Retnakaran R et al. 2006. Risk factors for renal dysfunction in type 2 diabetes. Diabetes, 55, 1832–1839

4. Wilcox M. 2013. Updated guidance on the management and treatment of Clostridium difficile infection. Public Health England

5. Glauser T et al. 2013. Updated ILAE evidence review of antiepileptic drug efficacy and effectiveness as initial monotherapy for epileptic seizures and syndromes. Epilepsia, 54, 551–563

6. SIGN. 2005. Diagnosis and management of epilepsy in adults. (Guideline currently under review)

7. NICE. 2012. The epilepsies: the diagnosis and management of the epilepsies in adults and children in primary and secondary care. NICE clinical guideline 137. www.nice.org.uk/guidance/cg137

8. Benson D. 2004. Genetics of atrioventricular conduction disease in humans. The Anatomical Record Part A: Discoveries in Molecular, Cellular, and Evolutionary Biology Special Issue: The Cardiac Pacemaking and Conduction System Volume 280A, 934–939

Index

The material in chapters 1 to 15 is indexed as chapter number.question number. The practice examination questions (chapter 16) are indexed as PE1 to PE65.